Oculoplastic Nursing Care: Key Concepts

For the full range of M&K Publishing books please visit our website:
www.mkupdate.co.uk

Oculoplastic Nursing Care: Key Concepts

John Cooper

Oculoplastic Nursing Care: Key Concepts
John Cooper

ISBN: 978-1-905539-81-9

First published 2020

All rights reserved. No part of this publication may be reproduced, stored in a retrieval system, or transmitted in any form or by any means, electronic, mechanical, photocopying, recording or otherwise, without either the prior permission of the publishers or a licence permitting restricted copying in the United Kingdom issued by the Copyright Licensing Agency, 90 Tottenham Court Road, London, W1T 4LP. Permissions may be sought directly from M&K Publishing, phone: 01768 773030 or email: publishing@mkupdate.co.uk

Any person who does any unauthorised act in relation to this publication may be liable to criminal prosecution and civil claims for damages.

British Library Cataloguing in Publication Data
A catalogue record for this book is available from the British Library

Notice
Clinical practice and medical knowledge constantly evolve. Standard safety precautions must be followed, but, as knowledge is broadened by research, changes in practice, treatment and drug therapy may become necessary or appropriate. Readers must check the most current product information provided by the manufacturer of each drug to be administered and verify the dosages and correct administration, as well as contraindications. It is the responsibility of the practitioner, utilising the experience and knowledge of the patient, to determine dosages and the best treatment for each individual patient. Any brands mentioned in this book are as examples only and are not endorsed by the publisher. Neither the publisher nor the authors assume any liability for any injury and/or damage to persons or property arising from this publication.

To contact M&K Publishing write to:
M&K Update Ltd · The Old Bakery · St. John's Street
Keswick · Cumbria CA12 5AS
Tel: 01768 773030
publishing@mkupdate.co.uk
www.mkupdate.co.uk

Designed and typeset by Mary Blood
Printed in Scotland by Bell & Bain, Glasgow

Contents

Foreword vii
Acknowledgements viii
Introduction ix
Glossary xi

1. Advanced and specialised roles within ophthalmic and oculoplastic nursing in the UK 1
2. Ectropion and entropion 9
3. Assessment and management of upper eyelid blepharoptosis 35
4. Floppy eyelid syndrome 69
5. Eyelid lesions and their management 75
6. The eyelashes and trichiasis 101
7. Blepharitis, meibomian gland disease and dry eye disease 109
8. The lacrimal system and dacryocystorhinostomy 119
9. Thyroid eye disease 143
10. Enucleation and evisceration 159
11. Exenteration and socket wound management 171
12. Emergency oculoplastic care 185
13. Facial palsy and related care 211
14. The orbit and related disorders 221
15. Oculoplastic surgical competencies 243

Further reading 324
Index 325

Foreword

I am very pleased to write this foreword for *Oculoplastic Nursing Care: Key Concepts* by John Cooper.

John has devoted many years to developing and advancing the role of the specialist oculoplastic nurse practitioner. His book will contribute further to this important development. The oculoplastic nurse practitioner plays a vital role in the care of patients undergoing oculoplastic surgical procedures, both preoperatively, intraoperatively and postoperatively. The well-trained and competent oculoplastic nurse practitioner can vastly improve the efficiency and safety of oculoplastic surgical procedures and plays a very important role in liaison between members of the surgical, anaesthetic, and nursing teams. The importance of pre-operative counselling, post-operative monitoring, pain control, wound aftercare and patient education is often overlooked in standard oculoplastic surgery textbooks and John bridges this gap very well in his textbook. I have no doubt that his textbook will encourage others to continue to improve the overall care of the patient undergoing oculoplastic surgical procedures, recognising the specialised knowledge required by nurses caring for these patients.

Mr Brian Leatherbarrow, BSc MBChB DO FRCS FRCOphth
Honorary Consultant Oculoplastic & Orbital Surgeon
Manchester Royal Eye Hospital

Acknowledgements

Nothing is achieved in isolation and, consequently, I have many individuals to thank for their love, support and help in realising and creating the body of work on which this book is based.

Firstly, to all my colleagues and peers at the Manchester Royal Eye Hospital (MREH), both present and past, who have nurtured, developed and created the professional that I have become.

To all the Oculoplastic Nurse Practitioners at the MREH, who have been front and centre in the creation and onward fostering of the role over the last two decades, namely: Rachel Badham (who created the role at the MREH), Sarah Day, Marion Platts, Sheeba Putheen Danial, Anne Mullett and Natalie Pollitt.

To my oculoplastic consultant colleagues at the MREH who have endured my upward trajectory and have at the same time helped me on my journey: Brian Leatherbarrow, Sajid Ataullah, Anne Cook, Paul Cannon, Aruna Dharmasena and James Laybourne.

I must give a special mention to the late Professor Janet Marsden, who was my mentor and actively encouraged me to undertake this project. Janet represented ophthalmic nursing care the world over and she very sadly passed away during the writing of this book. Thank you, Janet, for everything. I (we) miss you. RIP.

Mary Shaw has also been a supportive figure in my development as an oculoplastic practitioner, especially in relation to the Royal College of Nursing Forum.

To all my friends and family, but especially to Mum and Peter, Dad and Cynthia. You have allowed me to grow and develop, with all your love and support.

To my boys, Sean and Kieran. I love you both so much. See what you can do if you put your mind to it.

And finally, to my darling wife Jo, without whom none of this would be possible. I love you and thank you for everything. X

This book represents 27 years of ophthalmic nursing care – and a lifetime of love and support.

Thank you, all.

Introduction

Once I qualified as a registered nurse in 1992, I knew I wanted to become an ophthalmic nurse. This was after a short placement on an ophthalmic ward as a student nurse. I was mesmerised by cataract surgery and overwhelmed by the intricate surgical techniques required. Equally, I understood the huge impact of sight-related issues on people's lives and how we, as nurses, could help support them.

Subsequently, I have embraced many wonderful opportunities within my career, and have found my niche within the sub-specialty of oculoplastics. I have worked in various capacities in this field, in theatre, daycase and outpatients, initially as an oculoplastic nurse practitioner and latterly as an advanced nurse practitioner, having gained my Master's degree from Salford University.

Having also gained a Master's degree in clinical research from the University of Manchester, I felt it was time for a new challenge. Reflecting on what I have achieved, I recognised that I have gained a lot of clinical knowledge and experience within the realm of oculoplastic care. I have also had the opportunity to work with some of the best oculoplastic consultants and nursing colleagues at the Manchester Royal Eye Hospital (MREH), who have nurtured my knowledge and clinical ability.

Within the context of clinical nursing and surgical care, I have embraced the chance to broaden my abilities. I presently undertake a minor operations theatre list, temporal artery biopsies and various surgical procedures, amongst other clinical activities.

Outside the MREH, I have been involved in various national committees and ophthalmic groups, and I am proud to have been the Chair of the Royal College of Nursing Ophthalmic Forum and main author of *The nature, scope and value of ophthalmic nursing* (RCN 2016). More recently, I have become the Vice-Chair of the International Ophthalmic Nursing Association (IONA).

During the course of my career, I have had several short articles published, but the idea of writing this book arose because I wanted to share my knowledge in a way that would be all-encompassing. I wanted to write a book that not only provided what you might expect (the essentials such as the anatomy and physiology of the eye) but also, more crucially, the personal nuggets of advice and information that any aspiring practitioner might find useful. In some ways, it will be my legacy to those who follow me in this field and I hope it will inspire others to consider going into ophthalmic nursing and, more specifically, oculoplastic nursing.

As a student, I was frustrated that no specific oculoplastic nursing text existed and that many medical books appeared to skirt around the nursing aspects or simply ignored them. Likewise, there are several very good ophthalmic nursing texts but, all too often, they merely touch on various aspects of oculoplastic care. I felt this needed addressing.

This book represents my personal perspective on oculoplastic care and I appreciate that not everyone will agree with everything in it, or be aware of all the approaches to oculoplastic surgery and care that I have outlined. I have not gone to outlandish lengths to reference every sentence, but I have taken wisdom and inspiration from several texts, which I would encourage anyone interested in oculoplastics and ophthalmic care to purchase. These publications are listed in the references in each chapter, and the key titles appear in the 'Further reading' list at the end of the book.

I hope this book provides useful information about an area of nursing care I am truly proud to work in. I have tried to make it as accessible as possible.

John Cooper
January 2020

Glossary

anterior lamella the outward aspect of the eyelid, composed of skin and muscle (orbicularis).

atherosclerosis a disease process by which plaque builds up in the arteries, occluding them.

autologous refers to tissue obtained from the same individual, e.g. a full-thickness skin graft harvested from a patient's arm to correct an eyelid defect.

bandage contact lens (BCL) a non-permeable soft lens that can be placed over the cornea to protect the cornea from mechanical rubbing.

Bell's phenomenon (palpebral oculogyric reflex) on eyelid closure, the eye rotates upward and outward as a defensive mechanism.

blepharitis inflammation of the eyelids, causing irritation, itchiness and crusting of the eyelashes, usually caused by bacteria and/or blockage of the meibomian gland.

blepharoplasty surgical removal of excess eyelid skin, usually due to dermatochalasis.

blepharospasm involuntary spasm and contracture of the eyelid muscles, causing twitching and uncontrolled closing of the eyes.

brow ptosis drooping of the eyebrow, usually as a consequence of weakening of the associated muscles over time or (more rarely) due to facial palsy.

canaliculus a small passageway or tube that leads from the puncta to the lacrimal sac and drains tears

canthal ligament ligament in both the inner (medial) and outer (lateral) aspects of the lids that attaches the eyelids to the bony orbit.

canthotomy/cantholysis two surgical procedures used to release the lower eyelid at the lateral canthus during eyelid reconstruction and also in emergency situations when the orbit is tense and the pressure needs to be relieved.

chalazion blockage of the meibomian gland, causing a swollen raised lesion that can be inflamed and mildly painful.

chemosis swelling (specifically oedema) of the conjunctiva

cicatricial scarring, often associated with the conjunctiva; this can cause contracture and malposition of the eyelids.

collarette a circular collar of debris around the base of an eyelash.

comedo blackhead or blocked hair follicle (plural comedones).

conjunctiva lining that involves the inside of the eyelids and covers the white of the eye (sclera); it provides protection and lubrication for the eye; there is a lid portion (palpebral) and an eye portion (bulbar).

contralateral pertaining or relating to the opposite side of the body from where the particular lesion or condition occurs

Cyst of Moll a small transparent lesion arising from the seat ducts of the eyelid.

Cyst of Zeis a small yellowish/white lesion arising from glands of Zeis on the eyelid.

dacryocystorhinostomy surgical procedure to create a new passageway for tears to drain by opening the lacrimal sac lining and joining it to the nasal mucosa.

dacryocystitis inflammation/infection of the lacrimal sac causing a swollen area in the medial lower eyelid.

dermatochalasis excess hooding of upper eyelid skin that may obscure vision.

demodex microscopic parasitic mites that live on hair/hair follicles (specifically eyelashes) and can cause irritation and itchiness.

distichiasis excessive growth of additional eyelashes which means that the individual has two or more rows of eyelashes.

ectropion an eyelid that turns outwards, away from the eye, often leading to exposure issues.

entropion an eyelid that turns inwards, causing the eyelashes to rub on the eye and resulting in irritation.

enucleation surgical removal of the whole eye, due to trauma, severe infection, tumour or a severely painful blind eye.

epiphora excessive tears, due to over-production of tears or blockage of the tear drainage apparatus, leading to watering eyes and tears running down the face.

erythema increased redness of an area of skin due to infection or inflammation.

evisceration surgical removal of the contents of the eye, leaving the sclera and extra-ocular muscles behind, usually due to infection, or a painful blind eye.

exenteration surgical removal of the contents of the orbit (including the eye and surrounding structures), usually due to a tumour.

exophthalmometry measurement of proptosis in millimetres (eye bulging forward out of the orbit), using an exophthalmometer.

floppy eyelid syndrome a triad of symptoms, including obstructive sleep apnoea, obesity and excessive floppy upper eyelids; lax lids cause irritation and soreness and often require a surgical procedure to tighten them.

Hering's law a law of equal innervation, usually associated with eye movement, but also related to ptosis: when a ptotic eyelid is lifted (or surgically corrected), the opposite upper eyelid drops.

Hughes flap reconstructive surgical procedure in which the upper eyelid palpebral conjunctiva and a section of the tarsal plate are used to fill a defect in the lower eyelid.

hyperaemia increased blood flow to a region or structure.

hyperglobus upward displacement of the eye within the orbit.

hypoglobus downward displacement of the eye within the orbit.

iatrogenic condition or increase in symptoms, due to the inadvertent intervention of a physician or therapy.

inferior low or lower in position

ipsilateral pertaining to, or occurring on, the same side of the body.

Ishihara test a colour vision test that uses a series of coloured, dotted plates showing a number or path.

keratitis inflammation of the cornea.

lacrimal gland an almond-shaped exocrine gland located supra-temporally just under the orbital rim that produces tears.

lacrimal sac the upper aspect of the nasolacrimal duct which connects the canaliculi and conveys tears into the nasal cavity.

lagophthalmos inability to close the eyelids completely, causing eye exposure.

lateral pertaining or extending to the right/left side, away from the medial axis.

Lester Jones Tube (LJT) pyrex glass hollow tube that is placed (during a surgical procedure) in the medial canthal region to drain tears from the eye to the nasal cavity.

levator muscle muscle that elevates the upper eyelid.

lid lag where the upper eyelid is higher than normal when the eyes are looking down; commonly associated with thyroid eye disease.

madarosis loss of eyelashes, typically associated with a disease process.

medial towards the middle or the midline of the body or organ.

meibomian gland series of vertical meibum-producing exocrine glands located within the tarsal plates in the eyelids.

mucocele swelling of a sac, due to its distention with mucus; commonly associated with the lacrimal sac and, more rarely, with the frontal sinus swelling within the orbit.

Müller's muscle smooth muscle in the upper eyelid that helps to lift it and also holds the eyelid once lifted; it lies between the levator muscle (anteriorly) and the palpebral conjunctiva (posteriorly).

orbicularis muscle sphincter muscle that circumferentially covers the orbit and has three parts: orbital, pretarsal and preseptal; its function is associated with forcible closure of the eyelids.

orbital decompression surgical procedure to remove orbital bone and fat in order to alleviate proptosis associated with thyroid eye disease.

orbital implant circular man-made implant that is used to fill the void left by eye removal surgery.

orbitotomy surgical procedure whereby a section of the zygomatic bone is temporarily removed in order to access the posterior part of the orbit, usually in relation to an orbital mass.

ocular coherence tomography non-invasive imaging technique that uses light waves to take cross-sectional pictures of the retina.

pedunculated being on a 'stalk'; normally associated with skin lesions.

photophobia intolerance and discomfort due to being exposed to bright light.

posterior lamella the inner aspect of the eyelid, composed of the tarsal plate and the palpebral conjunctiva.

ptosis drooping of a structure; in ophthalmology ptosis is usually associated with the upper eyelid as well as other structures, including the brow and eyelashes (adjective ptotic).

pre-/post-auricular pertaining to the area either in front of (anterior) or behind (posterior) the ear.

pretrichial surgical incision just in front of the hairline.

proptosis abnormal protrusion of the eye anteriorly out of the orbit, associated with intra-orbital mass/lesion and thyroid eye disease.

pseudoptosis small group of disorders that create the illusion of an upper eyelid ptosis rather than a 'true' ptosis.

puncta small circular apertures in the upper and lower eyelid margin medially that collect tears from the lacrimal glands and transfer the tears into the canaliculus and nasolacrimal duct.

resect surgically draw tissue back/away from its normal position.

resection surgical removal of tissue, organ or structure.

retractor muscle lower eyelid muscle that originates from the inferior rectus muscle, which acts to depress the eyelid in downgaze.

rhomboid flap surgical reconstructive technique that uses a rhomboid shape as a basis to rotate skin to fill a defect.

Rundle's curve representation of the clinical course of thyroid disease in graph form, based on the work of Australian surgeon Frank Rundle.

seborrheic keratosis benign lesions, often pigmented brown or light tan, which appear slightly raised and waxy and give the impression that they are 'stuck on'.

selenium essential trace element which offers several health benefits and has also been shown to be valuable in preventing thyroid eye disease.

sessile flat, fixed in one place and immobile; normally associated with lesions.

stenosis narrowing of a tube, commonly associated with the canaliculus, which causes restriction of tear drainage.

superior above and/or over the top of.

supra-clavicular above the collar bone (clavicle), associated with harvesting full-thickness skin grafts.

synkinesis where usually unwanted involuntary contraction of the eyelid muscles is associated with simultaneous movement of other muscles (e.g. when smiling causes the eyelids to close), typically in facial palsy.

tarsi (tarsal plates) thin plates of dense connective tissue in both the upper and lower eyelids that give the lids support and form.

tarsorrhaphy procedure that closes the eyelids, either permanently or semi-permanently, in order to prevent exposure of the eye; in many cases this procedure can be reversed once the underlying problem has resolved.

telangiectasia small dilated blood vessels often associated with malignant lesions such as basal cell carcinoma.

Tenzel flap surgical procedure that involves rotating and advancing a small lateral semi-circular flap of skin from the temporal region to fill a lower eyelid full-thickness defect.

trichiasis misplaced in-growth of eyelashes that may rub against the eye, causing irritation and discomfort.

tylosis thickening of the tarsal border of the eyelid.

Whitnall's ligament fibrous band in the upper eyelid that acts as a pulley for the levator muscle and is also considered a surgical landmark.

xanthelasma yellowish/white subcutaneous lesions that commonly occur medially in the upper and lower eyelids; associated with lipid deposits.

1

Advanced and specialised roles within ophthalmic and oculoplastic nursing in the UK

Introduction

The concepts of advanced and specialised nursing roles have been embedded within healthcare in the UK for several decades. This is especially true of ophthalmic nursing, in which sub-specialisation has led to extended roles within vitreo-retinal, corneal, macular and oculoplastic nursing.

Within secondary and tertiary general acute care settings, advanced nurse practitioner roles have grown exponentially, especially in areas such as Accident & Emergency (A&E), acute medicine and intensive care (ICU). This growth has been driven by many factors, including financial, political, quality improvement, consumer accessibility, local strategic and operational issues (Lewis & Dixon 2005). As has been well documented, the reduction of junior doctors' working hours, combined with a predicted decrease in the overall number of doctors and changes to their training, have also been significant drivers for change (NHSME 1991, European Parliament and Council 2000, Bellman 2003, Por 2008). As a consequence, legislation and changes in boundaries have paved the way for new job opportunities and role expansion (Czuber-Dochan *et al.* 2005).

What is advanced practice?

Fundamentally, the advanced nurse practitioner (ANP) should be able to 'examine, investigate, diagnose, treat and refer patients independently' (Livesley *et al.* 2009, p. 586). These roles are also commonly associated with, and undertaken by, the junior doctor.

However, there is much confusion concerning the competence and role boundaries of advanced practice (AP) roles, partly due to the lack of national standards. Consequently, the boundaries of practice attributed to the role are varied (Czuber-Dochan *et al.* 2005).

It is difficult to discern the difference between specific titles in association with roles, especially those relating to nurse practitioner, advanced nurse practitioner and specialist nurse practitioner. The definitions of nurse practitioner and advanced nurse practitioner appear to be interchangeable, with some indication of increased knowledge and skill attributed to the latter. However, according to NHS Scotland's *Advanced Nurse Practitioner Toolkit* (2008), a specialist practitioner operates at a particular point on the novice–expert continuum – a level 6 functional role.

According to the International Council of Nurses (ICN 2006, p. 12), the advanced practitioner is 'a registered nurse who has acquired the expert knowledge-base, complex decision-making skills and clinical competencies for expanded practice'. Advanced nursing has been related to a degree of professional maturity and, significantly, working at 'higher' levels of practice over all aspects of various extended roles (Christensen 2011). However, Castledine (2004) exercises a degree of caution by suggesting that nurses working within a 'higher' level of practice have been conditioned to believe that a title will ultimately convey authority, but they have not necessarily assimilated the appropriate competence or knowledge to support their role. Por (2008) reiterates this point, suggesting that advanced nursing practice involves more than being an 'expert' in any given specialty merely by experience. Marsden & Shaw (2007, p. 121) state 'what is clear from the literature is that although some nurses undertaking advanced practice roles may be perceived as lacking adequate educational preparation they perform well', which is not reassuring, given the level of practice. And, as Christensen (2011) outlines, whilst the attributes and clinical abilities underpinning AP roles are widely appreciated and understood, there is less clarity about what exactly comprises advancing practice.

This problem is intensified by the debate about what constitutes 'advanced practice' versus 'advancing practice' (Por 2008). Livesley *et al.* (2009) expand upon this by suggesting that advanced practitioners may be wrongly perceived as 'mini doctors', thus creating varying degrees of misunderstanding, under-utilisation of skills, peer envy and organisational failings that may ultimately contribute to the role's loss of impact. Conversely, those tasked with 'advancing practice' may be perceived as mavericks who may work beyond their areas of responsibility. Concern has also been expressed in situations where the core of advanced nursing practice is fundamentally underpinned by what is essentially a medical model (Donnelly 2003).

Some might argue that all these concerns are really questions of semantics or individual interpretation, but my own view is that they apply irrespective of whether one is considering advanced or advancing nursing care.

Based on the literature, it would seem that the AP should have excellent decision-making skills, critical thinking, effective clinical judgment, high levels of self-awareness and reflective ability (Verger *et al.* 2002). Whether some of these attributes can be taught, or to what degree they are in fact personal traits possessed by an individual who is able to function at the advanced level, is difficult to discern and indeed the two types of attributes are closely interlinked. Furthermore, the models discussed in the literature are based on significantly varying healthcare settings in several different countries.

What is clearly essential, however, is the regulation and appropriate recognition and unification of advanced practice across the various specialist parameters. A learning programme that constitutes a formal level of education within a regulatory framework is also required. For instance, Livesley *et al.* (2009) describe an educational collaboration which provided the basis for a Master's level (7) degree programme to provide train advanced nurse practitioners.

Any Master's course should provide the individual practitioner with the tools needed to function at an advanced level, with specific taught units on applied anatomy and physiology, clinical examination, etc. and an important work-based clinical aspect that necessitates the examination and assessment of patients. For someone like me (coming from a background in ophthalmology), the most interesting aspect of such a course is the generic application of broad skills, such as clinical examination.

Advanced practice in ophthalmology: a brief overview

Kirkwood (2012), and previously Marsden and Shaw (2007) and Czuber-Dochan *et al.* (2005), have described the positive impact of advanced nurse practitioner roles within ophthalmology in the UK (and Australia and New Zealand).

APs have been involved in ophthalmology for a number of years, across various sub-specialties. In his comprehensive review, Kirkwood (2012) highlighted 19 areas, especially emergency care, within which AP roles were most prevalent. Other areas included: vitreo-retinal, glaucoma, cataract and oculoplastics.

However, much of the associated evidence described service-level evaluations, with few or no anecdotal findings. Only one randomised control trial was described. All the other bodies of work were cohort studies, which were either underpowered and/or had small samples. However, many of the findings appeared to either support and/or benefit patient care, through increased quality (Kirkwood *et al.* 2005, Gibbons & Frossell 2001, Marsden 1999), cost-effectiveness (Kirkwood *et al.* 2006, Slight *et al.* 2009) or patient satisfaction (Waterman *et al.* 2002, Bradshaw 2009, Davies 2005, Burlew-Quartey 2009, Hume & Abbott 1995, Dunlop 2010, Khan *et al.* 2010).

A considerable proportion of these papers described how nurse practitioners were at the core of facilitating and delivering service provision to specific groups within ophthalmology. Many of the authors described themselves as nurse practitioners, advanced nurse practitioners and specialist nurses. In many respects, the lead authors represented a rather homogenous group, with the same names appearing repeatedly in the literature. A considerable number of these papers were published in relatively low-impact journals.

Furthermore, some of the articles were based on healthcare systems that were not directly comparable with those of the UK, especially the ones written in Australia and New Zealand. Interestingly, there was hardly any literature from the USA, which boasts of having conceived nurse-practitioner roles in the mid-1960s (Duffield *et al.* 2009). This makes one suspect that such roles, particularly related to ophthalmology, may be less than equitably distributed.

In many instances, higher-level nursing practice (whether it be YAG laser treatment, Botulinum toxin injections or minor surgery, which often represent exceptionally specific treatments) was shown to be valuable and beneficial, even if the evidence to support the findings was weak. More profound consumer benefits were probably related to ophthalmic A&E services where, in several cases, most of the diagnosis, treatment and follow-up care was entirely undertaken by nurse practitioners. However, even these activities were limited to certain parameters, such as the anterior part of the eye (i.e. any presenting symptoms pertaining to the retina were taken up by the medical team).

Without doubt, there were some notable positive developments as a direct consequence of advanced nursing practice. However, many were produced in an ad-hoc manner and some, arguably, were developed more in order to meet service needs than to advance nursing practice (Marsden & Shaw 2007).

Evans (2011) interviewed several APs in ophthalmological roles and concluded that no two posts were the same, and particular attributes were essential to be able to perform at this level, including enthusiasm, willingness to self-direct learning, perseverance and humility.

Preparation for these roles was largely underpinned by experience and 'natural progression' (Evans 2011). This research project used interviews to ascertain the views of the participants. Even though the sample was small (n=5), this research did raise some interesting and recurring themes, particularly related to peer/medical support being poor at times, certain roles still being perceived as subservient, and a general lack of clarity regarding particular roles.

Czuber-Dochan *et al.* (2005) produced probably the most robust survey of advanced practice (despite now being more than 10 years old), with 117 respondents.

The authors also statistically compared their results with those from previous surveys carried out in 1997 and 1994, providing further interesting insight into the changes that have taken place. Essentially most nurse practitioners (83% of those surveyed) had an ophthalmic qualification (ENB 346 or, more recently, the renamed ophthalmic module) and the highest proportion (43%) were working at grade F (now band 6), mostly (23.9%) with the title of nurse practitioner (or variations of this title). Interestingly, there were no advanced nurse practitioners in the extensive list of potential titles, and much of the advanced practice was related to investigatory tasks and/or to particular treatments such as laser or minor surgery.

The paradox is that there is very little evidence, in all the information I've been able to elicit, of Master's degree-level ophthalmic advanced practice. The only examples were glaucoma APs (Manchester Metropolitan University) and an exceptionally small number of other individuals involved in vitreo-retinal surgery and oculoplastics. There are a significant number of nurse practitioners working within a plethora of ophthalmic settings, with some educational and experiential justification for their roles, but also with a mind-boggling array of underpinning qualifications and titles.

Perhaps most surprisingly, I was unable to find evidence of any nurse practitioner in the field of ophthalmology having accessed a course based on the advanced practice model that I have undertaken at MSc level. If we are to raise the bar and provide a basis for career progression, I believe ophthalmic providers need to explore the benefits of having advanced nurse practitioners pushing the boundaries of ophthalmic care and practice within their departments. We need to harness the ambitions of nurses who want to embrace and improve clinical practice while incentivising the next generation of practitioners.

What of the future? Well, I still believe that ophthalmic nursing is important and medical advances in the field make it interesting and exciting. However, with the lack of specific ophthalmic courses and seemingly reduced enthusiasm amongst higher education institutions about providing such courses, we may need to look at other ways to gain the specific knowledge required to provide the highest level of practice. In many cases this may come full circle and in-house training may again play a fundamental role in delivering the bespoke training that ophthalmic nurses need and want. It is certainly cost-effective, accessible and flexible. Moreover, collecting course credit points is no longer important in itself; and occupational educational requirements are now met with practical and individualised learning and development.

Certainly, I see nurses at all levels accessing ophthalmic nursing without specific ophthalmic-related qualifications. Does this matter? Well, yes and no. In some ways, it is refreshing to see new faces bringing new perspectives, but fundamental opththalmic knowledge is obviously still paramount. I would argue that we can be more imaginative in the way we provide it; and moreover we can make more effort to tailor the training to the specific needs of the departments and individuals involved.

Ophthalmic nursing is important and it is vital that it keeps its identity and its purpose, but not if it means 'dumbing down' our knowledge and skills. No matter what level we work at as ophthalmic practitioners, we must continue to explore new ways to practise, consider the wider needs of a financially restricted NHS, embrace audit and research, and ultimately provide the best care we can.

Within oculoplastic nursing care, this especially relates to patients' psychological and physical wellbeing and care. Many oculoplastic interventions (such as enucleation surgery, with its complex requirements) can be quite dramatic and life-changing for patients. We have a responsibility to stay abreast of these needs and broaden our knowledge and skills to meet them. In order to do this, we may just have to find new ways of accessing this knowledge.

References

Bellman, L. (2003). *Nurse-led Change and Development in Clinical Practice.* London: Whurr Publishers.

Bradshaw, J. (2009). An intensive nurse-led occlusion therapy programme. *Paediatric Nursing.* **21**(6), 37–39.

Burlew-Quartey, J. (2009). Registered nurse-led group medical appointments for pre-operative cataract patients. *Insight.* **34**(2), 28–31.

Castledine, G. (2004). 'The development of advanced nursing practice in the UK'. In: McGee & Castledine (eds.) *Advanced Nursing Practice.* 2nd edn. Oxford: Blackwell.

Christensen, M. (2011), Advancing nursing practice: redefining the theoretical and practical integration of knowledge. *Journal of Clinical Nursing.* **20**, 873–81.

Czuber-Dochan, W.J., Waterman, C. & Waterman, H. (2005). Atrophy and Anarchy: third national survey of nursing skill-mix and advanced nursing practice in ophthalmology. *Journal of Clinical Nursing.* **15**, 1480–88.

Davies, M. (2005). Nurse Practitioner-led consent in day case cataract surgery. *Nursing Times.* **40**(1), 30–32.

Donnelly, G. (2003). Clinical experience in advanced practice nursing: a Canadian perspective. *Nurse Education Today.* **23**(3), 168–73.

Duffield, C., Gardener, G., Chang, A. & Catling-Paull, C. (2009). Advanced Nursing practice: A global perspective. *Collegian.* **16**(2), 55–62.,

Dunlop, N. (2010). Advancing the role of minor surgery for nurses. *British Journal of Nursing.* **19**(11), 685–89.

European Parliament and Council (2000). *Organisation of working time (basic directive) 2003/34/EC.*

Evans, P. (2011). Ophthalmic advanced practice: The 'lived experience'. *International Journal of Ophthalmic Practice.* **1**(2), 80–84.

Gibbons, H. & Frossell, S. (2001). Ophthalmic nurse practitioner performing Nd:YAG laser capsulotomy. *Ophthalmic Nursing.* **5**(1), 12–15.

Hume, J. & Abbott, F. (1995). Setting up a shared care glaucoma clinic. *Nursing Standard.* **10**(11), 34–36.

International Council of Nurses (ICN) (2006). *Definition and Characteristics of the Role.* Genevan: ICN.

Khan, S., Wong, S., Gorrod, R., Gangat, I., Hiles, S. & Deane, J. (2010). Diabetic Retinopathy: Role of the diabetic specialist eye nurse. *Journal of Diabetic Nursing.* **14**(8): 292–301.

Kirkwood, B. (2012). Alternative Pathways to Ophthalmic Care: Advanced Nursing Practice. *Insight.* **37**(3), 5–10 (Summer).

Kirkwood, B., Pesudows, K., Loh, R. & Coster D. (2005) Implementation and evaluation of an ophthalmic nurse practitioner emergency eye clinic. *Clinical & Experimental Ophthalmology.* **33**(6), 593–97.

Kirkwood, B., Pesudows, K., Latimer, P. & Coster, D. (2006), The efficacy of a nurse-led pre-operative cataract assessment and post-operative care clinic. *Medical Journal of Australia.* **184**(6), 278–81.

Lewis, R. & Dixon, J. (2005). *NHS Market Futures. Exploring the impact of the health service market reforms. A discussion paper.* London: King's Fund.

Livesley, J., Waters, K. & Tarbuck, P. (2009). The management of advanced practitioner preparation: a work-based challenge. *Journal of Nursing Management.* **17**, 584–93.

Marsden, J. (1999). The nurse practitioner role in a United Kingdom ophthalmic accident and emergency department – 10 years of progress. *Insight.* **24**(2), 45–50 (Spring).

Marsden, J. & Shaw, M. (2007). The development of advanced practice roles in ophthalmic nursing. *Practice Development in Health Care.* **6**(2), 119–30.

National Health Service Management Executive (NHSME) (1991). *Junior Doctors – The New Deal.* London: NHSME.

NHS Scotland (2008). *Advanced Nurse Practitioner Toolkit: Definitions.* http://www.advancedpractice.scot.nhs.uk/ (last accessed 25.11.2019).

Por, J. (2008). A critical engagement with the concept of advanced nursing practice. *Journal of Nursing Management.* **16**, 84–90.

Slight, C., Marsden, J. & Raynel, S. (2009). The impact of a glaucoma nurse specialist role on glaucoma waiting lists. *Nursing Practice in New Zealand.* **25**(1), 38–47.

Verger, J., Trimarchi, T. & Barnsteiner, J. (2002). Challenges of advanced practice nursing in paediatric acute and critical care: education to practice. *Critical Care Nursing Clinics of North America.* **14**(3), 315–400.

Waterman, H., Mayer, S., Lavin, M., Spencer, A. & Waterman, C. (2002). An evaluation of the administration of sub-Tenon local anaesthetic by a nurse practitioner. *British Journal of Ophthalmology.* **86**(5), 254–256.

2

Ectropion and entropion

Introduction

Arguably the most common lower eyelid malpositions that the practitioner is likely to encounter in clinical practice are ectropion and entropion. Both these presentations can be very irritating and debilitating for the patient, causing redness, blurring of vision and repeated infections.

Essentially, an eyelid that turns outward, away from the globe, is known as an ectropion; and conversely an eyelid that rotates inwards is called an entropion. In a slightly laboured way, I remember the 'n' in entropion as 'in' (the eyelid turning in) and therefore the opposite must be ectropion.

The management and surgical treatment of these two presentations largely depends upon gaining a good background history and undertaking a meticulous clinical examination in order to distinguish the underlying cause of the alteration in eyelid position. It is therefore crucial for the practitioner to appreciate the importance of a thorough history and examination prior to treatment.

There are various causes for both morbidities and we will explore these below, but crucially the main physiological causes of all such alterations are:

- Horizontal laxity of the eyelid
- Shortening of the lid structures
- Lengthening of the canthal ligaments.

Anatomy of the lower eyelid

It is helpful to consider the anatomy of the lower eyelid to gain a fuller understanding of the mechanism that leads to the change of position of the eyelid. The key anatomical parts include:

Orbicularis muscle

This is a sphincter muscle that completely surrounds the eye, with fibres that radiate circumferentially outwards from the eyelid edges, covering the orbital rim. It is composed of three parts: orbital, pretarsal and preseptal portions. The orbital portion's main function is to (forcibly) close the eyes, whereas the pretarsal and preseptal are associated with involuntary blinking. The orbicularis muscle is innervated by the facial nerve.

Tarsal plate

These are two plates of fibrous tissue, the larger being in the upper eyelid, measuring 10mm in height (compared to the lower eyelid which is 4–6mm), approximately 1mm thick and 29mm long. The tarsal plates provide the eyelid's structural integrity, giving it form and structure. Modified sebaceous glands lie within the body of the tarsal plates, and these are more commonly known as meibomian glands.

Retractor muscle

The lower eyelid retractors are an extension of the tendon and fibres of the capsulopalpebral fascia, which wrap around the inferior oblique muscle, split into two arms and continue anteriorly to attach to the inferior edge of the tarsal plate. The two anterior arms (the inferior tarsal muscle and the capsulopalpebral fascia) are collectively known as the lower eyelid retractors.

Canthal ligaments

The medial and lateral canthal ligaments attach the eyelids to the bony orbital rims. They are tendons, which are extensions of the orbicularis muscle and its attachment to the periosteum. The lateral canthal ligament has two arms (associated with the upper and lower eyelid respectively). As it attaches to the orbital rim, the two arms become one. The medial canthal ligament is approximately 2mm lower in its attachment compared to the lateral canthal ligament.

The medial canthal ligament also has two limbs (posterior and anterior), between which lies the lacrimal sac. This is noteworthy, as the limbs of the medial canthal ligaments contribute to the 'lacrimal pump' mechanism, aiding the movement of tears through the lacrimal sac. Through blinking, the compression and expansion of the lacrimal sac by the limbs of the medial canthus enables the sac to fill and empty in a pump-like action.

It may be easier to visualise the lower eyelid (Figure 2.1) as two layers of a sandwich, with the terminating orbital septal fibres as the filling in the middle. The outer layer is called the anterior lamella and the inner is the posterior lamella. The border of the two lamellae, at the eyelid margin, is known as the grey-line and it is here that the layers can be physically separated (surgical landmark).

The anterior lamella essentially consists of the outer skin and the circumferential orbicularis muscle, whereas the posterior lamella is seen as the tarsal plate (and retractor muscles) and the palpebral conjunctiva. If there is shortening of the anterior lamella associated with skin disorders such as eczema or trauma (a skin burn, for example), this will mechanically pull the posterior lamella forward and cause a cicatricial ectropion.

Similarly, if the same mechanism is applied to the posterior lamella by shortening of the palpebral conjunctiva through scarring (which may occur in a condition such as ocular cicatricial pemipigoid – OCP), this would create a cicatricial entropion.

In order to appreciate the key nursing considerations, we need to discuss the various types and manifestations of ectropion and entropion.

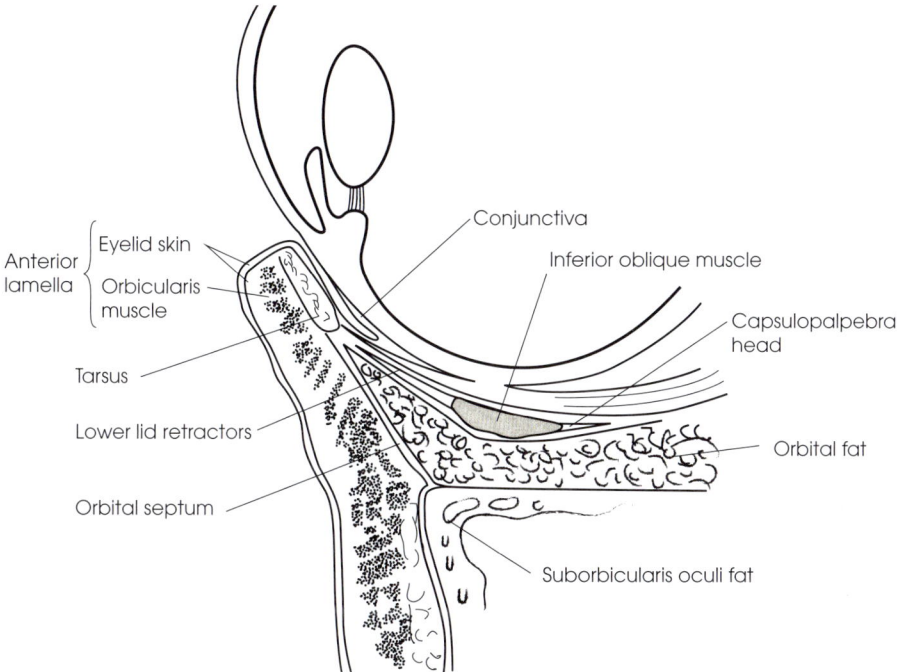

Figure 2.1: Lower eyelid anatomy

Ectropion

Generally, ectropion is the term associated with the eyelid being turned or pulled away from the globe (see Figure 2.2). It is generally seen in older patients and in men. There is some suggestion that it is more common in men because men generally have larger inferior tarsal plates. The extent of the ectropion can vary from involving the medial part of the lower eyelid or implicating the whole eyelid. The ectropion can involve a total eversion of the eyelid, leading to exposure and dryness of the tarsal palpebral conjunctiva, which in turn can lead to erythema, infection and discomfort. Or it may involve a laxity in the eyelid which doesn't sit snuggly against the globe, causing epiphora and dry eyes.

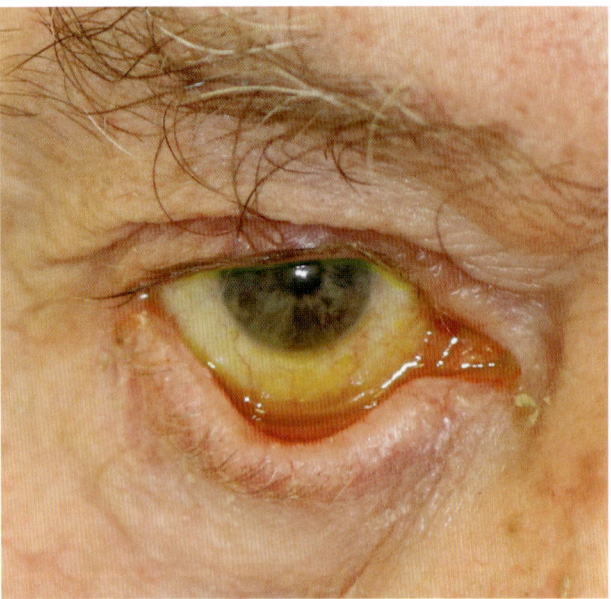

Figure 2.2: Ectropion

There are various causes that lead to an ectropion and from a treatment and nursing care perspective, it is important to understand which type of ectropion is presenting, as the treatment options will vary accordingly. Proper assessment and a thorough history are key to identifying the nature and cause of the ectropion.

Most importantly, the practitioner needs to ask:

- How long has the problem existed?
- Is there an underpinning history of a trauma or skin condition?

As part of the assessment of the lower eyelid, there are a few key tests that will aid diagnosis:

- Distraction test: The lower eyelid is pulled distally and anteriorly away from the globe, between the forefinger and the thumb. You shouldn't normally be able to distract the eyelid more than 10mm from the globe.
- Snap-back test: The lower eyelid is pulled down inferiorly toward the orbital rim and then released. The eyelid should briskly return to its normal position. However, any laxity in the eyelid would reduce this and it may take several 'blinks' for it to return back into position.
- Horizontal laxity: The lower eyelid is pulled horizontally and laterally and the position of the inferior puncta observed. It shouldn't be possible for the puncta to travel more than 2mm laterally – this would indicate medial canthal muscle laxity.

Types of ectropion (lower lid)
There are five main underlying types/causes of ectropion:
- Involutional
- Paralytic
- Cicatricial
- Mechanical
- Congenital

Involutional ectropion
This is usually due to a combination of weakness of the canthal ligaments and a mechanical effect of the preseptal muscle overriding the tarsal plate, causing the lower eyelid to turn outwards (lamellar dissociation). It can also be associated with a weakening of the capsulopalpebral fascia. The canthal muscle weakness may be associated with a reduction of elastic and collagen fibres (Damasceno *et al.* 2011). There may also be retractor disinsertion, which is represented clinically as a deep inferior fornix, no or very little movement of the lower eyelid when the patient is asked to look down.

Involutional ectropion is associated with aging and an associated loss of laxity in the lower eyelid. It is important to ascertain that there is no shortening of the anterior lamella, which is likely to be associated with cicatricial changes.

Paralytic ectropion
This type of ectropion is caused by VII cranial nerve palsy, due to the loss of orbicularis tone, and may be associated with an upper eyelid lagophthalmos.

Cicatricial ectropion
Scarring of the anterior lamella in conditions such as chronic dermatitis, ichthyosis, eczema, or due to trauma, can lead to a shortening and contracting of the skin, which pulls the eyelid down and away from the globe. The ectropion can be accentuated by asking the patient to open their mouth. It may be necessary to treat the underlying cause first, before considering surgical options.

Mechanical ectropion
This is a secondary ectropion caused by the mechanical action of a related problem, such as tumour or neurofibromatosis. In the first instance, removal of the causal factor may reduce or eradicate the mechanical ectropion.

Congenital ectropion
This is a very rare type of ectropion which is present at birth and may be associated with conditions such as Down's Syndrome (Pereira *et al.* 2007).

It is also worth mentioning 'floppy eyelid syndrome', as this condition can also be associated with lax eyelids. It is associated with middle-aged, obese men and nocturnal exposure (whereby their eyelids may evert in their sleep and be irritated by the pillow), leading to symptoms of irritation and keratoconjunctivitis.

Presentation

The most common presentation of ectropion is a combination of epiphora, lid swelling, pain, red eye and ocular irritation. This is turn can cause secondary exposure issues, including punctal epithelial erosions (PEEs) and keratopathy. Over a long period of time, the tarsal conjunctiva can become irritated and chronically thickened and may eventually become keratinised, leading to crusting.

The symptoms of epiphora occur as a consequence of poor eyelid position and eye exposure. The eyelid relies upon good muscle tone to keep it opposed to the globe, which in turn assists the lacrimal pump mechanism through blinking. These functions are diminished if the lower eyelid is not in the correct anatomical position.

Remember, there may be varying degrees of ectropion. The condition is usually progressive and may start with simple laxity, then punctal, followed by medial and eventually complete lid eversion. Also, the lateral canthus is slightly higher than the medial canthus. Considering this, any medial disengagement of the lower eyelid may lead to tearing from the medial canthus. This may be a clue when taking the patient's clinical history.

Non-surgical treatments

Conservative options to reduce or treat ectropion essentially include lubricants, steroid treatment, massage and possibly eyelid taping. It is unlikely that these treatments will completely resolve the ectropion, but they may reduce its debilitating effects and create an optimal environment for surgery. Eyelid massage can, to some extent (if executed well), reduce the degree of ectropion and therefore reduce the need for surgical input. For instance, it may decrease the skin-graft size required to lessen the deficit caused by corrective surgery. (See Figures 2.3a and 2.3b, massage technique.)

Treatment of underlying cause

Shortening of the anterior lamella may be a consequence of underlying skin problems such as dermatitis or eczema. It may therefore be necessary to coordinate concurrent therapy to simultaneously treat these problems and protect the eye. Liaising with the patient's GP and possible referral to a dermatologist (in order to treat the skin-related issues) may be required.

It may also be necessary to treat the eye with topical antibiotics if there is any suspicion of infection. In this case, bacterial swabbing may be needed to identify the bacterium involved.

Lubricants

The correct and effective application of lubricants on the eye and the lower eyelid (if completely everted) will help to reduce exposure-related symptoms. These treatments may well include viscous lubricants, administered at night-time and regularly during the day. It is important for the practitioner to assess the patient's (or helper's) drop instillation technique. Poor application could lead to further damage or infection – don't assume the patient will be proficient at it. It also important to keep the lids clean and remove excess debris/ointment, which may increase the chances of further infection or irritation. Again, it may be necessary to assess the patient's eye cleaning technique. Some of the more viscous ointments will also blur vision and this may cause problems for individuals with already reduced vision. Again, consider the patient's visual capacity and their social circumstances. For example, do they live alone? Or are they required to negotiate stairs? Similarly, for an individual who works and operates machinery or regularly drives, it is important to stress the impact the lubricants may have on their vision whilst undertaking such activities.

Steroid treatment

In some cases, a short reducing course of steroid therapy (ointment) may be necessary to treat the more severe forms of ectropion and help reduce inflammation prior to surgery.

Similarly, when treating mechanical ectropion (caused by scarring or the contracture of a full-thickness skin graft post-operatively), steroid injections can help reduce inflammation. This treatment, combined with massage, can help reduce contracture and reduce the scarring.

Steroid injections can be difficult to perform and are often painful to administer due to being infiltrated into thickened scar tissue. Therefore it is important for the practitioner to prepare the patient for this procedure and gain their consent. It is sometimes advocated that local anaesthetic cream should be applied to the skin prior to treatment. However, the use of topical local anaesthetic creams should be avoided around the eyelids and they are not usually licensed for such use, so don't be tempted to use them to reduce injection discomfort.

Remember that prolonged use of steroids can raise intra-ocular pressure (IOP) and cause cataracts.

Massage

In cases where there is complete ectropion, or there is a mechanical element caused by contracture or scarring of skin, massage of the eyelid may reduce the ectropion. However, the massage has to be done correctly for it to be effective, and patients will have varying levels of manual dexterity. Just as you might assess drop instillation technique, it is equally important to evaluate massage technique.

The purpose of lower eyelid massage is to make the skin more supple and counter the effects of the underlying cicatrising process. It should therefore work against the everted eyelid, moving upwards. It is easier if the index finger is used, and only ever with some form of lubrication between the finger and the eyelid skin. Various ointments can be considered for massage and most of them include liquid paraffin as an emollient base.

A suggested technique for lower eyelid massage

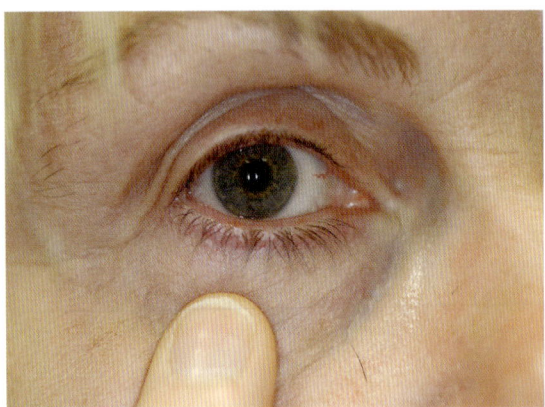 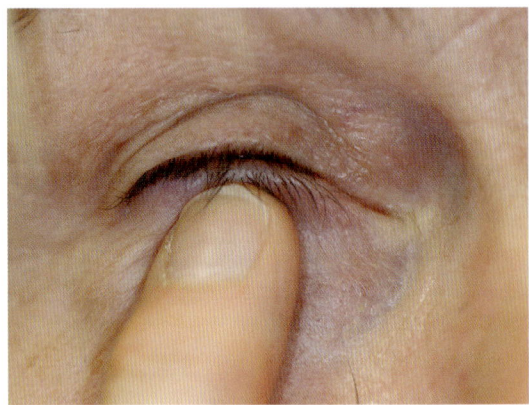

Figure 2.3a: (left) Lower eyelid massage technique – starting position
Figure 2.3b: (right) Upward massage of lower eyelid

Firstly check index fingernails are clean and not too long, so as to avoid damage to the eye. Wash hands prior to massage. It may be necessary to use a mirror or the guidance of a relative/friend whilst undertaking the massage. Then apply a small quantity of lubricant on index finger and gently spread over fingertip. Start the massage centrally below lower eyelid on the inferior bony orbital margin. Whilst applying firm pressure, slowly move index finger upwards, pulling/stretching the lower eyelid over the eye. Be careful not to poke the eye and ensure that the lower eyelid is between your finger and the eye. Hold and stretch the lower eyelid skin for 3–5 seconds and then let go. Repeat the process for 10 minutes, 5–6 times a day. This technique should be assessed by the practitioner and modified as necessary.

Massage technique is subjective and open to interpretation by the patient, especially in relation to how much pressure needs to be applied. It may therefore be necessary to demonstrate so that the patient fully appreciates the amount of pressure required. It is no use the patient having great technique if they are not applying the correct pressure – the outcome will be poor and time will be wasted. For this reason, it is important to check that the patient's massage technique is correct and that the appropriate degree of pressure is being applied.

Inevitably, massage will be difficult for some individuals to carry out, e.g. due to arthritic fingers, a tremor or poor vision. It may then become the responsibility of another individual to undertake the massage. Essentially, the same rules apply, in that the practitioner needs to check technique and pressure prior to the massage being commenced. If a relative or friend is applying the massage, it is easier for this to be undertaken from a position above and behind the patient, with the patient recumbent and looking up. This also reduces the risk of inadvertent contact of a fingernail with the patient's cornea.

Rarely, it simply isn't possible for a safe, reliable and regular massage regime to be adopted (or properly assessed or supervised). In this case, it has to be accepted that it may not be possible to undertake massage and other options may therefore need to be considered.

Temporary suture tarsorrhaphy

In order to protect the eye, it may be necessary to physically close the eyelids temporarily, using a stitch/suture. It will be important to gain consent for this procedure and prepare the patient accordingly.

- Discuss procedure with the patient (and relatives) and get written consent
- Wash hands
- Topical anaesthesia may be applied
- Infiltrate local anaesthetic (via subcutaneous injection) into upper and lower eyelids
- Clean skin, using antiseptic
- Usually a non-dissolvable 4/0 nylon suture and bolster is used (usually a short piece of silicon tubing)
- The initial pass of the suture is through the lateral part of the bolster
- Using needle holders and forceps, the suture is then passed through the lower eyelid approximately 3–4mm from the lash-line towards and through the grey-line
- Then the suture is passed through the opposing upper eyelid, initially through the grey-line and out of the skin 3–4mm superiorly
- The suture is now passed through another superior bolster
- Then the reverse is executed, approximately 10mm horizontally from the initial pass, by passing the needle back through the upper eyelid skin and grey-line and through the opposing lower eyelid
- The needle is removed and the suture tied up to the bolster, tightening as required
- The temporary suture tarsorrhaphy can be opened to apply drops or to examine the eye as required, and then closed again.

Hyaluronic acid injections

The use of hyaluronic acid (HA) dermal fillers injected into the lower eyelid to treat ectropion has been described in the literature (Romero *et al.* 2013). However, the duration of treatment required is uncertain and it may have to be repeated. HA also appears to have a more specific role in the management of patients with *ichthyosiform dermatoses* (rare genetic skin disorders characterised by thickened, dry and scaly skin), where treatment options are limited. Nevertheless, in selected cases, the results achieved using HA dermal fillers to treat ectropion have been reasonably good.

Surgical options

Once the underlying cause of the ectropion has been determined (most commonly involutional or cicatricial), and the conservative treatment options have been applied or exhausted, surgical treatment options may be considered.

For involutional ectropion (no anterior lamellar shortening), the options include:

- A complete tarsal ectropion – lateral tarsal strip procedure and posterior approach inferior retractor reinsertion
- Entire lower eyelid with no retractor dehiscence – lateral tarsal strip procedure and medial spindle procedure
- Punctal ectropion with horizontal laxity – lateral tarsal strip procedure or medial wedge excision and medial spindle procedure
- Punctal ectropion with no horizontal laxity – medial spindle procedure.

Lateral tarsal strip procedure (LTS)

This surgical procedure shortens the lower eyelid at the lateral canthus and may be undertaken in association with other procedures, such as an inferior retractor reinsertion (IRR) – see entropion (p. 29). Typically, the LTS procedure can be undertaken under a local anaesthetic (occasionally with sedation). Caution has to be applied with patients who are on blood-thinning medication (e.g. Aspirin or anti-coagulants), as the risk of an intra-orbital post-operative haemorrhage can be increased (see 'Key nursing considerations' below).

The LTS procedure involves releasing the lower eyelid from the orbital rim (lateral canthotomy) and then cutting the lower limb of the lateral canthal tendon (cantholysis). The lower eyelid will be freed and the lateral edge separated between the anterior and posterior aspects. A small strip of posterior lamella is then refashioned at the newly released free edge of the lateral lower eyelid and this is used to reattach the eyelid to the orbital periosteum at the suitable height. Prior to this, however, the surgeon estimates how much shortening of the eyelid is required (usually 3–5mm) and excess tissue is removed. The redundant anterior lamella is removed (including eyelashes) and the lateral canthal angle reformed.

Lower eyelid wedge excision

As a possible alternative to the LTS procedure, it may be possible to perform a lateral lower eyelid wedge procedure. This involves completely excising a pentagonal section of the eyelid (usually laterally). The eyelids are then approximated and sutured back together. According to Nerad (2001), the wedge excision procedure is, for various reasons (including scarring and difficult lid realignment), an inferior procedure compared to LTS. However, this is not always the case, as it would be far safer, for instance, in a single-sighted patient who is taking anticoagulants. A medial wedge has the advantage of removing a thickened area of eyelid with chronic conjunctival exposure (Leatherbarrow 2019).

For some patients, the wedge excision procedure is a viable alternative, especially for those who are unable to stop taking blood-thinning medications. It is also used in the upper eyelids in patients with floppy eyelid syndrome. The important point to remember is that in involutional ectropion the problem is related to lateral canthal tendon laxity and the appropriate treatment is therefore LTS; a lower eyelid wedge excision will not address this underlying fundamental cause.

Medial spindle (MS) procedure

This is a relatively quick procedure to correct a medical ectropion and reposition the inferior punctum. It involves cutting a small diamond of palpebral conjunctiva (and underlying inferior retractor) approximately 3–4mm below the inferior punctum (and tarsal plate). Vertical closure of the diamond causes the punctum to turn inwardly by shortening a small area of inferior retractor; this is usually undertaken by using a double-armed half-circle polyglycolic-acid dissolvable suture. If it is being performed in conjunction with an LTS, the MS procedure should be carried out first, as it will be difficult to perform once the lower eyelid has been tightened. The suture usually dissolves and falls out within approximately 3 weeks, but it may be better to remove it earlier to reduce scarring.

Key nursing considerations with LTS/MS procedures

1. Pain and discomfort: The lateral canthal area where the LTS suture is attached to the periosteum can be painful for several weeks following the procedure. Firstly, the patient needs to be warned about this and the reasons why. Secondly, appropriate analgesia will be required, especially in the first few days following the LTS. It is important to remember that the pain should be mild to moderate. Any suggestion of severe pain should cause suspicion and may indicate an intra-orbital bleed.

2. Potential for orbital bleed: There is a very rare possibility of a potentially sight-threatening post-operative bleed within the orbit (haematoma).

Pre-operative assessment is crucial in order to identify patients who are at risk of intra-operative and post-operative bleeding: those on anti-coagulants/antiplatelet medications such Clopidogrel, Dipyridamole, Apixaban, Rivaroxaban, Heparin, Warfarin and Aspirin. These medications may need to be altered or temporarily stopped prior to surgery (if possible), but only with appropriate guidance from the patient's anti-coagulant team and/or GP. It is also important to consider other herbal remedies and dietary supplements that can affect blood clotting and increase the potential for bleeding, including (but not limited to) chamomile, garlic, ginger, ginkgo biloba, ginseng, licorice root, parsley and turmeric.

It may be necessary to consider a bridging anti-coagulation therapy with a low-molecular weight heparin (short-acting blood thinner) if the Warfarin treatment is to be interrupted (and its anti-coagulant effect is outside the therapeutic range). If indicated, the Warfarin is stopped 4–5 days prior to surgery and the bridging therapy is commenced and stopped several days after surgery (with a brief hiatus immediately prior to and post surgery). This will have to be carefully coordinated with the haematologists and anti-coagulation team.

It is also important to emphasise to the patient, even if they don't take anti-coagulants, that they must avoid other anti-inflammatory drugs both pre- and post-operatively (for about two weeks prior to surgery and least one week after surgery). These anti-inflammatory drugs include Ibruprofen, Aspirin, Nurofen and Diclofenac, as they can predispose the patient to bleeding.

Some patients identified as being on an anti-coagulant regime may be unable to stop or alter their therapy and it may then be necessary for the oculoplastic team to consider other surgical options.

Post-operatively, if the patient complains of sudden onset of pain, increased swelling, diplopia and reduction of sight, this could be related to a retrobulbar bleed and should be treated as an ophthalmic emergency. It may be necessary to perform an urgent lateral canthotomy and inferior cantholysis to decompress the orbit and take the patient to the operating theatre to drain the haematoma.

3. Awareness of a lump at the lateral canthus: This is usually associated with the lateral canthal reattachment suture and can be initially uncomfortable. The lump should be small and will dissipate over time. The practitioner should observe for signs of infection such as erythema, discharge, increased temperature at the wound site and increased pain. It may be possible for a suture granuloma to form and this may necessitate the removal of the offending suture and treatment with antibiotics.

4. Over-tightening of the lower eyelid: The LTS procedure is performed to tighten the lower eyelid, but initially this can be uncomfortable and feel strange to the patient, especially if the lid has been lax for a long period. The tightening can lead to conjunctival chemosis (swelling) and irritation so it is important for the patient to be aware of this prior to surgery. It may be necessary to consider lubricants to protect the cornea in the short term. Usually the eyelid will become less tight over time and allow for a less restricted feeling.

5. Post-operative topical antibiotics: Following the LTS procedure, the patient will need to apply topical antibiotic ointment in the operated eyelid. The important point here is that the patient must not pull the lower eyelid down to insert the ointment, as this may undo the surgery and lead to detachment of the lower eyelid. Instead, they should apply a small amount to the inner corner of an open eye whilst looking up and not manipulating the eyelid. The practitioner should always, where possible, supervise and assess the patient's drop instillation technique before they are discharged.

Simple tips can help the patient apply the ointment more easily – for example, getting someone else to help install the drop. Likewise, warming the ointment up in one's hand a few moments before application can make it easier to squeeze out of the bottle.

6. Asymmetry: Given that the lower eyelid has been tightened, there may be an obvious difference in its position, compared to the lower eyelid of the un-operated eye. This may improve over time, leading to better symmetry.

Cicatricial ectropion

The management of a cicatricial ectropion is very different from that of an involutional ectropion, so it is important to differentiate between these two classic presentations. For example, performing an LTS procedure (in isolation) for a patient with a cicatricial ectropion would probably not be beneficial as the eyelid would likely be pulled back by the cicatricial process. This would happen because the underlying mechanical counter-tension of the cicatricial element would still pull the lid down and, as has been mentioned above, it may be important to manage or treat the underlying cause first. A vigilant practitioner is likely to recognise and identify the key indicators, such as underlying skin conditions or previous trauma. In extreme circumstances, a lower eyelid with cicatricial changes will be completely everted and it won't be possible to manipulate it back into its normal position.

In some cases, it may be necessary to treat the underlying skin problem before attempting to undertake any surgical correction and referral to a dermatologist may be required.

Remember, cicatricial ectropion is a shortage of anterior lamella (the outward part of the lid). Undertaking a procedure to lengthen this will therefore help to return the lower eyelid to a normal position. The most common surgical approach is to undertake a procedure that releases the scarred eyelid skin. An anterior skin deficit will be created as a consequence and then may be covered with a full-thickness skin graft (FTSG). This may often be performed with an LTS procedure to tighten the eyelid as well.

Typically, the surgical approach is to make a subciliary lower eyelid skin incision – that is, just below the lash-line, horizontally across the eyelid. This can be done using a blade or a cutting mono-polar cautery device with a narrow tip.

Full-thickness skin grafts can be harvested from several accessible areas, the most common being:

- Upper eyelid – it is important to measure upper eyelid skin to ensure there is enough excess skin to utilise (see p. 48). Essentially this skin can be harvested in a similar way to a blepharoplasty procedure. The upper eyelid skin is the thinnest in the body and it also provides a good colour match so it is often seen as the best choice.
- Pre-auricular – this is the area just anterior to the ear, between the tragus and the hair-bearing sideburn area. It is a reasonable colour match and is easy to access.
- Post-auricular – conversely, this area (being behind the ear) is harder to access but does again provide a reasonable colour match.
- Upper inner arm – there is often excess skin to harvest in this area and any potential scar is well hidden. However, the skin may not be a good colour match and can be hair-bearing.
- Supra-clavicular – being just above the collarbone, this is relatively easy to access, but will leave a visible scar, which may be unacceptable for individuals who often wear low-cut tops.

A FTSG is a section of skin harvested that includes both epidermis and dermis. The subcutaneous fat and deeper dermis will need to be removed and trimmed back prior to being sutured into position. This is because it could hinder the graft's ability to adhere and acquire a blood supply. If the FTSG doesn't gain a blood supply, it will become necrosed (die), so it is important that the graft is laid on an appropriate vascular 'bed', usually an underlying layer of muscle.

At the time of surgery, and once harvested, the FTSG will need to be debulked, prior to being sutured into place within the defect. This will require carefully trimming of the dermis layer from the underlying epidermis with Westcott Scissors to a point where the *rete-pegs* are revealed – these are epithelial extensions from the dermis into the underlying connective tissue (lamina propria) which are thought to reduce the shearing effects of the overlying skin. The rete-pegs can just be seen with the naked eye as multiple tiny raised areas on the underlying dermis. This is important as it provides a key indication of the correct amount of debulking of the skin graft – any more and it will be too thin, any less and it will be harder for the graft to survive.

Once the skin graft has been harvested, its edges are trimmed to fit the defect and sutured into place. Either dissolving or non-dissolving sutures can be used for this. However, most dissolving sutures are associated with increased risk of post-operative inflammation and therefore scarring. For this reason, it is recommended to use nylon non-dissolving sutures, to reduce the risk of scarring, and then to remove them at about 7–9 days. Alternatively, some surgeons may use a combination of surgical glue and (fewer) sutures to tack-down FTSGs. This is reasonable but the area needs to be kept dry for several days post-operatively so as to not disturb the glue.

As a surgical practitioner I harvest full-thickness skin grafts and my surgical competency for the procedure appears on p. 314.

Care of full-thickness skin grafts and the donor site

FTSGs are a relatively easy way of covering a defect, but they do come with a number of post-operative care considerations. These will need to be discussed with the patient prior to surgery, as they will need to appreciate their role in caring for both the graft and the donor site.

Firstly, FTSGs have a tendency to contract over time. This is a real problem and may even cause another ectropion if left untended. Post-operative massage is the key strategy to counter the effects of contraction but, as has already been highlighted above, this requires the patient to be able to carry it out effectively. Massage can be started from as early as the second week post-operatively although it should be relatively gentle to start with.

It is best to use a technique that counters the effects of gravity and mechanical contracture. Essentially in most patients this will be an upward motion, using the (clean) index finger and lubrication. I would stress that this should be entirely an upward motion, not up and down or circular. It may be useful to use the middle finger to help 'pin down' the cheek skin at the same time so as to provide a counter-tension. Lubrication should be with an ointment that is non-harmful to the eye.

As each day goes by, the massage applied can become firmer and it is important that the patient is aware that it needs to be really quite firm. I sometimes demonstrate this on the back of a patient's hand so they appreciate just how hard it should be. It is difficult to describe how firm this method should be as the concept of relative firmness is subjective; but I try to get the patient to imagine that they are trying to 'break down' the links the scar tissue is forming. If the massage is applied too gently, it will be largely a waste of time.

Massage is tiring so short, regular sessions are preferable, maybe 5–10 minutes every couple of hours. It is important for the practitioner to supervise and/or modify the patient's technique at subsequent outpatient visits if there are signs that the graft is contracting. Sometimes, in their efforts to get good results, the patient may overdo the massage and irritate the skin. In this case, it may be best to encourage them to reduce the amount of massage and allow the graft to recover.

Despite the best efforts of the patient and the practitioner, the graft may still contract and may need further input to cease the contracture process. One way is to inject corticosteroids directly into the graft. This is a difficult procedure, as it is hard to perform and can be painful for the patient. It is important to get full verbal and written consent for the procedure and the patient needs to be made aware of the potential adverse effects of injecting steroids into the graft, especially the slight risk of tissue necrosis (death), infection, blanching/discolouring of the skin (hypopigmentation) and the discomfort associated with the injection.

Other extrinsic factors can also affect wound healing and it is important to emphasise these to the patient and for the practitioner to assist in optimising them, where possible. These factors include: maintaining a healthy well-balanced diet, smoking cessation, control of underlying medical conditions and maintenance of psychological wellbeing.

It is also important not to forget the donor site. The sutures will need to be removed (if they are not dissolvable) after 10–12 days. At this stage, it is important to keep the site clean and to apply antibiotic ointment if prescribed. Thereafter, gentle massage may again be helpful in certain sites and the application of anti-scarring agents may also be advocated. Silicone-based treatments have been found to be useful in reducing long-term scarring, although the exact mechanism of their action is not fully understood (Bleasdale *et al.* 2015, Gold *et al.* 2014)). These cannot be prescribed on the NHS and need to be purchased by the patient and they are not cheap. Also, they do not work for everyone, so it is important to emphasise this.

Table 2.1: Post-operative care of the patient with an ectropion – lateral tarsal strip

Issue	Nursing input	Rationale	Evaluation	Comment
1. Pain and discomfort following surgery	Pre-operative information regarding post-operative pain associated with procedure at pre-assessment.	To ensure patient is aware of the potential for pain – but this should be mild to moderate.	Daycase procedure – patient will be discharged with information. Make sure patient has the appropriate contact details and/or is aware of what to do if concerned about pain.	Post-operative pain should be mild to moderate and confined to area of the surgery. A post-operative bleed is highly unlikely but the patient should be aware of the extremely low potential for a bleed and the need to act fast if there is any suspicion of a bleed. Staff should also be aware of the potential signs of a periorbital bleed.
	Post-operative analgesia – paracetamol should be enough to control pain.	To reduce pain associated with the procedure.	Ensure patient is either discharged with analgesia or has access to analgesia. Contact patient first day post-op to check.	
	Awareness of signs of periorbital bleed. Sudden moderate to severe pain, associated with: • Possible swelling • Reduction of vision • Tense orbit. Provide contact details and/or encourage patient to attend A&E immediately with these symptoms.	**Ophthalmic emergency – may require surgical input.** Contact ophthalmic consultant and liaise with theatre. Consider urgent canthotomy/cantholysis (get appropriate surgical instruments) and perform immediately. Urgent admission.	Mild to moderate symptoms are likely to subside over the days immediately following surgery.	
2. Potential for orbital bleed post-operatively	At pre-assessment highlight any potential anti-coagulants/anti-platelet regimes. Identify any herbal or dietary supplements that may affect bleeding. Encourage the patient to avoid anti-inflammatory medications.	To reduce the risk of peri- or post-operative bleeding, it may be necessary to stop or alter the anti-coagulant regime	Can usually restart anti-coagulation or anti-platelet therapy the day after surgery, with clinical guidance.	If anti-coagulant and anti-platelet therapies are stopped, this can dramatically reduce peri-operative bleeding, but this requires close management and monitoring, plus follow-up by the anti-coagulation team.

	Some patients are unable to stop or use alternative arrangements for anti-coagulation.	These patients may have to continue their anti-coagulant regime, which will increase peri- or post-operative bleeding. May need to alter surgical approach – wedge resection.	Post-operative care of wedge resection – topical antibiotics and wound hygiene.	
3. Awareness of lateral canthal lump	Lump at the lateral canthal/orbit, may be tender to touch. Be aware of signs of infection: • Redness • Erythema • Increased pain.	Associated with the lower eyelid tightening. The eyelid is stitched to the periosteum, the lining over the orbital rim bone. The periosteum has a good nerve supply – hence the discomfort often experienced for several weeks after the surgery.	The lump will reduce in size and discomfort over 2–4 weeks.	
4. Over-tightening of lower eyelid		Patient complains of discomfort and there is increased chemosis and/or conjunctival exposure. Treat with lubricants if necessary.	Over-tightening of eyelid constricts the conjunctiva, causing swelling. To protect the palpebral conjunctiva from exposure and drying.	Over time the lower eyelid will slacken and thus reduce the swelling. Very occasionally the procedure will need to be redone, due to over-tightening.
5. Post-operative prevention of infection	Use antibiotic ointment for the first 1–2 weeks on the wounds following the procedure. Assess drop regime with the patient or relative undertaking application of drops.	To reduce the chance of infection.	Occasionally the patient is allergic to antibiotics and this treatment needs to be altered or stopped.	Do not pull down on the eyelid on the operated side, as this could affect or undo the surgery.
6. Cosmetic appearance after surgery	There may be asymmetry following the surgery.	The operated eyelid will be tighter than the opposite eyelid.	Over time the operated eyelid will slacken slightly and it may be necessary to tighten the opposite lower eyelid.	

Entropion

When the eyelid turns and rotates inwards, this is defined as entropion (see Figure 2.4). Mechanically, this involves a shortening of the posterior lamella, affecting the palpebral conjunctiva and/or the tarsal plate and weakening the inferior retractors. If this occurs, both the eyelid margin and the eyelashes will be inverted. This will cause the eyelashes to rub against the eye, potentially causing irritation and infection. Again, it is important to identify the underlying cause of the entropion, as this will dictate the surgical treatment.

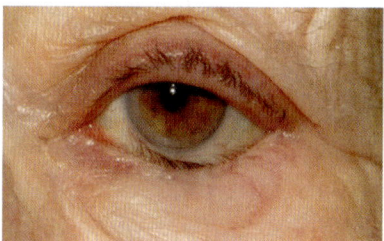

Figure 2.4: Entropion

There are three main types/causes of entropion:
- Involutional
- Cicatricial
- Spastic.

Involutional entropion

Due to the lower eyelid becoming more lax over time, the retractor muscle complex becoming weakened and an associated over-ride of the orbicularis muscle, the lower eyelid turns in. The cause is multifactorial but is typically associated with an age-related decrease of tensile collagen strength within the lid.

Presentation

The presentation is much the same as that of ectropion, with the patient complaining of tearing, irritation, discomfort and discharge. Interestingly, the entropion may only be intermittent – i.e. occurring either sporadically and/or if the patient is asked to forcibly close their eyes. You may need to ask the patient to do this in order to elicit an entropion, as it may not be obvious at first.

Conservative treatment options

Once the practitioner has identified the cause and extent of the entropion (and inspected the corneal surface), it may be possible to provide temporary relief with simple interventions. Firstly, the use of topical lubricants will reduce friction and provide some comfort. It is important to assess the patient's competence in applying the lubricants. This can be quite tricky and may need supervision at first. Many patients complain about the more viscous ointments causing blurring of vision, so timing of the application is important; don't apply the ointment just prior to driving, for example. Some patients simply misunderstand the purpose of the various ointments and drops they are asked to use and this leads to mistakes. It may be helpful to write key elements down and provide an information sheet that explains what to do. Never assume that the patient knows or understands the process or will necessarily read an information leaflet.

Eyelid taping can be useful but can be difficult to apply. The action of the taping is to simulate a tightened lower eyelid position not dissimilar to what would be achieved by performing an LTS procedure. I find paper tape the best to use, the 10mm diameter version especially. A short length is cut off (approximately 4cm) and this is firmly applied to the affected lower eyelid, starting just at the midline of the eyelid, and 2–3mm below the lash-line. The tape is then firmly pulled upwards and laterally to manifest the tightening effect, which is anchored temporarily to the skin. It is vital to check the positioning and ensure that the tape isn't interfering with the surface of the eye. It also important to protect the skin, as in older patients it may be friable and susceptible to damage, especially when removing the tape. Slow and careful removal of the tape is important under these circumstances.

It may be necessary to undertake the taping in front of a mirror and/or with the help of a relative or friend. It is important that the practitioner observes the patient undertaking the taping procedure before they leave the clinic to ensure safe practice. Unfortunately, in some instances, it may be too tricky for the patient to do themselves, but it can still be useful for the healthcare professional to undertake the taping in order to briefly show how an LTS procedure might help with correcting the entropion in clinic.

Everting sutures (Quickert's procedure)

A relatively simple procedure to correct an involutional entropion is everting sutures – otherwise known as Quickert's procedure. This is usually performed in the operating theatre, but can, if warranted and safe, be undertaken in a treatment room. The procedure involves passing 2 or 3 double-armed polyglactin (910) dissolvable sutures through the lower eyelid, incorporating and tightening the lower eyelid retractors, causing the eyelid to turn out.

The procedure is carried out under a local anaesthetic. Once this has been administered into the lower eyelid, the skin should be prepped using antimicrobial solution such as aqueous iodine. The double-armed suture (usually a half circle 4/0 with reverse cutting needle) is loaded back-hand into the needle holders. Using a pair of toothed forceps, such as Paufique forceps, to hold and lift the lower eyelid, the suture is initially passed from within the conjunctival fornix anteriorly toward the skin. As the needle is passed through the eyelid, it will pick up the lower lid retractors, and then it is passed superiorly to exit the skin approximately 2–3mm inferior to the lash-line. The process is repeated with the other arm of the suture, exiting adjacent to the first pass. Then the suture is tied on the skin whilst observing the degree of eversion achieved. Typically, a central suture is passed, with a medial and lateral suture alongside it.

In some cases, the entropion might be quite minimal and in this instance transverse sutures may be enough to stabilise rather than evert the eyelid. This is effectively the same procedure as above but the sutures are passed in a crosswise manner through the eyelid and thus provide a more stabilising effect, rather than everting the lid..

The everting suture procedure does not correct the horizontal laxity of the eyelid so, in cases where the lid is very lax (floppy), undertaking everting sutures may be futile, as the lid may just be too lax for the eversion to have any real effect .

Usually the sutures are removed at 3 weeks – if they have not already dissolved and fallen out. (In my experience, it can take anything up to 6 weeks for them to dissolve or fall out, so it is usually better to remove them.) While they are in place, the sutures should be kept clean and antibiotic ointment should be applied to them, as this will not only protect them from infection but also start to soften them. The localised scarring created by the everting sutures helps to hold the eyelid in position, so taking the sutures out too early could be detrimental to the success of the procedure.

Everting sutures are not usually intended to be a long-term option for entropion correction, but they can sometimes last for several years. However, it may often be necessary to perform a more definitive LTS procedure (with an inferior retractor reinsertion) to correct the problem, especially if the eyelids are overly lax.

For some individuals, everting sutures may a better and safer option than an LTS, especially if they have particularly complex co-morbidities that would make longer surgical procedures potentially risky. This is also a procedure that the nurse practitioner can learn to undertake as part of a minor-op procedure list (see surgical competency on p. 294).

Occasionally, some patients get a stitch granuloma (localised inflammatory reaction around the stitch). In this instance, the stitch would need to be removed and further topical antibiotics may be required.

Inferior retractor reinsertion (IRR) or advancement

The main procedure of choice for correction for involutional entropion is an inferior retractor reinsertion (IRR) and this is often undertaken in conjunction with an LTS procedure (see above) if there is an associated laxity. The purpose of the LTS is to stabilise the eyelid, while the IRR procedure is to shorten the fascia and reattach to the tarsus.

The IRR procedure starts with a subciliary skin incision, often using a handheld monopolar cautery (or a surgical blade). The dissection continues through the orbicularis oculi muscle and the orbital septum. Eventually the inferior eyelid retractors are identified and dissected from the overlying preaponeurotic fat and underlying conjunctiva. The retractor muscle is then shortened by removing a small strip of fascia (approximately 1mm) and reattaching it to the inferior edge of the tarsus.

The post-operative instructions for the care of the wound (i.e. cleaning and application of antibiotic ointment) are the main considerations after the IRR procedure. It is important to remind the patient not to pull on the lower eyelid, especially if they have to apply other drops into the eye. If the patient uses contact lenses, it is best not to put them in for 2 weeks after the procedure.

The patient needs to be vigilant for the early signs of post-operative infection and this should be explained to them prior to the surgery. Emphasise that symptoms such as pain, swelling, redness, discharge and lid malposition need to be reported as early as possible.

Cicatricial entropion

Conjunctival scarring and contracture may cause a lower eyelid entropion by the mechanical action of pulling the eyelid towards the eye. It is important to recognise this when assessing the patient and/or suspect potential contracture in patients who have had trauma or may suffer from associated ophthalmic conditions such as ocular cicatricial pemphigoid or Stevens-Johnson Syndrome (SJS).

Ocular cicatricial pemphigoid (OCP)

Ocular cicatricial pemphigoid (OCP) manifests as a chronic inflammatory conjunctivitis – over time the associated subepithelial fibrosis causes cicatrisation of mucous membranes. The chronic inflammatory process most commonly affects the mucous linings of the mouth and the conjunctiva, but it can also involve the oesophagus and the trachea, making it potentially life-threatening. Progressive scarring of the conjunctiva can cause entropion, symblepharon, conjunctivitis and corneal neovascularisation. Histopathological diagnosis is usually required.

Stevens-Johnson syndrome (SJS) and toxic epidermal necrolysis (TEN)

Stevens-Johnson syndrome (SJS) and toxic epidermal necrolysis (TEN) are due to a severe hypersensitivity reaction that is often associated with various drugs or infectious agents. In its acute phase the reaction can be very severe, with associated symptoms of rash, malaise, fever and cutaneous lesions leading to the detachment of the skin. Ocular features may include pain, photophobia, severe conjunctivitis, bullae and corneal ulceration.

Ocular treatment will involve topical steroids, lubrication, and lysis (breaking down) of the developing symblepharon, using glass rods or a symblepharon ring to break down adhesions.

Assessing and treating cicatricial entropion

When reviewing patients with suspected conjunctival shortage, it is important to pull the lower eyelid down and look for signs of scarring within the fornices. These will be in the form of attachments between the bulbar and palpebral conjunctiva which sometimes prevent or restrict eye movement. While the eyelid is pulled down, it is important to get the patient to look in various directions and especially upwards to reflect potential signs of contracture.

In some cases, the shortening of posterior lamella and conjunctival contracture can be quite restrictive and obvious. In other cases, it can be quite subtle so careful observation may be required, even when using a slit lamp.

In this instance, any attempt to correct the eyelid deviation with horizontal eyelid tightening will be ineffective and inappropriate. Essentially, when trying to correct cicatricial entropion, the main consideration is to release the scarring and to extend the amount of tissue available. This may in turn include deepening the inferior fornices. In order to achieve this, supplementary tissue will be required to bridge the deficit created by releasing the scarring, in a similar way to using a full-thickness skin graft to correct cicatricial ectropion. In this instance, however, a mucous membrane will be necessary and this is commonly harvested usually from the lower lip (oral labial).

Mucous membrane graft

Harvesting an oral labial mucous membrane graft in theatre involves exposing the lower lip and appropriately preparing the area using antiseptic. Access is often difficult and retracting the lip using Babcock's retractors will allow for better exposure without damaging the tissue.

Once retracted, the required area is marked and local anaesthetic is administered; this provides some immediate post-operative comfort. Adrenaline in the local anaesthetic acts as a vasoconstrictor and should reduce potential bleeding during surgery.

It is important for the surgeon to avoid the frenulum (small fold of tissue between lip and gum) and vermillion border, which is the junction of the mucous membrane with the anterior lip skin. Using a 15 blade and scissors, the surgeon carefully lifts and dissects the mucous membrane from the underlying fat. Once harvested, the mucous membrane graft is placed into the inferior fornix and sutured into place to cover the deficit created by releasing the scarred conjunctiva. The lip donor site wound can be closed with dissolving sutures, depending on the size of the defect, but usually the wound is left to heal by secondary intention.

Once the harvested mucous membrane graft is stitched in place, over time and whilst healing there is a risk that it will contract and therefore cause the inferior fornices to shallow and contract. To prevent this and to help deepen the fornices, at the same surgery a silicone band (usually used in vitreo-retinal surgery – 240 band) can be sutured horizontally deep into this pocket, with dissolvable sutures known as fornix-deepening sutures. This usually helps maintain the pocket while the graft heals in place, and prevents it contracting and adhering together.

Several weeks after the surgery, the silicone band is released in clinic (or operating theatre) by cutting the sutures that hold it in place and gently removing the band. This can usually be done using local anaesthetic drops, but it may be a little uncomfortable so it is important to support the patient and prepare them for the procedure.

Care of mucous membrane donor site

Initially, within the immediate post-operative period, the patient may well require appropriate analgesia. Avoidance of hot food and drinks will also be important for the first 48–72 hours. The patient may only be able to tolerate a soft diet. Oral cleanliness where possible, to prevent infection, will also be a priority and therefore an anti-inflammatory mouthwash such as Benzydamine, which also has anaesthetic properties, can be recommended for 2 weeks following surgery. The lip may swell in the first few days, and this is to be expected as a natural part of the wound healing process.

The patient should be warned that their lip area may be numb for a period following the surgery. This is important, as they could cause inadvertent damage to the wound or lip due to the numbness.

The patient should be vigilant in checking for early signs of infection, such as discharge, increased pain, increased temperature, increased redness, etc. The lip wound often recovers very well after the procedure but may take several weeks to heal completely.

Even though the lip wound can appear (and often is) very sore immediately after harvesting a mucous membrane graft, it usually heals remarkably well with the appropriate care.

References

Bleasdale, B., Finnegan, S., Murray, K., Kelly, S. & Percival, S. (2015). The use of silicone adhesives for scar reduction. *Advanced Wound Care.* **4**(7), 422–30.

Damasceno, R., Osaki, M., Dantas, P. & Belfort, R. (2011). Involutional ectropion and entropion: clinicopathologic correlation between horizontal eyelid laxity and eyelid extracellular matrix. *Ophthalmic Plastic Reconstructive Surgery.* **27**(5), 321–26.

Gold, M., McGuire, M., Mustoe, T. *et al*. (2014). International Advisory Panel on Scar Management. Updated international clinical recommendations on scar management (part 2). *Dermatological Surgery.* **40**(8), 825–31.

Leatherbarrow, B. (2019) *Oculoplastic Surgery*. 3rd edn. USA: Thieme.

Nerad, J. (2001). *Oculoplastic Surgery: The Requisites*. New York: Mosby.

Pereira, F., Trindade, S. & Cruz. A. (2007). Congenital ectropion: three case reports and literature review. *Arquivos Brasileiros de Oftalmologia.* **70**(1), 149–52.

Romero, R., Sanchez-Orgaz, M., Granados, M. & Molia, P. (2013). Use of hyaluronic acid gel in the management of cicatricial ectropion: results and complications. *Orbit.* **32**(6), 362–65.

3

Assessment and management of upper eyelid blepharoptosis

Introduction

One of the more common referrals the oculoplastic practitioner is likely to encounter is 'a droopy upper eyelid'. The clinical presentation of a lowered upper eyelid is known as a ptosis (silent 'p') and is derived from the Greek word meaning 'falling'. A ptosis can obstruct the vision by directly impeding the visual axis due to the eyelid falling over the cornea. Some patients will try to compensate for this by lifting their chin or brows. Some individuals refer to a ptosis as a 'lazy eye'. This may not relate to the eyelid but to the eye itself by way of astigmatism.

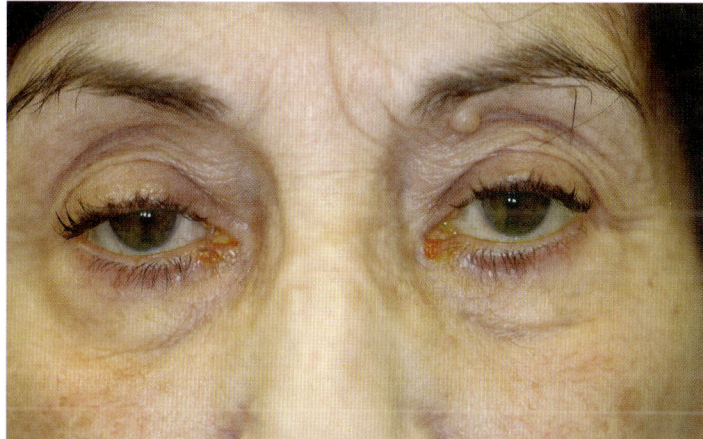

Figure 3.1: Ptosis

The cause of a ptosis is multi-factorial and it is important for the practitioner to recognise the underlying reasons for the eyelid to droop, as this can affect treatment and choice of surgical intervention. The most common causes can be grouped under one of the following headings:

- Myogenic
- Neurogenic

- Aponeurotic
- Mechanical
- Congenital.

Other, much rarer, secondary causes include drugs, orbital lesions and exposure to toxins. A ptosis can be either unilateral or bilateral and is more common in the elderly. Typically, it occurs due to a dysfunction of the muscles that lift the eyelid. The two main muscles involved in raising the eyelid are the levator palpebrae superioris and the Müller's muscle.

Often an eyelid that is drooping may be referred to as 'ptotic'. This is a generic term that can be used in relation to any organ or body part that is abnormally lowered.

Upper eyelid anatomy

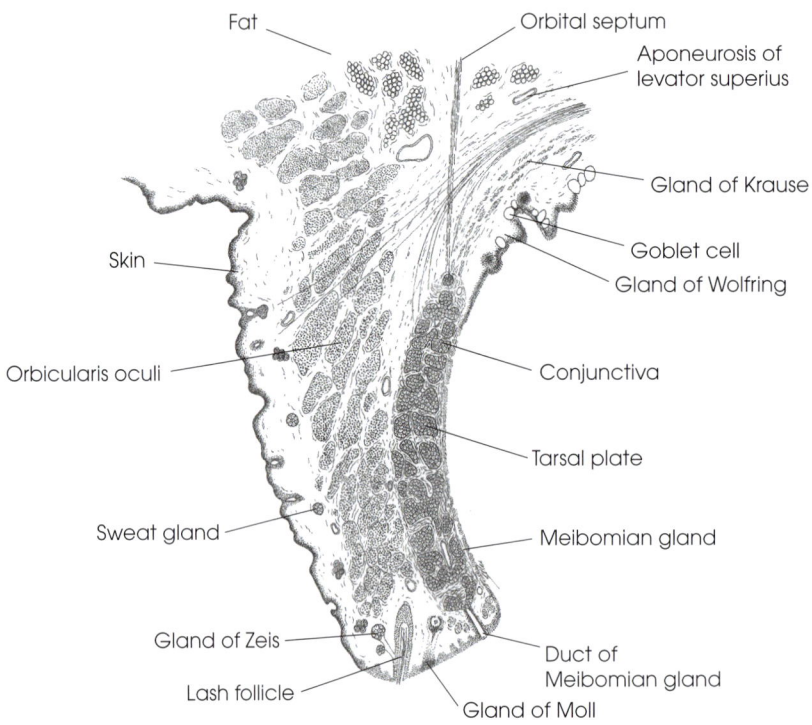

Figure 3.2: Upper eyelid anatomy

The eyelids have a horizontal length of approximately 26mm in females and 27mm in males, and they can shorten with age. The inner corner, towards the nose, is known as the medial canthal area; the outer corner, towards the ear, is the lateral canthal area. The point where the upper and lower eyelids meet laterally is known as the commissure. The lateral angle (canthus) is supported and attached to the bony orbit just behind the orbital rim (at Whitnall's turbercle) by the lateral canthal tendon which is an extension of the orbicularis muscle.

Medially, at the inner corner of the eye, the eyelids are supported by the medial canthal tendon, which is attached to the orbital rim at the bony lacrimal crest and the frontal process of the maxilla. The medial canthal tendon has two limbs which lie on either side of the lacrimal sac.

Both the upper and lower eyelids have an area of dense connective tissue known as tarsal plates; these provide a structure for the eyelids. The upper eyelid has a semilunar or D-shaped tarsal plate which at its broadest is approximately 10mm in width. The upper eyelid tarsal plate is also 25–29mm in horizontal length and 1mm thick. The lower eyelid also has a tarsal plate, but it is much smaller, with a vertical height of 5mm.

Skin layer of the eyelid

The eyelid skin, particularly in the upper eyelid, is the thinnest in the body. It is 0.04–0.06mm thick, although this varies very slightly between genders, races and age groups (Lee & Hwang 2002). The further it is away distally from the eyelid margin, the thicker the skin, and as it reaches the brow it is 2.8 times thicker than the eyelid (Ha *et al.* 2005).

The outer epidermis of the eyelid skin consists of keratinised stratified squamous epithelium and comprises five layers:

- Stratum corneum
- Stratum lucidum
- Stratum granulosum
- Stratum spinosum
- Stratum basale.

The epidermis layer contains no blood vessels and is nourished by the deeper layers and underlying dermis. The epidermis contains keratinocytes which are produced at the basal layer and act as a barrier to heat, UV radiation, pathogens and bacteria. This layer also contains melanocytes which absorb UV-B light and provide skin colour.

Beneath the epidermis is the dermis, which is largely composed of connective tissue, collagen and elastic fibres. Also within the dermis are sweat glands, nerves, blood vessels, lymphatics, sebaceous glands and hair follicles. The collagen and the elastic fibres provide the skin's integral strength and elasticity. Over time, these relax and allow the skin to form wrinkles.

The orbicularis muscle

The orbicularis oculi muscle is associated with closing the eyelids. It concentrically encircles the orbit and arises from the medial canthal area (nasal component of the frontal bone), encompassing the eyelids and the temporal/cheek areas of the face. The upper fibres medially merge into the corrugator muscle and centrally into the frontalis muscle. The orbicularis is largely a voluntary striated muscle and is innervated by the VII cranial nerve (facial). The orbicularis muscle is also anatomically subdivided into pretarsal (over the tarsal plate), preseptal (over the septum) which together are responsible for involuntary blinking, and an orbital segment that is associated with forced blinking (Nerad 2001).

Levator palpebrae superioris muscle

The levator SM is a skeletal muscle that lifts the upper eyelid. It originates from the inner surface of the lesser wing of sphenoid and just above the optic foramen at the back of the orbit. It transects anteriorly and superiorly over the eye, becoming progressively thinner. This narrow band of muscle eventually broadens and inserts into the superior tarsal plate. Some fibres continue and extend forward and insert into the skin of the eyelid, effectively creating the upper eyelid skin fold or skin crease. Assessing and measuring the skin crease height can provide information as to the cause of the ptosis. This is a measure from the upper eyelid inferior eyelid margin to the skin crease in the midline. Normally in males this is 8–10mm and in females it is 9–11mm.

The levator muscle overrides the superior rectus muscle within the orbit and is in very close proximity to it. The levator muscle is innervated by the oculomotor nerve (CN III), which provides motor function to lift the eyelid. It gains its blood supply from the ophthalmic artery.

Müller's muscle (or superior tarsal muscle)

At the upper border of the tarsal plate and inferior to (and originating from) the levator palpebrae superioris muscle is the superior tarsal muscle. This is approximately 20mm of smooth muscle that helps to keep the eyelid lifted (once opened by the levator muscle). It also synergistically provides a small proportion of the lift of the eyelid along with the levator palpebrae muscle (Esperidião-Antonio *et al.* 2010). It is innervated by the sympathetic nervous system with nerve fibres originating from the superior cervical ganglion.

It is more commonly referred to as 'Müller's muscle', named after the German anatomist Heinrich Müller (1820–1910) who first described the muscle in 1858.

Whitnall's ligament

Whitnall's ligament is an important surgical landmark and acts as a 'pulley' for the levator muscle. It extends transversely as a fibrous band from the lacrimal gland supero-laterally to the trochlea of superior oblique medially. It is often visualised during levator advancement surgery when correcting ptosis.

Blood supply

The eyelids have a very good blood supply which comes from branches of the ophthalmic, temporal and facial arteries. These arteries then supply several groups of vessels, including the marginal (and inferior), medial (peripheral), superior and inferior arcades. Most of the venous drainage is associated with the superior and inferior ophthalmic veins.

Innervation of the eyelids

The eyelids are innervated by the sensory and motor nerves.

Sensory

The ophthalmic (CN V – trigeminal) has three major branches:

- Ophthalmic (V1) branches to form the frontal nerve and then subdivides into supraorbital (forehead and scalp) and supratrochlear branches (upper eyelid and superior medial canthus)
- Ophthalmic (V2) branches to form the nasociliary nerve which then subdivides into infratrochlear (inferior medial canthus) and external nasal branches (nose)
- Ophthalmic (V3) branches to form the lacrimal nerve (lacrimal gland) maxillary (V2) divisions of the trigeminal nerve.

The infra-orbital nerve innervates the lower eyelid, cheek, upper gingiva and teeth.

Motor

The oculomotor (CN III) has two divisions. The upper supplies the levator palpebral muscle which lifts the eyelid (and innervates the superior and medial rectus muscles). The lower division supplies the inferior rectus and oblique muscles.

The facial nerve (CN VII) innervates the orbicularis oculi muscle, which is responsible for shutting the eyelids. The nerve has five branches, two of which are directly associated with the eyelids:

- Temporal – orbicularis, procerus, corrugator and frontalis muscles
- Zygomatic – orbicularis of the lower eyelid and the lacrimal gland
- Buccal – mouth
- Mandibular – mouth
- Cervical – neck.

The functions of the eyelids and the blink mechanism are to:

- Provide protection and comfort to the eye

- Contribute to tear drainage
- Spread lubricants and tears over the eye
- Assist in the removal of debris
- Cover the eye while asleep
- Control the amount of light entering the eye.

Causes and aetiology of upper eyelid ptosis

Myogenic

It is important to consider the various definitions of myogenic-related ptosis. The term 'myogenic' refers to a primary weakness of a muscle group. An impairment of the transmission of impulses at the neuromuscular junction, which causes a weakness of the muscle fibres when it affects the levator muscle, may cause a ptosis. This is known as a 'neuromyopathic' ptosis and is classed as 'neurogenic'. However, there does seem to be some crossover between myogenic and neurogenic ptosis. Similarly, a 'dystrophy' can be seen as a subtype of progressive myopathy and is defined as muscle degeneration leading to weakness. Various conditions are associated with these types of ptosis and they can either be acquired or inherited.

Myasthenia gravis (MG)

This is an autoimmune disease in which acetylcholine receptors at the neuromuscular junctions are either blocked or destroyed by antibodies so preventing nerve impulses and subsequent muscle contraction. It affects skeletal muscle and the onset can vary, sometimes being quite sudden. It can be associated with diplopia, due to weakness of the extra-ocular muscles. It is a very rare cause of upper eyelid ptosis and can be both unilateral and bilateral.

With this condition, it is important for the practitioner to consider other related muscle limitations such as those associated with swallowing and speaking as well as facial muscle weakness.

The diagnostic gold standard is to take a blood sample for acetylcholine receptor antibodies (AChR). If the result is positive, this may indicate MG. However, one does have to be slightly cautious as even those patients who have classic signs of ocular MG may have a negative AChR test. In this case, another uncommon blood test may be performed – antiMuSK (muscle specific kinase) – to aid diagnosis.

Chronic progressive external ophthalmoplegia (CPEO)

This rare disease typically affects young adults and is associated both with bilateral ptosis and an inability to move the eyes. Patients may tilt their heads to compensate for the lid droop. However, it is often diplopia that causes the patient most concern and this is often the presenting problem.

CPEO is a transmitted mitochondrial myopathy that is associated with mutations of the mtDNA that particularly affect the extraocular muscles. The disease requires diagnosis from muscle biopsy, and there are limited treatment options. These may include ptosis props mounted onto glasses to help lift the upper eyelid or surgical correction of the ptosis.

Myotonic dystrophy (MD)

This genetic disease is associated with debilitating gradual muscle loss and weakness. The condition can affect various systems within the body but is mainly characterised by muscle weakening, increased risk of cardiac defects, frontal hair balding, absent or depressed distal reflexes, difficulty in walking and cataracts.

There are two main classifications of the disease. Type 1 (sometimes known as Steinert disease) is the most common form and is associated with eyelid ptosis. Type 1 myotonic dystrophy symptoms overlap with those of type 2, but they are generally more severe and are associated with muscle weakness in the lower legs, neck, hands and face. Compared to type 2, they can shorten a person's lifespan.

Unfortunately, there is no cure for MD and there is a high risk of genetic transmission, so genetic counselling is necessary. Treatment usually involves management of the symptoms.

Neurogenic

The main cause of neurogenic ptosis is associated with innervational defects related to a major nerve.

Third cranial nerve (CN) palsies

The third CN (oculomotor) is entirely associated with motor function and innervates skeletal fibres of some of the extra-ocular muscles (superior, medial, inferior recti and the inferior oblique) and the levator muscle. It also includes axons of parasympathetic nature that enable constriction of the pupil.

The course of the third CN starts in the midbrain of the spinal cord and passes anteriorly and laterally to the posterior clinoid process. It then traverses through the cavernous sinus into the orbit via the superior orbital fissure. Upon entering the orbit, the nerve divides into two: a superior and inferior branch. The superior branch supplies the superior rectus and the levator muscles. The inferior branch, the larger division, then further separates into three branches: the first supplies the medial rectus; the second the lateral rectus; and the third supplies parasympathetic innervation via the ciliary ganglion to control the sphincter pupillae muscle (contraction) and the ciliary muscle (accommodation).

The symptoms of third CN palsies vary depending upon the position and nature of the contributory causative factors. However, the common clinical signs are:

- Complete ptosis, due to weakness of the levator muscle
- Abduction (outward – exotropia) movement of eye, due to unopposed antagonistic action of the lateral rectus muscle
- Weakness of medial rectus muscle
- Weakness of the superior rectus and inferior oblique muscles
- Limitation of elevation and depression
- Dilated pupil, due to palsy of parasympathetic effect upon accommodation.

This combination of related signs and symptoms produces the classic 'down and out' gaze of the affected side in a patient with a third nerve palsy.

The causes of acquired third nerve palsies are varied but can include the following.

Trauma
A subdural or extra-dural haematoma as a direct consequence of a trauma may cause pressure on the third nerve.

Aneurysm
An aneurysm of the posterior communicating artery near the junction of the internal carotid artery at the optic chiasm may cause a painful third nerve palsy. This is a medical emergency as the problem could progress to an intracranial aneurysm.

Diabetes
A microvascular palsy may be caused by diabetes (or hypertension) which does not involve the pupil but can be painful.

Tumour
A compressive tumour may cause third nerve palsy, e.g. meningioma's.

Idiopathic
As many as 25% of third nerve palsy cases can be associated with no obvious cause.

Vasculitis
Conditions such as giant cell arteritis may sometimes be attributed to a third nerve palsy, although these are quite rare.

As a consequence of some of the indications outlined above and the close physiological proximity of other cranial nerves, it is possible that there may be some involvement of other cranial nerves. This may mean, for example, that a particular combination of symptoms could be associated with third, fourth and sixth cranial nerve palsies.

Horner's syndrome
This uncommon condition represents a combination of symptoms all arising from the sympathetic nerve supply and the spinal cord. The ipsilateral symptoms are caused by various disease processes including tumour, carotid aneurysm, internal carotid dissection

and even trauma. One of the symptoms is ptosis (usually mild to moderate) and this can also be associated with anhidrosis (lack of sweating), miosis (constriction of the affected side), upside down ptosis (lower eyelid raises) and conjunctival haemorrhage.

The syndrome is caused by a deficiency of sympathetic activity and can be identified by the following tests:

- Cocaine – instilled into both eyes: The affected eye would not dilate (unlike the normal pupil). Cocaine actively blocks the re-uptake of noradrenaline at the nerve endings and therefore accumulates, leading to dilation of the unaffected eye. However, in Horner's syndrome there is no noradrenaline secreted at the nerve endings and cocaine consequently has no effect.
- Apraclonidine [Iopidine] – instilled into both eyes: This is a glaucoma medication that elicits a similar reaction to the cocaine test. It is easier and cheaper to acquire than cocaine and is more dependable. Apraclonidine is an alpha-agonist, causing the normal pupil to be unaffected, but the eye associated with the Horner's syndrome will dilate.

Aponeurotic

This is the most common cause of acquired upper eyelid ptosis and is associated with stretching or partial (or total) dehiscence of the levator muscle, or its attachment tissue, known as aponeurosis. It is sometimes referred to as senile or involutional ptosis, as it is more commonly associated with the elderly. Aponeurotic ptosis may occur as a result of repeated eye rubbing or eyelid manipulation during the insertion or removal of corneal contact lenses. It is also linked to the effects of aging and gravity, and can be associated with chronic inflammation, intraocular surgery or trauma.

The aponeurosis is a layer or sheet of fibrous tissue that attaches muscles to the body parts they manoeuvre. It is typically white and shiny in appearance and has a reduced number of vessels and nerves. There are various other examples of aponeurosis in the body, including epicranial (frontalis muscle to the occipitalis) and intercostal (membranes between the ribs). In the upper eyelid, the levator aponeurosis is attached to the levator superalis muscle at the posterior end and the upper tarsal plate and dermis at its anterior end.

Many individuals who present with a ptosis, regardless of the cause, try to compensate by lifting their brow (frontalis overaction). Also, in a patient with an acquired ptosis, the skin crease height may be high or even absent.

Mechanical

A ptosis can be due to the muscles being unable to elevate the eyelid the eyelid being pushed down because it is overcome mechanically (weighed down). This is commonly associated with a secondary cause such as orbital fat prolapse, eyelid tumours or blepharochalasis (inflammation of the eyelids). In this case, it may be necessary to remove or treat the causative factor and this may alleviate the ptosis.

Congenital

Some infants are born with a ptosis or it may manifest in the first few years of life as a hereditary chromosomal defect. The cause of congenital ptosis is largely unknown and idiopathic. However, in these cases, the levator muscle is described as 'dystrophic' (wasted), due to defects in the muscle which is infiltrated with fibrous tissue or fat. On examination, the upper eyelid skin crease is found to be absent and there is poor levator function.

Ptosis in a child may cause astigmatism and therefore needs to be treated as early as possible.

Other causes of congenital ptosis

These may include the following.

Blepharophimosis

This condition is associated with upper eyelid ptosis and raised lower eyelids, causing a narrowing of the palpebral opening (fissure). This is also related to a flattened nasal bridge and altered orbital bony rim.

Marcus-Gunn jaw-wink

In this condition there is an altered motor nerve signalling of a branch of the mandibular division of the fifth cranical nerve. When the patient chews or opens their mouth, the ipsilateral ptotic upper eyelid opens.

Third nerve palsies

As explored above (see p. 41).

Pseudoptosis

It is worth mentioning that several conditions may appear to resemble a ptosis but they are not associated with a drooping of the eyelids. The practitioner needs to be aware of these potentially deceptive presentations and understand how to differentiate between them. An example may be upper eyelid retraction in one eyelid, giving the impression that the opposing eyelid is ptotic. Similarly, patients with asymmetrical upper eyelid skin creases can also give the mistaken appearance of ptosis.

Dermatochalasis

This condition is hooding of excessive upper eyelid skin over the lid margin, giving the appearance of a drooping lid (see Figure 3.3). During assessment, if the lid skin is gently lifted, it will often be found that there is no underlying ptosis. If the dermatochalasis affects vision, the excess skin can be removed with a blepharoplasty procedure.

Asymmetry

This is not a cause of ptosis but can give the mistaken impression that there is a ptosis. The opposing upper lid is actually retracted, rather than drooping. It may therefore give the impression that the contralateral eyelid has a ptosis when it is in fact in the correct position.

Hypotropia or a squint

In this condition, the affected eye looks down when in the primary position, which may create the illusion of a ptosis, due to its effect on the superior rectus and the levator muscle.

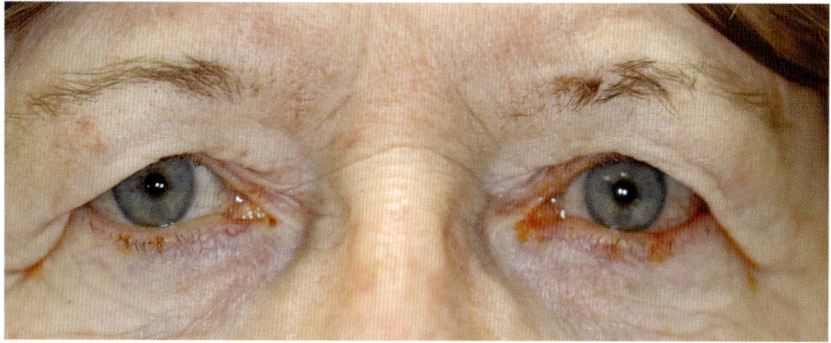

Figure 3.3: Bilateral Dermatochalasis

Ptosis examination and assessment

An important part of diagnosis and treatment of ptosis is to undertake a good clinical examination and obtain a thorough history. As a practitioner you may have to undertake these examinations, and come across some of the terminology, so it is important to understand what these tests mean.

A good clinical history should aim to discover when the patient recognised the onset of the ptosis; it can be helpful to ask them to look at old photographs to identify when changes occurred. It may also be important to establish any predisposing factors such as muscle weakness, trauma or family history. This will include an ophthalmic history, especially contact lens wear or ascertaining any previous surgery.

In order to determine the degree of ptosis, several measurements can be taken and appropriately recorded. Therefore, one of the practitioner's most important 'tools' is a small, plastic, see-through ruler, typically 15cm (6 inches) in length.

As the examiner, it is important to sit directly in front of the patient and to have a pen torch handy for some of the tests. The ruler should be placed vertically next to the upper eyelid in the midline and used to make the following measurements.

Vertical palpebral aperture (PA) or palpebral fissure (PF)

This is the distance between the upper and lower eyelid margins in millimetres in the primary position and at the widest point. In adults this typically measures 9–10mm (Figure 3.4).

Marginal reflex distance (MRD)

In order to gain a better understanding of the degree of upper eyelid ptosis, the MRD provides a fairly accurate and reliable measure of lid malposition (Nemet 2015a). Marginal reflex distance is commonly split into three distinct measures which are related to each other and to the PA. To elicit the most precise measurement, as outlined above, the practitioner sits directly in front of the seated patient and shines a light into their eye they are assessing in the primary position. The light should reflect the central cornea – the light reflex. From the central cornea light reflex, the distance is measured as follows:

- MRD_1: The distance between the central cornea light reflex and the upper eyelid margin at the widest point; this typically measures 4–5mm (Figure 3.5).

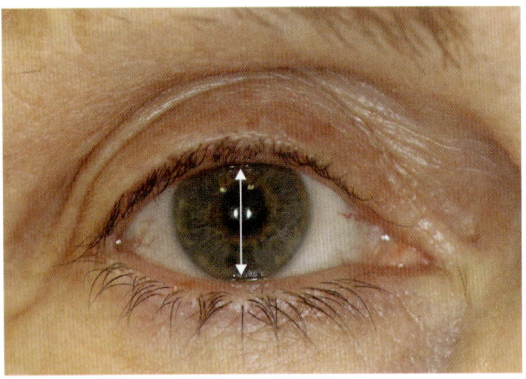

Figure 3.4: Palpebral aperture (PA)   Figure 3.5: MRD_1

- MRD_2: This is the distance between the central corneal light reflex and the lower eyelid margin at the widest point and is approximately 5mm. If you add the MRD_1 to the MRD_2 you should get the PA. In other words, $MRD_1 + MRD_2 = PA$.
- MRD_3: This is a more uncommon measure, but it may be referenced in some instances. It is the distance of the ocular (not light) reflex to the central upper eyelid when in extreme up gaze, and a normal result may be 7mm.

Levator function (eyelid excursion)

Determining how well the levator muscle works is essential, as this will directly affect any potential surgical correction. In patients with neurogenic or myogenic ptosis, the levator muscle function is likely to be diminished so it is important to understand the underlying aetiology of the ptosis.

To measure the functionality of the levator muscle, the practitioner first needs to negate the frontalis muscle's involvement (in lifting the eyelid) by firmly pressing on the brow, on the side they wish to measure, to limit its movement. Then ask the patient to look down to the floor (without moving their head) and place the ruler vertically next to and in the midline of the eye. Align the zero point of the ruler (with the numbers going upwards) with the margin of the upper eyelid in downward gaze (see Figure 3.6). Then ask the patient to look up as high as they can and measure again in up gaze (see Figure 3.7). The distance between the two measures will be the levator function (LF) and is classified as follows (although there is slight variation between references):

- \> 15mm: Normal
- 10–15mm: Good
- 5–9mm: Fair
- < 5mm: Poor
- 0mm: Absent.

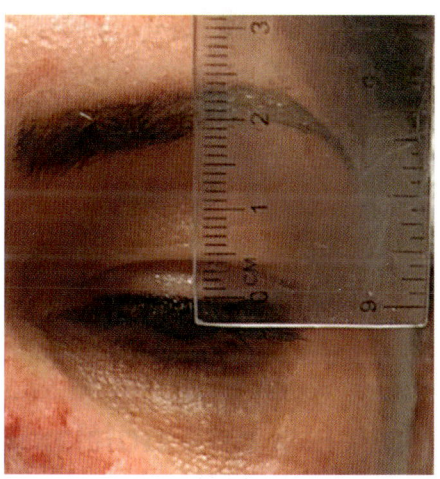 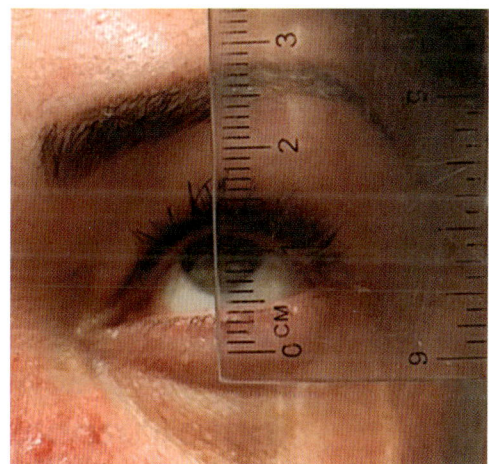

Figure 3.6: Levator function A   Figure 3.7: Levator function B

Skin crease

As discussed earlier, the levator aponeurosis and some of its fibres extend forward to the orbicularis and skin. In many individuals, the traction this exerts creates a natural skin crease horizontally across the upper eyelid. There is a slight difference in skin crease height between genders and it is usually higher in women (8–10mm) than men (6–8mm). It may also vary with age, as other extraneous factors may affect the height such as fat prolapse or brow ptosis. In certain circumstances the upper eyelid skin crease may be almost absent, particularly in children or in congenital ptosis. Conversely, a high skin crease might suggest an aponeurotic defect.

To measure the skin crease, again use the ruler in the vertical position and in the midline, and measure the distance between the upper eyelid margin and the skin crease whilst the patient looks slightly down. It may be necessary to apply gentle upward pressure to the lid edge to accentuate the crease if it isn't immediately obvious. It may not always be obvious and some patients may have more than one skin crease, making it more difficult to differentiate.

The upper eyelid skin crease is often used as a surgical landmark as the crease can mask the wound. This is especially the case in levator correction surgery or blepharoplasty.

Upper eyelid skin

It is also important to assess the amount of lid skin and this can be measured from the upper eyelid margin (vertically and in the midline) to where the skin changes to brow skin. This measurement is approximately 30mm. However, it can be slightly difficult to assess it accurately, as it isn't always entirely obvious where the demarcation between the lid and brow skin actually is. Measuring the upper eyelid skin is especially useful if the surgery to correct the ptosis is combined with a blepharoplasty.

Apart from basic but important measures there are several other important key observations, which are listed below.

Hering's law of equal innervation

This law, originally proposed by Edwald Hering (a German physiologist), suggests that in relation to eye movements, innervation is equal to the dependent extraocular muscles in order to maintain conjugacy (unity). This law also applies to upper eyelid movement, due to the close relationship between the superior rectus and the levator muscle and their shared embryogenesis.

In practice, Hering's phenomenon is significant, in that if a unilateral ptotic eyelid is lifted the opposing eyelid may droop (Nemet 2015b). This can be demonstrated in the clinical assessment by using a finger to gently lift the ptotic eyelid and simultaneously observe the contralateral upper eyelid. The opposing lid may immediately fall a couple of millimetres, but the occurrence may be subtle.

In some, but not all, patients with a ptosis the Hering's phenomenon may mean that both upper eyelids will require surgical correction. It is therefore essential that this is identified prior to surgery so that the patient can be consented and counselled for a bilateral procedure.

Phenylephrine test

Phenylephrine is an adrenergic drug that can affect smooth muscle. Müller's muscle is sympathetically innervated smooth muscle. When phenylephrine is inserted into the eye, this muscle is stimulated and can in turn lift the upper eyelid a couple of millimetres. This is a useful tool for assessment of the potential eyelid lift that might be achievable by undertaking a surgical resection of Müller's muscle (see below).

When assessing ptosis at pre-operative assessment, administering a drop of phenylephrine 2.5% into the affected side can elicit a temporary simulated lift of the ptotic eyelid within approximately 5 minutes of insertion. It also has the effect of dilating the pupil – it is therefore important to warn the patient to arrange for someone else to drive them to and from the appointment. It is also prudent to check beforehand that the patient has no history of angle-closure glaucoma if using dilating drops, due to the risk that the drops could significantly raise the intra-ocular pressure. The practitioner should also get a clinical photograph prior to insertion for a baseline and in order to compare once the drop has been inserted and also post-operatively.

An alternative to phenylephrine is Apraclonidine (Iopidine), which takes longer to work but can also simulate a lid lift.

Fatigue test

A common pre-operative test is to ask the patient to look up at a fixed point for 30 seconds. Individuals with myasthenia gravis (MG) are unable to hold this sustained gaze and the eyelids begin to droop. This is known as the fatigue test and is attributed to Scottish neurologist John Simpson – it is therefore also sometimes known as the Simpson test.

Another well-recognised, but more subtle, test is Cogan's lid twitch test. In this test, the patient is asked to rapidly move their eye from downgaze to the primary position; in patients with MG the eyelid briefly overshoots before returning to its original position. This twitch sign may provide further evidence of the underlying MG.

A further 'bedside' test is to apply an ice pack over the closed ptotic eyelid for 2–5 minutes because the activity of acetylcholine is inhibited by cooling the muscles. (The practitioner should be careful to protect both the eyelid and the eye from damage or burns by placing a gauze between the ice and the skin.) Once the ice pack is removed, the ptosis will temporarily vanish.

Bell's phenomenon (palpebral oculogyric reflex)

As a defensive mechanism, the eye moves upwards and outwards under the eyelid when an attempt is made to close the eyes and this is known as Bell's phenomenon.

This reflex can also be elicited when patients are asked to forcibly close their eyes, against a practitioner who attempts to keep the lids open. Again, this reflex may not be present in about 30% of the population and may also be absent due to muscle or neurogenic wasting.

Corneal surface

It is vitally important to check the corneal surface on the slit lamp using fluorescein and ascertain whether the patient has a history of dry eyes (amongst other things). Any surgery to potentially lift the ptotic eye may exacerbate the symptoms of dry eye, due to increased surface area exposure. It is therefore important to make the patient aware of the need to use regular lubricants.

Evert the upper eyelid

Checking under the eyelid will enable the practitioner to eliminate any other potential mechanical reason for a ptosis. It is good practice to check under the palpebral eyelid for abnormalities such as lesions or any evidence of trauma that might contribute to a ptosis.

At the slit lamp, and using a cotton tip, with one hand gently hold the upper eyelid eyelashes between finger and thumb (see Figure 3.8). At the same time, use the cotton tip to lever the tarsal plate and flip the lid (see Figure 3.9).

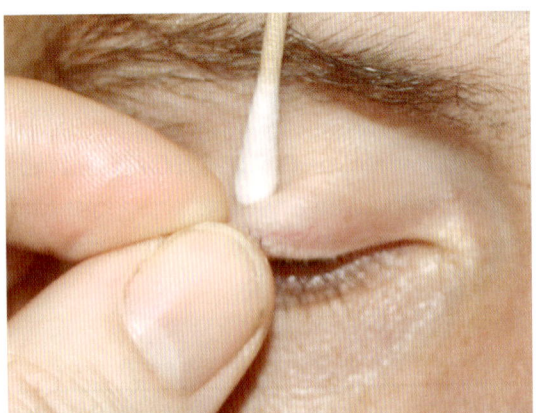
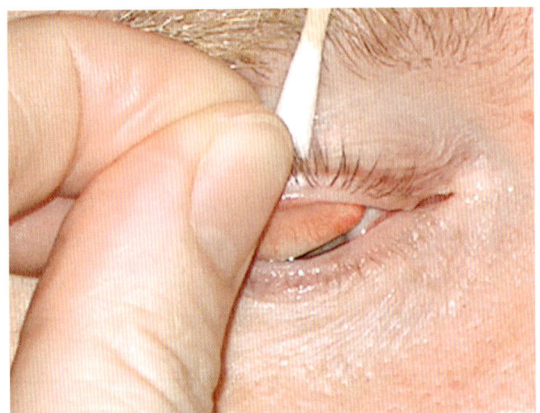

Figure 3.8: Eyelid eversion *Figure 3.9: Flipping the lid*

Ptosis treatment and management

Generally, upper eyelid ptosis can only be corrected using surgical intervention. However, in specific cases, a possible alternative is the use of ptosis props. These are attachments added to glasses that physically lift the eyelid. They are not always suitable and can be restrictive, but for some individuals they offer a non-surgical option.

Otherwise surgery is advocated to correct upper eyelid ptosis and the choice of procedure is dictated by the degree of levator function. The nursing care will also vary slightly, depending on the approach taken. The three main surgical approaches will be discussed below.

There are several points that need to be considered pre-operatively. The most important one is whether the surgery is actually needed to help with vision or is associated with cosmesis. In the United Kingdom, the National Health Service has become quite strict about the criteria for upper eyelid ptosis correction. and in mild ptosis it may not be eligible for surgical correction. A clinical photograph taken prior to surgery will provide a baseline and comparison post-operatively for both the patient and the clinician.

Pre-operative nursing considerations

It is easy to underestimate the personal and social effect of living with ptosis, particularly when it is bilateral and especially for women (Richards *et al.* 2017). Patients may avoid social interaction or feel afraid of the perceived attitudes of others. Some individuals fear being perceived as 'dopy' or uninterested by casual observers. Also, when corrective surgery is considered to be cosmetic (rather than therapeutic), some individuals avoid seeking advice or help for fear of being seen as vain. This can be particularly true of those patients who have an underlying condition, such as myasthenia gravis, causing the ptosis. The practitioner therefore needs to support patients through the process, both from a physical and a psychosocial perspective.

It is also important to find out whether the patient is taking any medications that might impact on the surgery. This is especially pertinent in relation to anti-coagulants or anti-platelets (such as Warfarin or Aspirin). In some cases, it may be important to co-ordinate and briefly stop the medication prior to surgery in co-operation with the patient's GP or anti-coagulant clinic team (if it is safe to do so). Non-steroidal anti-inflammatory agents such as Ibruprofen need to be avoided at least 2 weeks before surgery.

As part of the consent and pre-operative information-gathering process, the patient should be made aware of the potential outcomes from the surgery. Lifting the eyelid will increase exposure of the eye so any problem with dry eyes may be exacerbated. In addition, the patient will be unable to completely close their eyelids after the surgery – lagophthalmos. Until the denervated orbicularis muscle recovers from surgery and regains normal function, the eyelid may struggle to close. It is important to assess the patient's lubricant medications (and drop technique) and it may be necessary to adjust these in relation to the increased exposure. This will be especially important at night-time where the risk of exposure is increased, and a liberal amount of lubricant will therefore be needed.

It is also vital to warn the patient of the risk of under- or over-correction of the eyelids. During ptosis surgery, the surgeon will endeavour to get the correct eyelid height, but extraneous factors (such as swelling or Hering's phenomenon) can affect the outcome. Some surgeons do aim to slightly over-correct as the lid is likely to drop post-operatively, and again it may be necessary to warn patients about this prior to surgery.

Surgical approaches to correction of upper eyelid ptosis

Levator aponeurosis advancement (LAA) procedure

In a patient with a significant ptosis and a good levator function, a levator aponeurosis advancement (LAA) procedure aims to reattach the dehisced/stretched muscle to the tarsal plate. The LAA procedure is commonly undertaken under a local anaesthetic, either with or without sedation. During the procedure some surgeons like to check lid height and may sit the patient up on the theatre trolley, but to do so they require the patient's co-operation. Anyone having the procedure under a general anaesthetic, particularly children, will obviously not be able to co-operate in this way.

The LAA procedure involves:

- Marking of the skin crease (in some patients a blepharoplasty may be performed at the same time to address dermatochalasis)
- Administration of subcutaneous local anaesthetic
- A lid skin crease incision – some surgeons prefer to use a hand-held monopolar cutting/coagulation device
- Cutting through the skin, orbicularis muscle and the orbital septum
- Preaponeurotic fat is dissected off the levator muscle
- The levator muscle is then dissected off the underlying Müller's muscle and the superior edge of the tarsus
- Commonly, using double-armed 5/0 Vicryl sutures, a stitch is passed through the tarsal plate centrally and then through the detached levator muscle at a higher point to create a suitable lift; this is the advancement part of the procedure
- At this point it may be necessary to check lid height and contour by sitting the patient up
- Any excess levator may be excised
- Once satisfied with lid height, further supportive sutures may be inserted medially and laterally to the central stitch
- The eyelid wound is closed, using interrupted Vicryl skin sutures.

Key nursing considerations with regard to the LAA procedure

After an LAA procedure there are several key post-operative issues, listed below.

1. Pain and discomfort

There may be mild to moderate discomfort after an LAA procedure and this can be managed with simple analgesics. However, if the pain is severe there must be some suspicion. Severe pain is most commonly associated with a corneal abrasion so the practitioner should check the cornea on a slit lamp. It will also be important to avoid keeping an eye-pad on for any substantial length of time after the procedure (certainly no longer than 48 hours) – to avoid the eye drying or the danger of creating a corneal abrasion.

2. Swelling and bruising

In the early stages after the procedure there may be some swelling and this can be reduced with the use of ice-packs (ensuring that the ice-pack is not directly in contact with the skin).

3. Protection for the eye and the use of lubricants

After the upper eyelid has been lifted, the key problem is corneal exposure and lagophthalmos, and so the concerted use of lubricants will be very important – especially at night-time. Some surgeons use a lower eyelid frost suture to temporarily close the eye to protect it. Very occasionally some surgeons also inject air into the lower eyelid to raise it and protect the eye.

4. Cleanliness of the wound and antibiotic ointment

It is important to keep the eyelid wound clean immediately post-operatively and carry out daily cleaning with sterile water or saline. If the patient has no access to pre-packaged saline, an alternative is to use boiled water from the kettle that has cooled.

For approximately one week following the surgery, the patient will usually need to apply antibiotic ointment (e.g. chloramphenicol or fusidic acid) on the wound.

5. Bathing and showering

After the surgery, the patient will be able to shower and bathe as normal but should take care not to get soap or shower gel into the eyes.

6. Sleeping at 45° incline and avoiding the side of surgery

In order to reduce swelling and damage to the operated eyelid, it is advisable for the patient to sleep at a 45° incline, i.e. using 2–3 pillows. The patient should also be advised not to sleep on the affected side. Immediately after the surgery there may be a degree of lid swelling which may be reduced to a degree by sleeping with the head up.

7. Sutures are likely to be dissolvable

Most surgeons are likely to use Vicryl sutures in the eyelid wound and these will dissolve and fall out after a couple of weeks. However, the longer the sutures are in place, the greater the risk of inflammation and scarring. It may therefore be best to remove the sutures at the first post-operative visit.

> **Terminology**
>
> **Resection** To surgically remove tissue, organ or structure
>
> **Recession** To draw tissue back/away from its normal position

Table 3.1:
Post-operative care following ptosis surgery – levator aponeurosis advancement

Issue	Nursing input	Rationale	Evaluation	Comment
1. Pain and discomfort following surgery	Pre-operative information regarding post-operative pain associated with procedure at pre-assessment.	To ensure patient is aware of the potential for pain – but the pain should be mild to moderate.	Daycase procedure, patient will be discharged with information. Make sure patient has the appropriate contact details and/or is aware of what to do if concerned about pain.	Post-operative pain should be mild to moderate and isolated to area of the surgery. A post-operative bleed is highly unlikely – but the patient should be aware that there is an extremely low risk of a bleed and of the need to act fast if there is any suspicion of a bleed. Similarly, staff should be aware of the potential signs of a periorbital bleed.
	Post-operative analgesia: paracetamol should be enough to control the pain.	To reduce pain associated with the procedure.	Ensure patient is either discharged with analgesia or has access to analgesia. Contact patient first day post-surgery to check on their pain level.	
	Awareness of signs of periorbital bleed. Sudden moderate to severe pain can be associated with: • Possible swelling • Reduction of vision • Tense orbit.	Contact ophthalmic consultant and liaise with theatre. Consider urgent canthotomy/ cantholysis (get appropriate surgical instruments) and perform immediately. Urgent admission.	Mild to moderate symptoms are likely to subside over the days immediately following surgery.	

	Provide contact details and/or encourage the patient to attend A&E immediately with these symptoms. Ophthalmic emergency – may require surgical input.			
2. Upper eyelid wound care	Initially a pad may be applied.	To protect the wound and reduce swelling.	The pad should be removed within 48 hours.	Cleansing of the wound should be introduced pre-operatively and the patient's technique evaluated. Wound cleansing should be a priority and the patient made aware of signs of infection and how to report it.
	Once the pad has been removed or if no pad has been used, simple wound care should be applied.	To reduce the risk of post-operative infection.	Use either sterile normal saline or cooled boiled water and sterile pads to clean wound.	
3. Exposure and lagophthalmos	Having lifted the eyelid, the eye (and specifically the cornea) is exposed; need to apply lubricants.	Need to avoid the eye becoming dry.	Apply regular lubricants and it may be necessary to review the patient at the slit lamp if there are any changes.	It may be necessary to assess the patient's drop technique. It is also important to understand how to measure/recognise lagophthalmos.
4. Removal of sutures	The sutures are likely to be dissolvable but may still need to be removed.	To reduce post-operative inflammation and scarring.	At first visit after surgery, consider removing sutures.	Use a magnifier with suture-tying forceps and Vanna scissors to remove the sutures.
5. Post-operative prevention of infection	The use of antibiotic ointment on the wounds for the first 1–2 weeks following the procedure. Assess drop regime with the patient or relative undertaking application of drops.	To reduce the chance of infection.	Occasionally the patient is allergic to antibiotics and this needs to be altered or stopped.	Do not pull down on the eyelid on the operated side, as this could affect or undo the surgery.

6. Reduction of post-operative swelling	Initially the application of an eye-pad or ice-packs. Sit upright and use extra pillows in bed.	Cooling and pressure can reduce the inflammation.	Cooling and pressure can reduce the inflammation. Use the eye-pad only for a short period after surgery to reduce risk of corneal abrasion. Ice-packs should be applied gently, and wrapped in gauze to protect the eye.	Be aware of corneal abrasion. If the swelling persists, ensure there is no other obvious cause.
7. Under- or over-correction of eyelid height or contour irregularities	The eyelid should be checked pre-operatively as follows: • PA • MRD1 • Skin crease • Upper eyelid skin. Similarly, a post-operative comparison should be made. The eyelid height might be distinctly under- or over-corrected or contour peaked.	Report to the surgeon or consultant. It may be necessary to correct surgically.	The sooner this takes place after the original procedure, the better the potential outcome from corrective surgery. It is important to make the patient aware of the potential need for corrective surgery at consent.	Other factors might contribute to the lid height, including swelling, so it may be beneficial to allow this to settle first.

Müller's muscle resection

The alternative surgical procedure to the anterior approach LAA is to resect the Müller's muscle, first described by Putterman and Urist in 1975. This muscle is sandwiched between the levator muscle anteriorly and the conjunctiva posteriorly. It is approached from the palpebral conjunctiva by everting the eyelid (usually using an instrument to support the eyelid such as a Desmarres retractor). The degree of lift required will determine how much of the Müller's muscle is resected; and several authors advocate using various formulae to gauge this. Resecting the Müller's muscle and reinserting it into the tarsal plate effectively shortens the muscle and in turn creates a small lid lift.

Typically, the Müller's muscle resection procedure is undertaken if the lift required is moderate (i.e. 2mm) and the levator function is good. Compared to the LAA, a Müller's muscle resection is arguably easier to perform, less destructive to tissue and doesn't leave an obvious scar.

Performing a Müller's muscle resection procedure

- Infiltrate local anaesthetic (with adrenaline) subcutaneously into the upper eyelid skin crease
- Insert an upper eyelid traction suture
- Evert the upper eyelid (using a Desmarres retractor)
- Further subconjunctival local anaesthetic is administered
- A horizontal subconjunctival incision is made with a 15 blade above the superior aspect of the tarsus
- A further incision is made with Westcott scissors through the Müller's muscle into the space between the Müller's and levator muscles. A plane is then dissected with Westcott scissors.
- Conjunctiva is then separated from the Müller's muscle
- A strip of Müllers muscle, approximately 5–6mm, is then resected (removed)
- Three 7/0 Vicryl sutures are inserted through the 'stump' of the Müller's muscle and tied, attaching the resected edge of Müller's to the superior edge of the tarsus, and ensuring that the sutures are buried.

Nursing considerations with Müller's muscle resection

All the same pre- and post-operative care outlined above for an LAA will be needed for a Müller's muscle resection. Some surgeons insert a bandage contact lens (BCL) into the eye post-operatively to provide short-term protection for the eye. If this is done, the patient will need to be made aware of the presence of the bandage contact lens. Use of a bandage contact lens can expose the patient to a small risk of sight-threatening bacterial keratitis and therefore is not advocated by some surgeons. The liberal use of lubricants in the eye will be necessary, along with antibiotic ointment.

There may often be eyelid swelling and bruising in the first week or two following surgery, and ice-packs (or even a bag of frozen peas wrapped in lint) may help with this. (Always ensure that there is no direct contact between the pack and the patient's skin, e.g. by using a layer of gauze.)

If the lift is too high, the patient may sometimes be post-operatively encouraged to gently pull the eyelid down by taking hold of their eyelashes between their thumb and forefinger. However, this may be slightly uncomfortable and may need to be supervised and monitored in the first instance. The patient may need to be warned about the possibility of bleeding.

Posterior approach levator aponeurosis advancement (sometimes termed white-line advancement)

The posterior approach advancement technique involves a palpebral conjunctival approach, starting with a horizontal incision along the superior tarsal plate using a 15 blade. A conjunctival-Muller's muscle flap is then dissected, using Westcott scissors, a few millimetres until it reaches the posterior aspect of the levator muscle. This is seen as a white line – hence the more recently coined 'white-line advancement'.

Once identified, a double-ended 5/0 Vicryl suture is passed through the 'white line' and subsequently full-thickness through the eyelid at the superior tarsal plate. The suture is presented at the skin and tied. The conjunctiva is draped over the wound and not sutured.

This approach can lift the lid up to 4mm. It is also minimally disruptive to surrounding structures (it doesn't breach the orbital septum, for example) and often provides a good contour, often all with just one stitch.

Post-operative care is quite straightforward, with some surgeons opting to use a bandage contact lens initially, but appreciating the potential risks outlined above. Chloramphenicol antibiotics may or may not be used, as they can cause conjunctival granulomas post-operatively.

Frontalis suspension

For patients with an upper eyelid ptosis (especially congenital) and poor levator function, adjusting lid muscle heights will be largely ineffective. It will therefore be necessary to undertake an alternative approach to lifting the eyelids. In patients with ptosis associated with a neuromuscular weakening, the frontalis muscle in the forehead is utilised, essentially using the brow lift to raise the lids. The frontalis muscle affords up to 1.5cm of potential action (Leatherbarrow 2019) which, if connected to the tarsus, can enable a significant eyelid lift.

Historically, several different materials have been used to create the suspension, but more recently either autologous fascia lata silicone bands or prolene sutures appear to be the main options. Both materials have advantages and disadvantages, as listed below.

Fascia is a layer of fibrous connective tissue that is bound to, and surrounds, muscles, stabilising and separating them. The fascia lata encloses the muscles of the thigh. Given its inherent strength and stable nature, this tissue is useful in various ways. In this context, thin strips can be used to lift the lid.

Fascia Lata

Advantages:

- Relatively easy to place

- Autologous so unlikely to cause a foreign-body reaction

Disadvantages:
- Bulkier than sutures and may be seen under the skin
- Requires extra theatre equipment/ time to harvest
- Creates a second wound with additional risks
- Once healed, very difficult to remove or adjust.

Silicone sling

Advantages:
- Easier to place and a viable alternative to fascia lata if the surgeon doesn't have access to the equipment to harvest this
- Easier to remove
- Cheap.

Disadvantages:
- Bulkier than sutures and may be seen under the skin
- Not autologous and therefore open to foreign-body reaction and extrusion
- Can slip or break due to the smooth nature of the sutures.

Prolene sutures

Advantages:
- Easier to place and less bulky
- Easier to remove if required.

Disadvantages:
- Not autologous and therefore open to foreign-body reaction and extrusion
- Can slip or break due to the smooth nature of the sutures.

The surgical procedure essentially uses two similar ways to lift the lid via the brow by passing the material subcutaneously between the eyelid and the brow. One technique is to use a pentagon (Fox) shape (see Figure 3.10) and the other is a (Crawford) double triangle (see Figure 3.11). There are others described in the literature, but these appear to be the two most common approaches. The Crawford technique using fascia lata is usually seen as the gold standard and provides the best surgical outcomes (Chung & Seah 2016).

The pentagon (Fox) procedure

This technique is preferably performed with non-autologous material:

- Two small incisions (2mm) are made 1mm above the lash line and medially/ laterally to the corneal limbus

- A further three brow 'stab' incisions are made medially and laterally, and centrally above the brow, creating the pentagon shape
- Using a Wright ptosis needle, the polypropylene suture material is passed between the five sites, initially engaging the lid incisions and the tarsal plate; then superiorly, being passed behind the orbital septum to the upper central brow incision
- Once the correct height has been achieved by pulling the sutures via the central brow incision, the suture material is tied
- The wounds are closed with 7/0 Vicryl
- The eye needs to be protected throughout the procedure using a lid-guard.

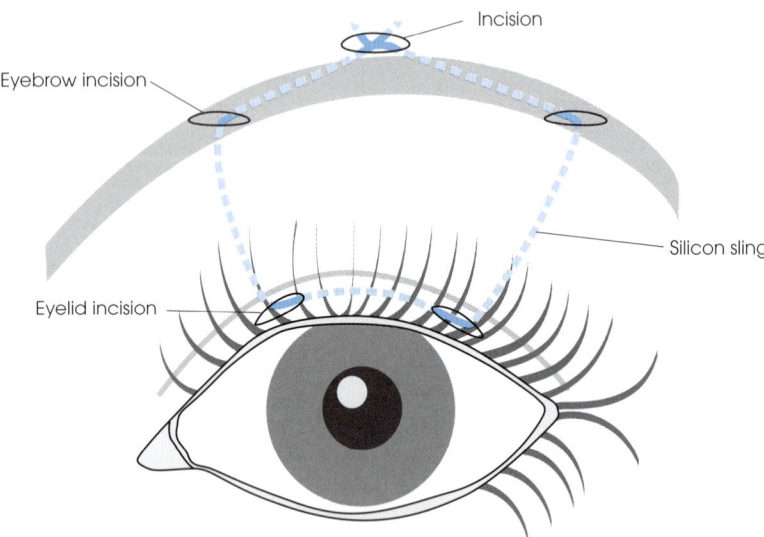

Figure 3.10: The pentagon (Fox) procedure

The double triangle (Crawford) procedure

This technique is used with autologous fascia lata harvested from the thigh.

- In a similar way to the Fox method, three small eyelid incisions are made, 1mm above the lash line and equidistant to one another, again corresponding to the corneal limbus
- The fascia lata material is passed subcutaneously, using a Wright ptosis needle, between the brow incisions and the eyelid as two separate triangles (isosceles)
- Again, the fascia lata is tied once the correct height is achieved
- The incisions are closed with 7/0 Vicryl.

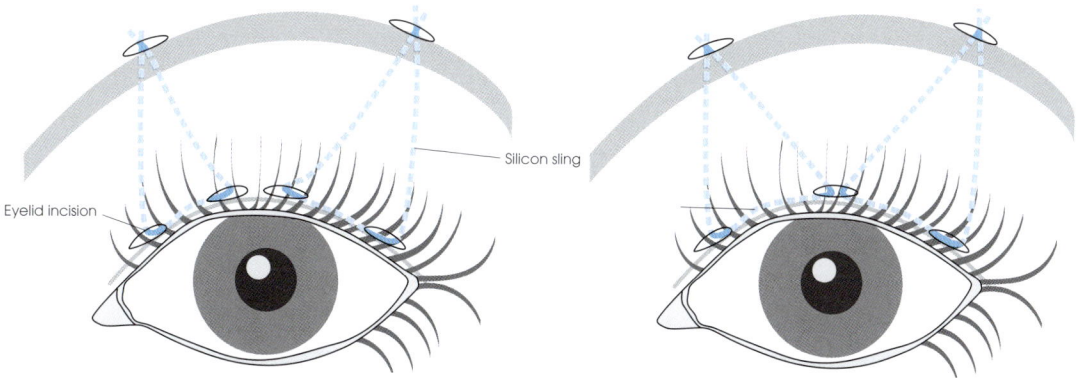

Figure 3.11: The double triangle (Crawford) procedure
L: Modified Crawford's technique   R: Mehta's modification of Crawford's technique

Care associated with harvesting of fascia lata

The fascia lata is harvested from the thigh, from the rectus femoris muscle. Fascia is a thin sheath of fibrous tissue that covers muscles. The section used overlies the musculature of the lateral thigh muscles. A line drawn from the head of the fibia to the anterior superior iliac spine provides the direction required. Two particular instruments, the Crawford stripper or the Moseley fasciotome, can be used to harvest the fascia. Approximately 1 x 15cm fascia is required to provide enough tissue to perform the lid lift.

The fascia is harvested through a 3–4cm wound on the thigh, which is closed with sutures. Once the fascia lata has been harvested from the thigh, direct pressure is required, to reduce bruising and swelling. A small dressing is used to cover the wound initially, and a pressure dressing is applied to the whole length of the leg, bearing in mind that the subcutaneous wound runs the length of the thigh. Once the patient is in recovery, it is important to monitor foot skin colour and pulses to ensure the bandage is not too tight.

Other care considerations related to eyelid ptosis surgery

The practitioner has to consider and manage the patient's post-operative pain and irritation caused by ptosis surgery. Whilst most of these procedures are arguably associated with mild to moderate degrees of pain, it is still important to address any pain-related issues. These are usually day-case procedures so the practitioner needs to ensure that the patient has sufficient access to analgesia at home. Any severe pain should be acted upon and may be due to some other underlying cause, such as a bleed.

Having lifted the eyelid, the increased exposure of the eye can be distressing and uncomfortable, and it is important to ensure that the operated eye has sufficient post-operative lubrication. It will also be necessary to check the patient's drop technique to ensure that they are delivering the drops safely.

The wounds will need to be kept clean using aseptic technique and antibiotic ointment applied for the first 1–2 weeks post-operatively. Ensure that the patient has clear instructions on how to apply the antibiotic ointment to the wound (otherwise they may put it in the eye unnecessarily).

There may be swelling and oedema for several weeks post-operatively and the practitioner will need to reassure the patient that this is normal after surgery and will dissipate over time.

Brow ptosis and dermatochalasis

As mentioned earlier, excess skin can hood over the upper eyelid margin and obstruct the line of sight – dermatochalasis. In such cases, it may sometimes be necessary to perform a blepharoplasty at the same time as the upper eyelid levator ptosis surgery. Eyelid ptosis may also be associated with brow ptosis (brow droop) and there may be underlying periorbital fat prolapse, often caused by ageing and weakening of the connective tissues. Brow ptosis is associated with a drop in the underlying sub-brow fat pad falling below the superior orbital rim.

Blepharoplasty may involve the removal of eyelid skin and underlying orbicularis muscle, which can debulk the fat pad. This procedure may be either functional or cosmetic. Similarly, the brow ptosis can be corrected by a brow lift procedure.

However, it is essential that the correct amount of eyelid and brow skin is removed, as any over-excision may lead to incomplete closure of the eyelids. This is known as lagophthalmos, and it may cause drying of the eye.

Applied upper eyelid anatomy

The eyelids have a horizontal length of approximately 26mm (in females) and 27mm (in males). The lateral corner of the eyelids, the lateral canthus, is slightly higher than the medial corner. Within the eyelid is the tarsal plate, which is a semilunar or D-shaped structure composed of dense connective tissue. The tarsal plate gives form and structure to the eyelid. It is approximately 10mm in diameter (at its widest) and 25mm in horizontal length. At its superior edge, the levator aponeurosis attaches to the plate.

The distance between the eyelid margin vertically (in the midline) to the start of the inferior edge of the brow is approximately 30mm (in down gaze).

This is important, because any removal of skin should leave a minimum of 20mm skin. There can be variation between individuals regarding the amount of upper eyelid skin so it is important to measure the distance pre-operatively, and record it in the notes. For example, if the measure of upper lid skin was 28mm, the maximum amount that could be excised would be 8mm (leaving the minimum 20mm).

The upper eyelid skin crease is another important surgical landmark and is approximately 7–8mm in females and 5–6mm in males. The skin crease may be absent in some individuals and and may vary according to ethnic background. Again, it is important to record the skin crease height, as it can vary slightly between individuals.

The eyebrows have three recognised parts: a head (medially), body and tail (laterally). The underlying brow skin is thicker than the eyelid skin. In males, the brow is lower and sits just on the orbital rim. In females, the brow (especially laterally) is slightly higher. Also, in females the brow is more arched, whereas in males it is flatter and arguably more prominent. The brow is physically lifted by the action of the frontalis muscle and is quite independent of the eyelids. These muscles are some of the most important for facial expression so any significant changes to the position of the brow over time may interfere with this.

Understanding the height and contour of the brow will be important and these details should be noted. A good example is a patient who is reviewed with an upper eyelid ptosis with associated brow lift (over-compensatory). Conversely, practitioners might come across an individual who presents with brow ptosis and dermatochalasis.

The blepharoplasty surgical procedure

With blepharoplasty surgery, the primary goal is to remove excess upper eyelid skin and underlying muscle if necessary. However, it is crucial that the appropriate information is gained prior to surgery, appropriate written consent is obtained and facial photographs are taken.

At surgery the excess skin will be carefully measured and the amount of skin will be marked out in relation to the skin crease.

The procedure is usually undertaken with local anaesthetic (with or without sedation). Then, once anaesthetised, the marked tissue will be removed, using either a monopolar cautery or Westcott scissors.

Once the desired tissue has been removed, the wound will be closed with interrupted Vicryl sutures. When the sutures are being placed, some of them will pick up a small bite of underlying levator muscle so as to form a new skin crease. When performing ptosis surgery, the upper eyelid skin crease is used to access the levator muscle.

Brow ptosis procedure – direct brow lift

The brow can be elevated by performing a direct brow lift, which involves removing an area of skin just above the superior edge of the brow and laterally. This is very much a functional procedure and sets out to physically lift the brow. It is important to note that this procedure can leave a noticeable scar above the brow which may not be acceptable for some individuals. This needs to be emphasised pre-operatively and as part of the consent process. In some patients a more lateral brow lift can provide a good functional lift and be more cosmetically acceptable.

The amount of tissue that is to be removed has to be carefully measured prior to the procedure. The surgeon will lift the brow to the desired position with their finger and, whilst using a ruler to measure, allow the brow to drop into a relaxed position. This distance will define the amount of skin to be removed. The surgeon also needs to allow for the brow contour, which varies between males and females. An over-exaggerated brow lift in a man, for example, could lead to an overly feminine-looking result.

The excess brow skin is excised using either a hand-held monopolar cutting device or scissors.

The wound is then closed using deep dissolving sutures, such as 5/0 Vicryl, and the skin is closed with subcutaneous prolene sutures. Obviously, these sutures will need to be removed at approximately 7–10 days; the earlier the better in order to reduce the potential for inflammation and scarring. Some surgeons use skin glue to close the skin wound.

Endoscopic brow lift

An alternative to the direct brow lift is to elevate the entire forehead and this can be undertaken in a couple of different ways. Direct brow lift, as outlined above, is effective for a solely functional elevation, but unfortunately scarring over the brow can be obvious. From a cosmetic perspective, this would be unacceptable. A brow lift incorporating the entire forehead, with the incision sites within the hairline, may therefore be a better option for some patients. Incisions are made within the hairline and the forehead is elevated from the frontal bone and all attachments released using an endoscope for direct visualisation. The elevated forehead is then secured, either using screws inserted within the wound or drill holes placed in the bone.

Pretrichial brow lift

This is another approach that avoids unsightly brow scarring. Incisions are made just anterior to the hairline (pretrichial) and, in a similar way to the direct brow lift, a section of skin and muscle is removed. In suturing the wounds closed, the lift is exhibited. . The results can be very good but there are some potential risks, including weakening of the frontalis muscle, trauma to motor/sensory nerves, haematoma and alopecia. These all need to be outlined during the consent process.

Internal brow lift

This surgical technique very rarely yields much of a brow lift and is reserved for brow stabilisation. If combined with a blepharoplasty procedure, the same upper eyelid skin crease incision is used to place a single supporting suture laterally that suspends the underlying lateral fat pad to the deep frontalis muscle above the orbital rim. This approach avoids the risk of an obvious scar that might be associated with a direct brow lift.

Endotine transblepharoplasty brow lift

This is a surgical brow fixation device which is placed into the bone of the brow using a drill. The 'tines' are small dissolvable hooked devices that are inserted into the frontal bone approximately 1cm above the orbital rim. Once they are placed, the brow muscle is lifted and suspended on the hooks.

This approach generally offers fair surgical results but in some patients the tines can be felt or seen under the skin. As a procedure it has fallen out of favour as the results are arguably no better than an internal brow lift.

Botulinum toxin brow lift

A brow lift can temporarily be elicited with botulinum toxin injections into the superior orbicularis, procerous and depressor supercilli muscles. The stronger action of the frontalis muscle will then override the weakened brow muscles and provide a small brow lift. However, this treatment is not available on the NHS and will be quite costly. It also needs to be repeated every 3–4 months. It is an alternative to surgery, but apart from being costly, there are side effects from botulinum toxin injections, including possible allergic reaction (very rare), but most commonly blepharoptosis or impaired reflex blink (which could exacerbate dry eye symptoms).

Nursing care considerations for blepharoplasty

Immediately after surgery, depending on the surgeon's preference, a Jelonet dressing and eye-pad may be applied. This will be useful in reducing swelling in the post-operative period, but there may be an associated risk of corneal abrasion. It is therefore important to advise the patient to remove the eye-pad if they feel any discomfort. Essentially, they should keep their eye closed under the pad whenever possible.

Once the eye-pad has been removed, or as an alternative to wearing it, the patient may be encouraged to use ice-packs to reduce swelling. In this case, it is important to ensure the ice-pack is not in direct contact with the eyelid/eye – gauze should be used in between.

Sitting up and sleeping in a slightly elevated position will help reduce swelling so the patient should be advised to use 2–3 pillows.

Keeping the wound clean is crucial, using either sterile normal saline solution or cooled boiled water. Using the cleaning process to soften the Vicryl sutures and to remove debris will be important in order to reduce infection and inflammatory reaction. After cleaning, applying Oc. Chloramphenicol antibiotic ointment onto the wounds can reduce the potential infection risk. Observation of the patient's application technique will be important.

The patient should be given advice regarding how to observe for signs of infection. These may include: redness, erythematous swelling, pain and discomfort and discharge.

One of the most serious post-operative complications following a blepharoplasty would be a bleed/haematoma. The patient should be given advice regarding how to observe for signs of infection. These may include: redness, erythematous swelling, pain and discomfort and discharge.

It is important to address this where possible pre-operatively by ascertaining whether the patient has any issues with hypertension. Also, careful management of anti-coagulants and anti-platelets will be necessary prior to any surgical intervention. Where possible, the patient should temporarily cease the use of these medications prior to surgery. However, this may need to be coordinated with the patient's GP or anti-coagulant team. In some cases, it is not viable or safe to stop anti-coagulant therapy prior to surgery; this will have to be seriously considered prior to any intervention and will need to be discussed with the patient's cardiologist.

It is important that the patient does not over-exert themselves following the procedure and this includes sports activity and gardening. It is a good idea to discuss these restrictions with the patient pre-operatively.

Other potential problems following blepharoplasty surgery may include asymmetry of the eyelid contour, bruising, swelling (which could lead to wound dehiscence), and numbness. These risks all need to be outlined as part of the consent process.

The patient will probably be reviewed 2–3 weeks post-surgery and it may be best to remove any remaining sutures at this stage. Even though the stitches may be Vicryl, in my experience they can take a while to dissolve and this can cause unnecessary scarring and irritation. Some surgeons prefer to use prolene sutures, and these need to be removed 6–8 days after surgery; the earlier the better, again to reduce scarring potential.

Removing sutures in the outpatient setting can be undertaken using a slit lamp if the practitioner is competent to do so, or using a magnifying unit that has a light. I usually use suture-tying forceps and Vanna scissors.

Some patients may be keen to apply make-up after blepharoplasty but this should be avoided over the wound site for at least a week. Similarly, the patient needs to avoid getting the wound wet (e.g. in the shower) or going swimming.

Nursing care following brow ptosis surgery
As with other surgical procedures the key factors to consider are immediate post-operative bleeding and swelling. The patient should be encouraged to keep the wound clean using either sterile normal saline or cooled boiled water.

The sutures should be removed 10–12 days after surgery. Some surgeons may use nylon subcutaneous sutures which will need to be pulled through.

The eye may be slightly more open and will therefore tend to dry more easily. The patient should therefore be encouraged to use lubricants.

Given that the brow wound is likely to scar, the patient should also consider using anti-scarring preparations, especially silicone-based topical products. Although the science isn't fully understood, silicone-based anti-scar treatments have a proven record in reducing some individuals' scars. The thinking is that silicone:

- Increases hydration and in turn regulates fibroblast production, with reduced collagen production
- Protects against bacteria
- Modulates the expression of growth factors that affect the wound.

Most silicone products come either as a topical gel, which is applied as a thin coat on the scar, or as sheets that can be reapplied. Examples of these include Dermatix© (Meda Pharmaceuticals), Kelo-Cote© (Alliance Pharma) and Cica Care© (Smith & Nephew).

References
Chung, H. & Seah, L. (2016). Cosmetic and functional outcomes of frontalis suspension surgery using autologous fascia lata or silicone rods in pediatric congenital ptosis. *Clinical Ophthalmology.* **10**, 1779–83.

Esperidião-Antonio, V., Conceição-Silva, F., De-Ary-Pires, B. *et al.* (2010). The human superior tarsal muscle (Mullers muscle): A morphological classification with surgical correlations. *Anatomical Science International.* **85**(1), 1–7. https://doi.org/10.1007/s12565-009-0043-0 (last accessed 28.10.2019).

Ha, R., Nojima, K., Adams, W. & Brown, S. (2005). Analysis of facial skin thickness: defining the relative thickness index. *Plastic & Reconstructive Surgery.* **115**(6), 1769–73.

Lee, Y. & Hwang, K. (2002). Skin thickness of Korean adults. *Surgical and Radiologic Anatomy.* **24**(3–4),183–89: Epub 2002 July 12.

Nemet, Y. (2015a). Accuracy of the marginal reflex distance measurements in eyelid surgery. *Journal of Craniofacial Surgery.* **26**(7).

Nemet, Y. (2015b) The effect of Hering's Law on different ptosis repair methods. *Aesthetic Surgery Journal.* **35**(7), 774–81.

Nerad, J. (2001). *Oculoplastic Surgery: The Requisites.* New York: Mosby.

Richards, H., Jenkinson, E., Rumsey, N. & Harrad, R. (2017). Pre-operative experience and post-operative benefits of ptosis surgery: A qualitative study. *Orbit.* **36**(3), 147–53.

4

Floppy eyelid syndrome

Introduction

This sounds like an unlikely name for an eyelid condition, but it couldn't be more descriptive of a difficult issue for a number of individuals. Floppy eyelid syndrome (FES) has to be taken very seriously, as the long-term effects can be life-changing and sight-affecting.

Commonly, the patient will present with reddened eyes (conjunctival injection) associated with pain, chemosis and epiphora. FES is also associated with other seemingly unrelated symptoms. Firstly, when questioned, they may reveal a poor sleep pattern, specifically obstructive sleep apnoea which causes them to wake several times during the night. The sleep apnoea may include breath-holding and heavy snoring during the sleep.

Secondly, the individual may have an increased body mass index (BMI) and possibly be obese. And, thirdly, FES is more common in men. So we have a triad of commonly presenting symptoms that can point to FES:

- More common in men
- Sleep apnoea
- Increased BMI and/or obesity.

Identifying floppy eyelids

If the patient has FES the eyelids are very lax, especially the upper eyelid. When manipulated during the investigation, the upper eyelid can easily be everted (see Figure 4.1). A normal eyelid is quite resistant, often requiring a cotton bud to help turn it. However, in FES the eyelid can literally be stretched and turned with ease, with minimal resistance. When the lid is everted, you may well see chronic papillary conjunctivitis, and large undulating papules on the inner eyelid surface. The patient may also complain of discomfort and continual mucous discharge.

FES and the extensive laxity of the eyelids are associated with a significant decrease in the elastin content of the eyelid, which enables the lid to become more flaccid. Due to the poor juxtaposition of the palpebral conjunctiva against the globe, the eye can often become irritated, causing papillary conjunctivitis and discharge. In extreme cases and when the patient is asleep, the eyelid can spontaneously evert and rub on the pillow, causing further irritation. This may be especially apparent if the individual sleeps on the same side every night (so it may be worth ascertaining if this is the case when taking the history).

As the individual finds the eye irritating, they may also rub the eye excessively and this will undoubtedly exacerbate the condition.

Furthermore, FES can also be associated with keratoconus, which may be a consequence of the mechanical effect on the cornea.

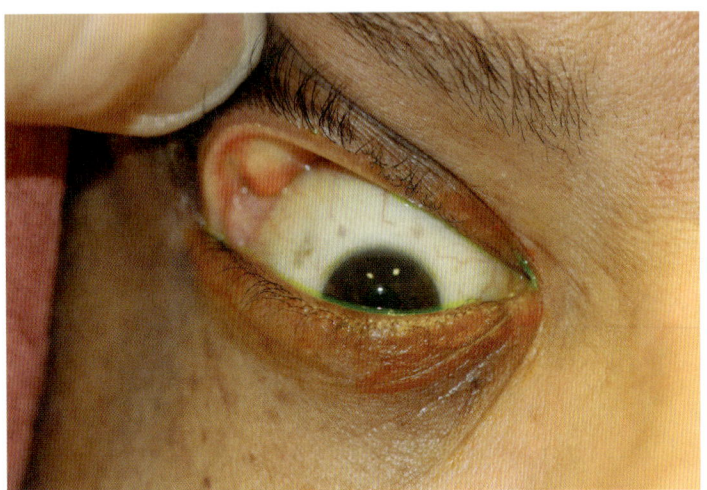

Figure 4.1: Manipulating a floppy eyelid

Assessment and history-taking

History is crucial when constructing a potential picture that might relate to FES. Usually the presenting symptoms will be the red eye and related discharge and irritation.

Whilst you are taking the history, you may notice that the patient is overweight or that they are particularly noisy breathers. However, it is important to remember that not all potential FES patients will exhibit the classic symptoms, so be wary.

You could ask questions to elicit potential clues, such as:

- Do you have a poor sleep pattern?
- Has your partner noticed you holding your breath or snoring excessively?
- Do you find that you are constantly tired and sleep a lot during the day?

Don't forget many patients may not realise that they have sleep apnoea and they are certainly unlikely to comprehend the connection between their reddened eyes and why you are asking about their sleep pattern. It may therefore be pertinent to explain, in a sensitive manner, the relationship between the two, once you have completed your history and examination.

Other presenting diagnostic features may include:

- Superficial punctate erosions (PEE) on the cornea
- Keratitis
- Dry eyes and blepharitis
- Ptosis
- Eyelash ptosis
- Chemosis.

Obstructive sleep apnoea

It is also worth considering obstructive sleep apnoea (OSA) because this is a potentially serious condition which, if suspected (but not actually diagnosed), will require further investigation.

Essentially OSA is a syndrome in which the upper airway collapses causing hypoxaemia (a low level of oxygen in the blood). It is caused by upper airway obstruction or narrowing, due to reduced muscle tone when asleep. Consequently, the patient will stop breathing (or breath-hold) during deep sleep and will then be aroused quite suddenly, waking with an audible gasp as they try to gulp air. This can happen several times an hour in more serious cases. The upper airway narrowing can be attributed to various factors including myopathy, obesity (especially in the neck), enlarged tonsils, hypothyroidism and alcohol; sedatives also contribute to the problem.

OSA is often associated with obesity, diabetes mellitus and hypertension, so it will be worth checking the patient's blood pressure. In the most severe cases OSA can lead to further very serious complications including pulmonary hypertension and even congestive cardiomyopathy (primary heart muscle disease where the heart becomes dilated and unable to pump blood effectively).

If OSA is suspected, the patient should be considered and referred for sleep studies, which will assess the sleep pattern, whilst measuring the oxygen levels with pulse oximetry.

The treatment may require surgical removal of potentially obstructive elements such as enlarged tonsils or more conservative weight-loss management. In extreme cases, the patient may require continuous positive pressure ventilation in the form of a CPAP machine. This means that, at night, the patient is connected to a machine and a firm-fitting face mask that delivers continual pressure to keep the airway open during sleep.

As a practitioner you may come across patients who have, or have not, realised they have OSA, and they may require support and help. Understanding the connection between the various symptoms and the manifestation of the problem can be useful. The need for further investigation and exploration of the symptoms may also need to be explained.

Treating FES

Due to the irritation caused by the floppy eyelid, the initial treatment regimens are usually conservative and take the form of lubrication and occasional steroids (to reduce inflammation). Lubricating ointments used just prior to going to bed can soothe the eye and provide a protective layer to prevent rubbing. This offers some protection but not if the eye is continually rubbing against a pillow or bed sheet. In this case, a more robust form of management may be required and the use of a plastic cartella shield over the eye can stop the physical contact between eye and bedding. Although this may not be very cosmetically attractive, it can offer very effective protection.

However, if the individual uses a CPAP machine, the mask can interfere with the positioning of a shield, either making it uncomfortable or affecting the seal between the face and the mask. Any potential leak is not helpful as it will affect the efficiency of the ventilation and leaked gases can also contribute to drying the eye (if it is partially open). This may mean that alternative measures (such as actually taping the eye closed) may be better than the cartella shield for some people.

If these approaches are not sufficient, or the eyelid becomes excessively lax, it may mean that surgery is required to correct the problem. Tightening of the eyelids will be the obvious approach and often the easiest method is to remove a section of the eyelid (Wedge excision). A wedge of eyelid tissue is effectively excised, usually from the lateral third of the eyelid, incorporating some (but not all) of the tarsal plate. If it is taken too medially, this can pull the puncta horizontally out of position. The wedge is a pentagonal shape and the amount taken has to be carefully assessed prior to excision.

Once it has been excised and cautery applied to prevent bleeding, the two opposing edges of the lid are anastomosed back together, using dissolving stitches to bring the deeper layers together. This may be augmented with a silk lid margin stitch to provide additional strength and better alignment of the lids. The lid margin stitch is placed like a vertical mattress suture (see Figure 4.2). Remember how this stitch is placed if you are involved in the removal. The stitch is placed via the grey-line, between the two new ends of the eyelids at the grey-line. Then it is returned from the ipsilateral side, back over to near the original insertion, and tied off. If positioned, a silk stitch is likely to be kept in situ for 2 weeks and removed in clinic.

It can be quite uncomfortable to take out, so be gentle. Using a slit lamp or magnifier (or loups) will make life a lot easier.

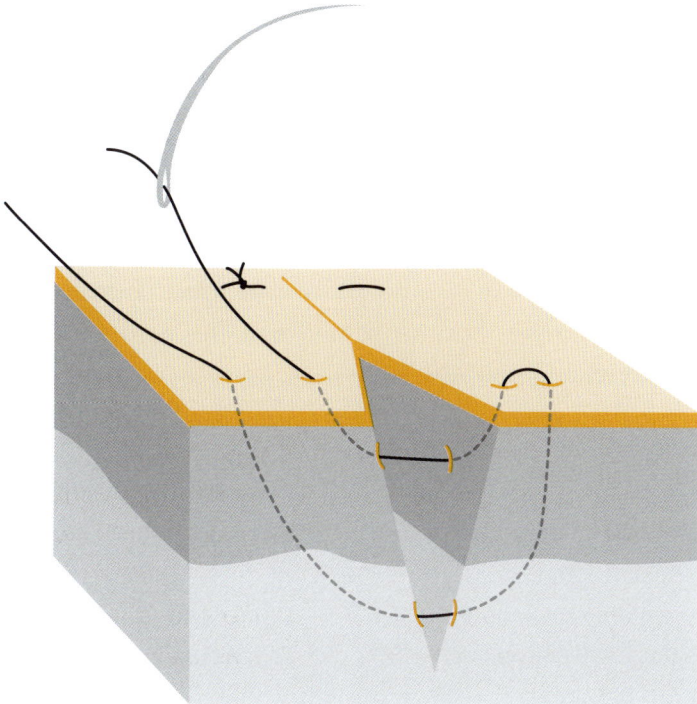

Figure 4.2: Vertical mattress suture

Unfortunately, there can be some post-operative complications and the most common of these is wound dehiscence. Obviously, the wound is under a small amount of tension, which can allow it to slip open if the underlying sutures come undone. In these circumstances, and if the wound is small, it can be left to granulate and may do very well. But occasionally the wound needs to be surgically re-closed and a brief return to theatre is required. If the wound edges are inflamed it may be necessary to wait a few days and treat the inflammation with steroid drops/ointment before re-closing. Suturing inflamed tissue can be difficult and may lead to the stitches tearing through the friable tissue and not holding.

Despite the initial good outcome of surgery, in some cases over time the lid may become lax again and some individuals may find themselves back in the same situation.

Other eyelid-tightening approaches can be used, such as a lateral tarsal strip, but this may not be as effective as this method doesn't effectively shorten the lid and therefore may have limited effect in overcoming the laxity.

Caring for patients with FES

Initially, the key points are to ascertain whether or not the individual has underlying OSA and to provide lubrication for the eyes. Identifying FES should lead you to question whether there is any potentially related OSA. Referral for further investigations and tests may provide reassurance. OSA can be serious if it is left undetected and untreated, so it is important to work with the patient to understand the related issues and investigate them as appropriate.

All these risks may be completely new to the patient and they will need reassurance, information and support. Time spent discussing the issues and explaining preventive measures will not only provide comfort but may also go some way towards reducing symptoms and irritation. Showing the patient how to safely tape the eyelid closed is important, as incorrect taping may cause damage to the eye or at worst lead to a corneal abrasion.

If surgery is required, the usual pre-operative work-up will be necessary. Most patients can undergo a wedge-excision procedure under a local anaesthetic (with or without sedation). Given that the patient may have other health risks (such as airway management, obesity, hypertension, etc.), a general anaesthetic may be riskier. Working collaboratively with the anaesthetist will ensure that the safest approach to surgery is explored. Some units now run anaesthetic-led clinics which aim to address some of the more complex anaesthetic issues associated with these patients.

Post-operatively, the patient will need at least one follow-up appointment and it will be necessary to remove sutures. Careful examination, looking for dehiscence or lid-notching, is important and, if present, these conditions need to be treated effectively.

Post-operative lid hygiene (with either saline or cooled-boiled water) will be required for the first 2 weeks. Ensure that the patient has been shown how to do this as well as how to apply the antibiotic ointment that will be required in the short term.

There may be eyelid swelling and bruising in the initial weeks following the surgery. It will be important for the patient to observe for signs of infection – redness, inflammation and discharge

Conclusion

Although FES may present as a rather innocuous disease, it clearly has some much more serious associated consequences. However, with careful management and treatment, complemented by meticulous investigation and work-up, the patient can significantly benefit from treatment. However, due to the nature of the underlying disease processes, they may well find themselves with similar issues at some later point.

5

Eyelid lesions and their management

Introduction

A considerable number of patient referrals to the oculoplastic team relate to various periocular skin/eyelid lesions and practitioners may have to review and manage such cases. In many units, nurse practitioners undertake clinics and minor-op theatre lists dealing with eyelid lesions. It therefore seems helpful to consider the various types of lesions the practitioner may encounter, and discuss management options, especially as any confusion or misdiagnosis could be detrimental to the patient. Furthermore, some lesions (such as tumours) will require further medical input and surgical involvement, which will also be discussed.

Chapter 15 provides an outline of surgical competencies in relation to the nurse practitioner undertaking the surgical management of several common lesions (as well as various other surgical aspects).

Examining eyelid lesions

As a practitioner presented with a lesion, the key initial goal is to rule out malignancy. When presented with a lesion (or several different types of lesion) in the clinic, the practitioner therefore needs to elicit certain crucial points – specifically when and how it appeared, how long it has been present, its growth rate and any changes in its appearance. It is also necessary to confirm whether the patient is experiencing any other specific issues associated with the lesion, including pain, discharge, epiphora, itchiness, crusting or bleeding. These aspects are important in helping to differentiate particular lesions and whether or not they may be tumorous.

A full medical history (including the presenting complaint, medications, allergies and social history) is required. This might seem like 'overkill' for a simple lesion but subtle clues may emerge that aid diagnosis. For example, if the patient has spent a lot of time working outdoors (UV skin damage), smokes or has underlying systemic conditions (such as the pox virus), this may predispose them to particular lesions (e.g. *molluscum contagiosum*). Also, there may be a previous history of other lesions. For example, some individuals may have had a basal cell carcinoma (BCC) removed in the past.

Examination of the lesion needs to include the following:

- Position – the location of the lesion needs to be outlined, with particular attention to whether it incorporates the entire eyelid or perhaps just sits adjacent to the puncta
- Size – the exact dimensions of the lesion need to be recorded if possible, bearing in mind that some lesions may be quite diffuse and therefore it may not be easy to determine the exact borders
- Is it diffuse or well defined?
- Colour – subtle colour differences can, for example, indicate that the lesion may be vascular bluish, or transparent like a cyst of Moll, or pearly in appearance (as in a basal cell carcinoma)
- Firm or soft to touch – is there evidence of induration, i.e. hardening or sclerosis of the lesion?
- Is it a single lesion or multiple lesions?
- Is it sessile or pedunculated? Some lesions are flat (sessile) and others are on a stalk like a skin tag (pedunculated)
- Nodular – is the surface uneven and irregular? This could be suggestive of a basal cell carcinoma
- Is it scaly or wart-like?
- Is there overlying crusting or evidence of bleeding – again suggestive of a tumorous growth?
- Has the lesion been destructive to surrounding normal tissue?
- Ulceration – is there obliteration of tissue associated with the lesion?
- Madarosis – any loss of eyelashes in the vicinity of the lesion?
- Telangiectasia – tiny blood vessels within the lesion?

A gross examination of the face in good light will indicate how the lesion(s) may be manifesting. They may be grouped together or causing a mechanical ectropion, or the practitioner may identify other similar lesions on another part of the face. With certain lesions, it is important to find out if the patient has any more anywhere else on their body, and examine them as well if necessary (remember to consider having a chaperone).

Once the practitioner has recorded this information, it is prudent to get a clinical photograph of the lesion (whether or not there is any medical or surgical input). It is also good practice to draw a picture in the notes of the location and extent of the lesion. Remember to measure the lesions and record the measurements in the notes.

Lesions can derive from different skin layers and it is useful to appreciate where these particular lesions originate. With regard to skin layers, lesions commonly either originate in the epidermis or dermis, or in appendages within the dermis, such as sweat glands or hair follicles.

It is also useful to classify lesions as benign or malignant, and the following characteristics may suggest a tumorous lesion:

- Local loss of eyelashes
- Change in shape or nature of pre-existing lesion
- Damage/obliteration of the eyelid or surrounding structures
- Pearly appearance
- Telangiectasia
- Induration (to harden)
- New enlarged pigmented lesion.

Related eyelid skin anatomy

The eyelid skin is the thinnest in the body, measuring a mere 0.04–0.06mm, although this can vary slightly between age groups and ethnic groups (Lee & Hwang 2002). The skin gets progressively thicker as it gets further from the eyelid margin towards the brow, where it is some 2.8 times thicker.

The epidermis

The outer layer of skin, the epidermis, is composed of five layers or strata:

- Corneum
- Lucidum
- Granulosum
- Spinosum
- Basale.

Nourished by the underlying dermis, the epidermis is largely made up of keratin (a fibrous protein that is found in hair and nails). The epidermis surface cells are mostly dead and are shed continually.

The epidermis contains specialist cells called keratinocytes that act as a barrier against UV radiation, heat, water loss, bacteria and viruses. There are also Merkel cells (receptor, touch-sensitive), Langerhans and melanocytes (skin colour and absorption of UV light) within the epidermis.

At the base of the epidermis is a stratum of cells called the basal layer. Not surprisingly, this contains basal cells which produce keratinocytes. This layer is significant because it is the basal cells that can be altered though UV damage and become tumorous, resulting in basal cell carcinoma (BCC).

The dermis

The underlying dermis layer is composed of collagen and elastic fibres, and within this layer there are sweat glands, nerves, hair follicles, blood vessels, oil glands and lymphatic vessels.

Various glands are found in the deeper dermis layer, including:

- Sebaceous glands – these are exocrine glands that are connected to eyebrow hairs and the caruncle. The glands secrete sebum, which is an oily substance that acts to waterproof and lubricate the skin. Sebum also contains a small quantity of acid which serves as a barrier to bacteria.
- Meibomian glands – these are a type of modified sebaceous gland that are found within the tarsal plate of both the upper and lower eyelids. There are approximately 25 vertical meibomian glands in the lower eyelid and 50 in the upper. The meibomian glands produce a substance called meibum that functions to lubricate the eye. Any blockage of the meibomian glands will lead to a reduction of meibum secretion, potentially contributing to dry eyes. There is further discussion of meibomian gland dysfunction and dry eyes in Chapter 7.
- Glands of Zeis – these are also modified sebaceous glands, which are at the eyelid margin and lubricate the eyelashes.
- Glands of Moll – sometimes referred as the ciliary glands, these are modified apocrine or sweat glands located at the base of the eyelashes and slightly anterior to the meibomian glands. If the glands of Moll get blocked, this can cause swelling and manifest as a stye.

Benign lesions associated with appendages/adnexa

Chalazion (meibomian cyst, meibomian gland lipogranuloma)

This is a common often self-limiting lesion, which is associated with a blockage of the meibomian glands of the eyelid (see Figure 5.1). They usually appear over the course of a few days and typically present as small nodules of erythema and inflammation. Chalazia are often firm and largely painless lumps that can affect either eyelid. They can cause a considerable amount of pre-septal swelling and can be quite disconcerting for the patient. Occasionally, they can be big enough to cause a slight mechanical drooping of the upper eyelid and they may also press on the cornea, disrupting vision.

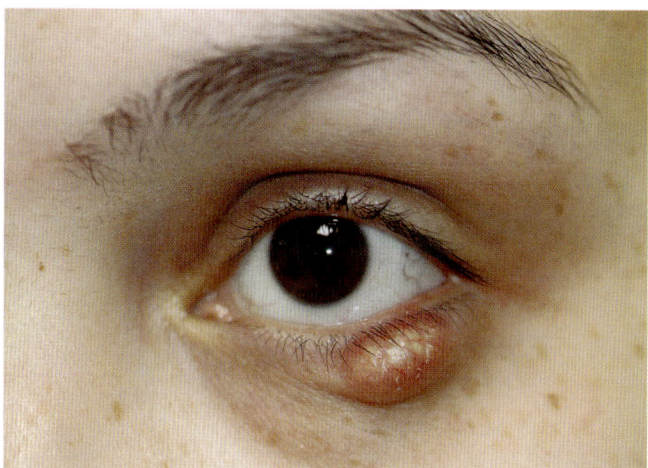

Figure 5.1: Chalazion

Usually the lesion is within the tarsal plate (where the meibomian glands are found) but the position of the chalazia may occasionally be more anterior. Sometimes there can be an associated granuloma which forms adjacent to the chalazion on the palpebral conjunctiva. A persistent chalazion in the same region of the eyelid should be biopsied, due to the very rare possibility of it being a tumour (a sebaceous cell carcinoma).

Treatment of a chalazion initially can be as simple as eyelid hygiene, regularly using eyelid wipes or specifically created cleaning solution. There are many eyelid-cleaning products available on the market or via a pharmacist. This cleaning programme can be augmented with hot compresses, using a microwavable 'heat-bag' to apply onto the face and provide constant and even warmth to the eyelids. This can help to liquefy the sebum and, along with eyelid massage and expression, can encourage drainage and unblock some of the glands.

According to NICE (2015) guidance, topical or oral antibiotic treatment is not recommended for chalazia, as they are usually sterile in nature and antibiotics would therefore have little or no effect.

Persistent chalazia may require more robust treatment, such as a steroid injection (Dexamethazone or Triamcinolone) into the body of the lesion to reduce it. However, if using Triamcinolone, the patient should be aware of the risks associated with this steroid, including depigmentation, skin atrophy, subcutaneous white deposits and (very rarely) tissue necrosis. The injection can be painful and should be administered with anaesthetic drops.

Alternatively, a chalazion that hasn't resolved may eventually require an incision and curettage (I&C) procedure, which is usually carried out in theatre. A steroid injection can be instigated at the same time as the I&C. An outline and competency for I&C of chalazion can be found in Chapter 15 (see p. 280).

Unfortunately, some patients have a particular propensity to develop chalazia and this is often associated with skin conditions such as acne rosacea and seborrhoeic dermatitis, which may need to be treated at the same time as the chalazia.

Stye (external hordeolum)

This is a small self-limiting lesion associated with an infection of an oil gland (Zeis) on the eyelid and the causative bacterial species is usually *staphylococcus aureus*. It presents as a small painful erythematous lump on the eyelid with a yellowish spot in the centre. In larger lesions, much like a chalazion, a stye can cause an upper eyelid droop.

Styes can be associated with, or secondary to, blepharitis. They can also be caused by eye-rubbing, poor nutrition, dehydration, sleep deprivation or lack of hygiene and they are also associated with diabetes. (The diabetes link may need to be explored and ruled out if this hasn't already been done.) Good eyelid cleaning, particularly when using and removing cosmetics, can help prevent such lesions. As styes are contagious, the patient should be advised to take measures to help prevent the spread of infection – i.e. not to share flannels or face towels and not to 'squeeze' the lesions.

In most cases, the lesion resolves in a couple of weeks but antibiotic ointment (such as Chloramphenicol) can have some limited effect in reducing the lesion. Very rarely, styes may require surgical drainage.

Cyst of Moll (hidrocystoma, sudoriferous cyst)

These are cysts associated with the sweat ducts of the eyelid (glands of Moll). They usually present as small transparent lesions which can have a bluish tinge, occurring commonly near the puncta.

The lesion can be left and is typically harmless, but they may cause more epiphora if they interfere with the puncta and tear drainage. Otherwise, the recommended treatment is usually to surgically excise the lesion – an outline and surgical competency can be found in Chapter 15 (see p. 289). However, simple needle aspiration may not be enough to completely drain the lesion and it may recur. In this case, 'de-roofing' and removing the encapsulated cystic bag may be a more effective treatment.

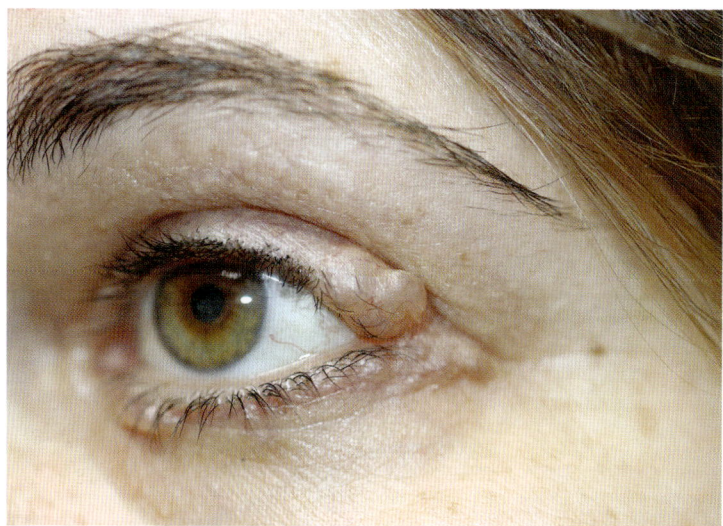
Figure 5.2: Cyst of Moll

Cyst of Zeis

This is a small painless cystic lesion arising from the gland of Zeis and presents as a small, firm lump filled with yellowish-white material. These cysts are usually harmless and can be left, but they may interfere with puncta and tear drainage, causing epiphora.

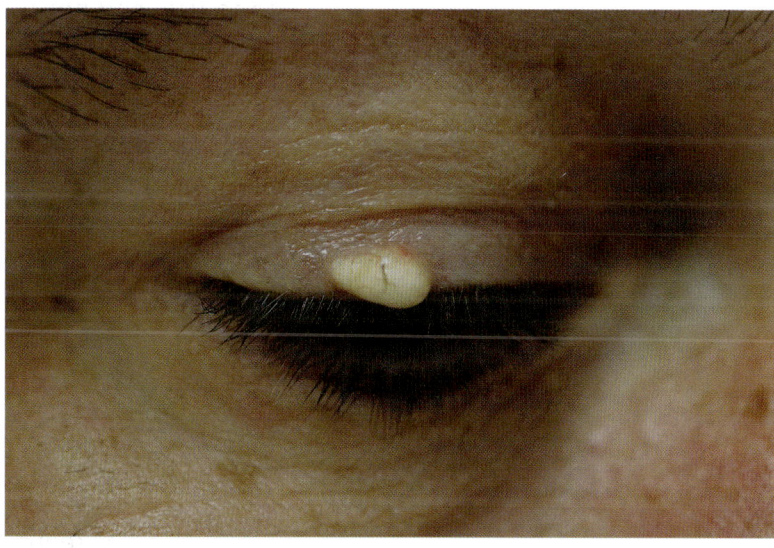
Figure 5.3: Cyst of Zeis

The treatment for these lesions is surgical excision and cautery. An outline and competency can be found in Chapter 15 (see p. 289).

Sebaceous cyst

Epidermal sebaceous cysts can often occur within the brow hair and may be quite large (10–20mm in diameter). Very rarely, they can occur on the eyelid. They are usually painless and relatively firm, with a yellowish colour. Typically, a small hole can be observed on the surface of the lesion, which represents the blocked gland opening.

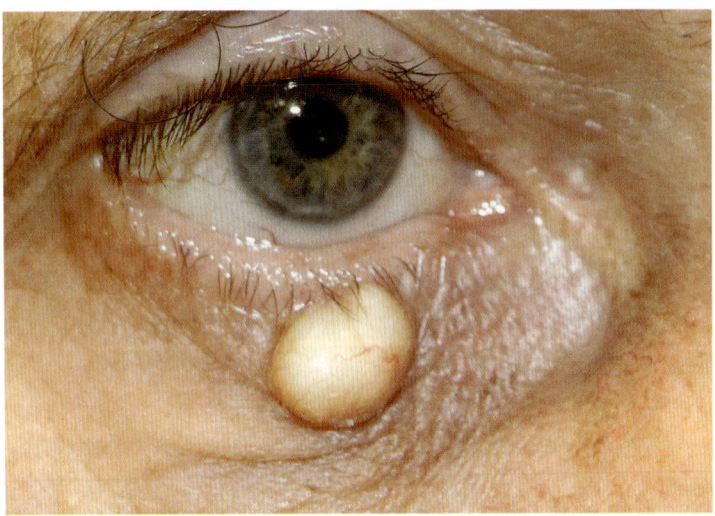

Figure 5.4: Sebaceous cyst

This type of lesion will require surgical excision, removing the whole encapsulated lesion. An outline and surgical competency can be found in Chapter 15 (see p. 289).

Comedo (comedone/blackhead)

This is a blocked hair follicle on the skin associated with keratin and other oils that occlude the opening. They can occur individually (comedo) or in varied numbers (comedones), and either open (the classic blackhead) or closed as raised small papules. There is also a small inflammatory component related to them, which may be attributed to various factors, including: excessive increase of testosterone, free fatty acids in the sebum, overhydrated skin, some chemicals in cosmetics, reduced salt in the sebum, smoking and certain dietary factors.

Topical agents, known as comedolytic medications, can be applied to the skin to reduce blackheads but the treatment may be needed over many years. Some notable topical treatment agents include benzoyl peroxide, azelaic acid, salicylic acid and glycolic acid, but these should all be used with care near the eyes.

Antibiotics may have a limited effect in reducing the inflammation associated with comedones. Otherwise there are some forms of prescribed hormonal therapy which may help. Isotretinoin (derived from vitamin A) can help reduce sebum production and the size of the glands, but conversely sometimes has quite notable side effects which can actually make the skin worse. However, in the form of accutane it does have good results with severe acne.

Fine needle extraction can be undertaken to remove the lesions. Cosmetic microdermal abrasion can also be effective in removing comedones.

Benign epidermal lesions

Squamous papilloma (acrochordon/fibroepithelial polyp/skin tag)

This is a common lesion caused by the human papilloma virus (HPV types 6 and 11) and is associated with the squamous cells within the epidermis. Squamous papilloma can be associated with various parts of the body and can be either sessile (flat) or pedunculated (on a stem/stalk). Occasionally the lesion can have a hyperkeratotic horn-like appearance or alternatively a broad-based sessile form with a raspberry-like surface. They are usually painless and can be left, but very rarely the base of the lesion can change and become cancerous and surgical removal is therefore an option.

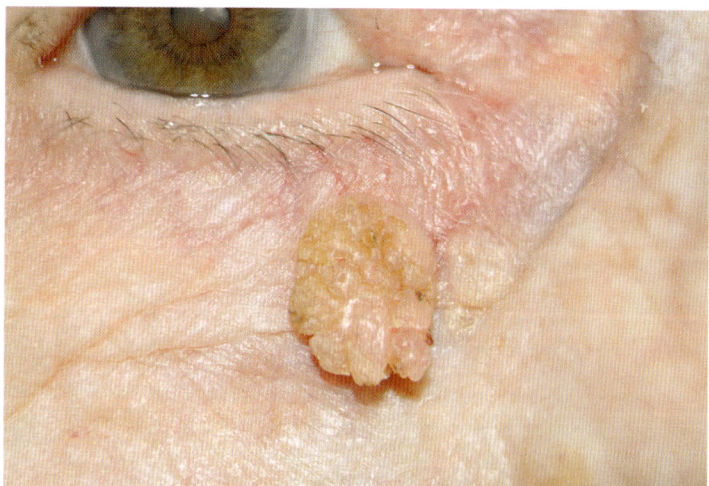

Figure 5.5: Squamous papilloma

An outline of the surgical procedure and competency can be found in Chapter 15 (see p. 289).

Seborrhoeic keratosis (basal cell papilloma)

This is a common lesion that presents as a painless brown growth and has a waxy and scaly appearance. It sometimes looks as though it has been stuck on to the skin. A proliferation of basal cells cases an extension of the squamous epithelium.

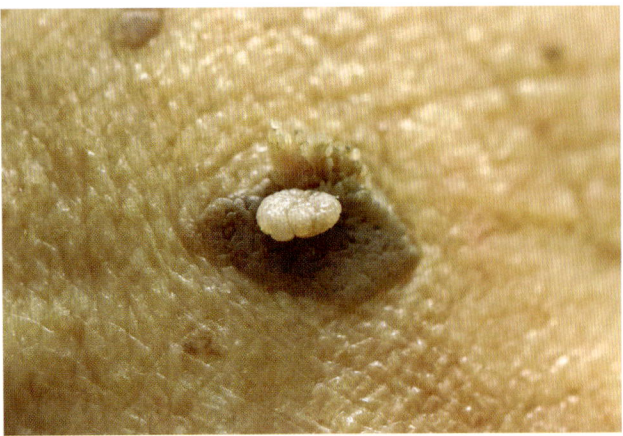

Figure 5.6: Seborrhoeic keratosis

This type of lesion may itch and become irritated and infected, particularly if it rubs against clothing. Surgical excision of the lesion may be indicated, but it can sometimes be left and cause no problems.

Milia

These present as crops of tiny (1–2mm), round, white lesions that are caused by occlusion of pilosebaceous units. Simple cleaning regimes such as mild soap, steam opening of the pores in the shower and exfoliation, can help reduce and prevent milia, and retinoids (vitamin A supplements) may also be helpful.

Milia can be removed using a hypodermic needle or careful excision under a local anaesthetic.

Actinic keratosis (solar keratosis)

This is a common pre-cancerous painless lesion that is caused by UV sun damage and appears as a solitary, sessile, scaly, slightly erythematous patch on the skin. Actinic keratosis can predispose the individual to squamous cell carcinoma, although it is very rare for these lesions to evolve into anything more serious.

Occasionally the lesion may develop into a cutaneous horn. The treatment regime may be to simply leave it alone. Alternatively, practitioners may utilise treatments such as 5-Fluorouracil, Imiquimod, photodynamic treatment or surgical removal.

Molluscum contagiosum (water warts)

Caused by a viral infection (the pox virus), molluscum present on the skin as small raised, painless pearly lesions with a slight dimple in the middle. They occur singly or in crops and can be itchy and slightly irritating. They are self-limiting and will disappear after approximately a year. The lesions can easily be spread and are very contagious, through sexual activity, using the same towels or interfering with the lesions.

The recommended treatment is often just to wait for the colonisation to resolve in its own time. Non-surgical options may include Cantharidin and Imiquimod, but the effectiveness of these agents is questionable. Occasionally it may be necessary to surgically excise some lesions, but this may cause scarring.

Benign dermal lesions
Neurofibroma

This nerve-sheath benign tumour affects the peripheral nervous system and can be divided into two distinct types: dermal and plexiform. Most of these cases present as individual stand-alone tumours that appear as small pea-sized lumps under the skin. These lesions are associated with an inherited disease called neurofibromatosis (NF1), which occurs in approximately 1 in 2,500 of the UK population (Nerve Tumours UK 2019).

Dermal neurofibromas originate from individual nerves in the skin and can be on the surface of the skin as sessile or pedunculated lesions, or reside under the dermis as deep nodular lesions.

Plexiform neurofibromas are often associated with internal nerve bundles within various layers in the body and may feel like a bunch of knots under the skin. This type of neurofibroma can sometimes develop into a malignant nerve sheath tumour.

Very occasionally individual lesions appear and after biopsies turn out to be neurofibroma. However this is rarely a surprise, as the patient will be known to have neurofibromatosis.

Some patients have extensive problems with multiple lesions over their entire body, especially the face, while others may only have very mild changes. Neurofibromatosis is also associated with an orbital component and may require extensive surgery to debulk them. The common presentation with the orbit is a proptosis and an associated S-shaped upper eyelid deformity. Pale spots can sometimes also appear. These may be coffee-coloured, known as 'café au lait' spots, and the individual may also have more abundant freckles.

These symptoms can lead to notable facial deformity and this can be difficult to manage. A very small minority of patients require surgical excision and recession of multiple neurofibromas, and in my experience this has been successful in terms of improving functionality but cosmesis is rather more difficult to attain.

Given that neurofibromatosis is a genetic condition in which there is a high chance of the affected gene being passed from parent to child, genetic counselling and screening are important, especially when dealing with couples who are considering having a baby.

Neurofibromatosis has other issues associated with it, including hypertension, pain and itching, learning and behavioural problems and self-image issues.

The nurse practitioner may be well placed to offer support and advice in such circumstances, and there are a couple of very useful organisations that can provide help: Nerve Tumours UK (www.nervetumours.org.uk) and Changing Faces (www.changingfaces.org.uk)

Capillary haemangioma (strawberry naevus)

This is a very rare condition, often presenting in childhood as an extensive bright red lesion that blanches on pressure and can swell on crying. These lesions more commonly occur on the upper eyelid and may cause a ptosis. Steroid injections can effectively reduce the lesions.

Xanthelasma

This is a common lesion that presents as a well-differentiated yellowish plaque under the skin. The plaques represent a deposition of abnormal lipids under the skin, especially particular lipid-laden histiocytes (foam cells) that commonly occur in the medial canthal region. These lesions (along with corneal arcus, a pale ring circumventing the cornea) are closely associated with raised serum cholesterol (hyperlipidaemia/hypercholesterolaemia and atherosclerosis of vessels). It is therefore necessary to refer the patient to GP to have this checked. Specific testing for apolipoprotein (A1) and (B) levels can be a better predictor of risk of lipid deposition, and this can be suggested as a blood test.

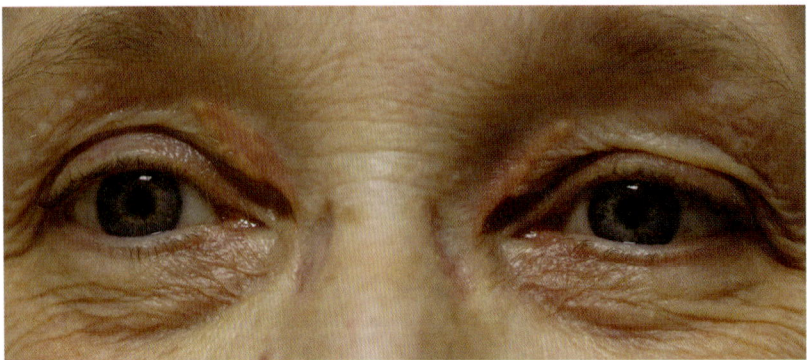

Figure 5.7: Xanthelasma

Possible treatments for xanthelasma are as follows:
- Application of tricholoacetic acid (TCA) – this powerful and destructive acid can be applied very minimally to the lesion with a fine-tipped applicator and may lead to a significant reduction in xanthelasmata. However, this treatment needs to be undertaken with a local subcutaneous anaesthetic and it may also require several treatments. Various strengths of TCA can be applied; in my

practice it is typically a 90% solution. Obviously there can be significant risks if the acid is allowed to migrate or is spilled from the treatment area, so considerable caution is required during its use and application. I'd encourage the practitioner to keep the bottle of TCA in the sink during use and only apply a very minimal amount on the tip of the applicator. Ensure that there are no drips from the tip of the applicator. TCA also causes quite significant hyper-pigmentation immediately after treatment which can be distressing for the patient. It should therefore be avoided in patients with pigmented skin. As a practitioner I have applied TCA on xanthelasmata with varied results over many years. An outline and competency can be found in Chapter 15 (see p. 298).

- Carbon dioxide ultra-pulse laser treatment – this treatment has been shown to be effective and causes minimal scarring and disruption to the surrounding tissue.
- Various lasers (argon, Nd:YAG, Er:YAG) – these treatments cause significant ablation/coagulation of xanthelasmata and are well tolerated. However, the recurrence rate can be quite high, especially with argon laser.
- Surgical removal – this can be very effective, particularly if the xanthelasmata are small. However, there can be the usual complications that come with surgery, especially scarring, bleeding, bruising, infection and eyelid malposition. This will be especially true of larger lesions, which can very difficult to excise without causing distortion of surrounding tissue.

There is no acknowledged gold-standard treatment for xanthelasmata, and certainly in the UK access to particular NHS treatments is variable and in some cases restricted. With all these treatments, the risk of recurrence can still be quite high, so it is important to counsel the patient appropriately for this.

Benign pigmented lesions

Naevus (acquired)

There are various forms of this relatively common cutaneous lesion depending upon their depth and position in the skin.

Intradermal naevus

This is the most common type of naevus, which presents as a poorly pigmented irregular papillomatous lesion with dilated blood vessels. It develops from the dermis within the skin. When associated with the lid edge, the lesion can incorporate the eyelashes. The lesion can be shaved off the lid edge and cautery applied. However, the patient may have to be prepared to lose some eyelashes and this could be permanent. A little tip for undertaking shave biopsies at the eyelid edge/margin is to use a chalazion clamp, as this can help control bleeding whilst removing the lesion. It is also helpful when applying controlled diathermy, and helps protect the eye.

Junctional naevus

This usually presents as a small raised brown area or plaque, often on the eyelid margin. There is a slight risk of these lesions becoming malignant and they therefore require monitoring, especially if the patient opts not to have them removed. These lesions develop from the junction of the dermis and epidermis, which is why they are called 'junctional'. The lesion can be left and monitored or the practitioner may perform shave excision and cautery. Occasionally, more robust surgical intervention is required, i.e. a wedge excision.

Compound naevus

This presents as a raised tan or brown-coloured pigmented lesion. It is not dissimilar to a junctional lesion and involves both the epidermis and dermis.

In all cases the lesions can be left and monitored over a lifetime. However, if there is any suggestion of change within the lesion or notable signs of malignancy, it should be excised/biopsied.

Naevus (congenital)

There is a congenital form of pigmented naevus, which is rare and histologically similar to the acquired form. There is also a very rare alternative form of congenital naevus which affects both lids laterally at the commissure. This is called a 'kissing naevus'.

Lentigo (Lentigines)

These are small, well-defined, pigmented lesions within the skin, which are generally harmless. They are associated with an increased number of melanocytes. These lesions typically do not require any intervention but can occasionally be removed with surgical excision for cosmetic reasons.

Malignant epithelial lesions

Basal cell carcinoma (BCC)

This is the most common eyelid malignancy and is associated with cumulative UV sun exposure (usually from sun beds), increasing age and paler skin types. It accounts for 90% of all eyelid tumours. BCC occurs most commonly on the lower eyelid, followed by the medial canthus, then lateral canthus, and is least likely to be found on the upper eyelid. Some patients and clinicians may still refer to BCCs as 'rodent ulcers', as the lesion gradually 'gnaws away' the eyelid skin (hence its association with the word rodent).

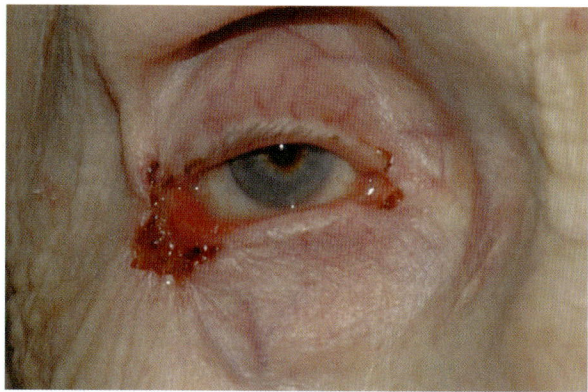

Figure 5.8: Basal cell carcinoma (ulcerative).

BCCs arise from the basal layer of the epidermis and can have a variety of clinical appearances. The most common varieties include:

- Nodular – this most commonly occurs on the sun-exposed areas of the face and head. It can present in various forms, but it is slow growing and generally has a nodular appearance with rolled-over edges. The surface of the lesion may be a little red and may have an area of ulceration and erosion or it may be pearly. There may be telangiectasia. The patient may experience itching, crusting and bleeding with the lesion.
- Ulcerative – this type of lesion may have a more erosive angry appearance with destruction of tissue and loss of lashes. It is also non-healing.
- Cystic – a lesion with a cystic appearance.
- Pigmented – a brownish lesion that may appear like a melanoma.
- Morphoeic – appears like an indistinct whitish scar and can have a deep involvement, especially at the medial canthus.
- Superficial – resembles eczema or psoriasis with scaly patching and can be confused with local inflammation.
- Or a mix of the above.

BCCs very rarely metastasise and are usually indolent and slow growing. However, if left, they can invade the orbit, causing several issues, including fixation/restriction of the eye movement, pain and destruction of tissue. In this case, orbital exenteration may be required. The invasion of the local tissue is three-dimensional, which means that it attacks both vertically and horizontally within the eyelid. This is important to consider, as the patient may only conceptualise the lesion spreading in one plane. The tumour will not only erode soft tissue but will also corrode bone.

An incisional biopsy of the lesion may be required to completely diagnose BCC but it can usually be diagnosed from clinical appearance. If an incisional biopsy is required, the patient will need to attend as a day-case patient and have a small piece of the lesion surgically removed (in theatre) and sent for histopathology. It is important to explain to the patient that a biopsy merely allows for diagnosis. It is unlikely that any attempt will be made to repair the incision, as the probable outcome will be further surgery to remove the lesion in its entirety. Post-operatively, the lesion is possibly going to bleed and the patient will therefore need to care for it and be gentle when cleaning.

Very small, well-defined, lesions can be completely excised. As long as a sufficient margin is allowed, this might be all the treatment that is required.

However, larger and less distinct lesions will require complete removal, once histopathological confirmation of high-risk BCC has been gained. British Association of Dermatologist (BAD) guidelines (Telfer 2008) recommend surgical excision and radiotherapy for extensive BCCs. The surgical options include:

- Mohs microscopic excision
- Staged excision
- Frozen excision and delayed reconstruction.

These will be considered below in more depth. However, the outcomes from surgical excision are generally very good.

Alternatively, radiotherapy may be considered for patients who are reluctant to undergo surgery or for whom it would be too unsafe. Radiotherapy requires multiple trips to hospital and may be exhausting for the patient. Clinically, radiotherapy may also be destructive to local tissue, including the nasolacrimal duct or the eye. It can also cause skin-related changes and cataracts, so the patient will need to be warned of the potential side-effects. A mask may need to be fabricated in order to protect the face from the radiation and this can be claustrophobic.

Squamous cell carcinoma (SCC)

This represents approximately 2% of all eyelid malignant tumours but has a greater risk of spread than BCC. Like BCC, SCC tends to affect the lower eyelid more often and occurs as a consequence of UV damage, increasing age and fairer skin types and can be associated with actinic keratosis. SCCs may be nodular, plaque or ulcerative and this type of lesion often presents as a thickened, scaly cutaneous formation with indurated (hardened, fibrotic) borders. There will be loss of eyelashes if the lesion incorporates the eyelid margin. It is faster growing than a BCC and can be more aggressive to local tissue. Metastasis is uncommon but can affect 20% of cases if the regional lymph nodes are involved. If a patient has biopsy-proven SCC, it may therefore be pertinent to undertake an examination of the lymph nodes for lymphadenopathy.

Treatment options include surgical excision and primary reconstruction or delayed reconstruction/excision with frozen section control and primary reconstruction/or Mohs excision and reconstruction (see below). There can be orbital spread and this might warrant extensive surgical removal – typically orbital exenteration and/or radiotherapy.

Sebaceous cell carcinoma (SGC)

Originating from the meibomian glands and (more unusually) the glands of Zeis and the caruncle, this particular type of tumour commonly affects the upper eyelid (unlike SCC and BCC). Most notably, in the early stages, it may resemble a chalazion or blepharitis. The practitioner should therefore always treat any non-healing meibomian cyst with suspicion, and biopsy it if in any doubt.

There is a significant mortality rate with this type of lesion, due to its widespread metastasis and frequent misdiagnosis. Clinically SGC can appear quite innocuous – either as a nodular lesion or a spreading erythematous diffuse infiltration.

A lesion biopsy (including conjunctival mapping biopsies) may be required in the first instance to provide a diagnosis. However, SGC may be misdiagnosed if the specimens are not appropriately prepared – fat stains will be specifically required and the pathologist should therefore be informed of the potential diagnosis. Lymph node examination will also be essential to rule out lymphadenopathy.

Wide surgical excision will be required and may include exenteration. Again, lymph gland spread may well mean radial neck dissection of the nodes.

Malignant non-epithelial lesions

Melanoma

This is a very rare, typically pigmented lesion that rarely develops in the eyelids (but bear in mind that not all melanoma are pigmented). A few forms are notable – lentigo maligna, nodular and superficial spreading melanoma. Chronic thickening, areas of pigmentation or a nodule may appear.

The treatment will include wide surgical excision (10mm margins) and radical neck dissection. Unfortunately, depending upon the degree of invasion, the prognosis can be very poor, with a mortality rate as high as 50% in some cases.

Merkel cell tumour

This is a very rare, malignant lesion, which presents as a fast-growing (within weeks, as opposed to months) painless, red or purple nodule. Again, the risk is increased by excessive UV exposure, a weakened immune system and fairer skin. The tumour is extremely malignant, with a poor prognosis: 50% of patients experiencing spread to brain, bones, liver or lungs.

Nursing considerations

If the patient presents with a malignant lesion, it will be necessary to undertake various investigations, including scanning and biopsies, and they will probably need to attend theatre to have the lesion removed. This may all come as a shock to the patient, especially when they possibly presented with a relatively small innocuous lesion. Over the years I have come across a handful of patients on my minor-op list who have had a lesion routinely biopsied with no overwhelming suspicion of anything unusual, only to then find that the histopathology report suggests something more sinister. More often than not, these turned out to be BCCs, which are treatable, but nonetheless an unwelcome surprise.

Discussion and consent

As part of the consent process for all my patients who are likely to have a biopsy (and sometimes even when they don't), I will warn them of the slight chance that the histopathology report will bring up something unexpected, however improbable that may seem. This can of course be worrying for the patient, but I think an honest approach is important and the risk must always be put into some sort of context. Some individuals will be reassured if, for example, you can express the probability of a cancerous lesion in terms of numbers, say '1 in 100,000'. Others respond to more qualitative terms, in which case you can suggest that the likelihood is 'rare' or 'negligible'. Whichever approach is adopted, there needs to be careful consideration of how these potential outcomes are conveyed to the patient.

There are some patients who will not be expecting to undergo any surgery, either to remove the lesion or to perform the subsequent reconstruction. Adjunctive therapies, such as radiotherapy, may also be required. If there is any suggestion of the patient having a suspicious lesion, the potential surgical or treatment outcomes should therefore be introduced as early as possible. Support from various groups and individuals can then be considered from the outset. The consent process is an opportunity to listen and answer any questions the patient may have. It is always good to go over aspects of the potential care pathway a couple of times, as patients often forget or simply do not take in the details. Patient information sheets are useful, as they obviously provide information the patient can refer back to if necessary. However, providing patient information sheets can also be a bit of a 'tick box exercise' and some of them may end up in the bin, not having been read. If you decide to offer a patient information sheet, it's therefore best to go through it with them.

Some patients may suspect that their lesion is related to cancer and will require significant input. They may also have preconceived ideas and concerns with regard to the diagnosis, so it is important to allay some of their fears. In the digital age, with access to various social media pages and websites, patients often plough through videos and web pages to gain information. This is of course acceptable if the information they find is both trustworthy and reliable. However, there is a danger that some of the information unearthed either doesn't relate to their particular condition or is simply wrong so it is important to have a number of trustworthy websites ready to suggest to the patient. I have therefore included references to various dependable websites and groups in this book relating to specific conditions.

In Chapter 11 (on orbital exenteration) I discuss the breaking of bad news and the impact upon all involved (see p. 173). If the prognosis is poor or the patient requires extensive surgery (such as an orbit exenteration or wide resection), the practitioner should clearly take time to prepare for the discussion and reflect on how it can be undertaken in a sensitive and appropriate manner.

Pre-operative assessment

If the patient requires surgery, they will need a pre-operative assessment. Most biopsy and subsequent reconstructive surgeries can be undertaken either under a local anaesthetic or a local with sedation. Very rarely, especially if the reconstruction is likely to be extensive, they might need a general anaesthetic.

Consider whether the patient can lie down for a long period, and assess how to access other parts of the body for potential donor sites for skin grafts, and how to make the patient comfortable. Remember, a reasonable proportion of patients will be elderly and may have specific needs.

During the surgery

Reconstruction surgery can take anything up to a couple of hours. In most patients, especially the elderly, it will therefore be important to check pressure points during the surgery and protect them. Keeping the patient at a comfortable temperature is also vital, as theatres can be cool, especially with air-flow systems moving the ambient air around, which can lead to hypothermia. There are various body warming devices that can be used to maintain an appropriate temperature.

Some surgeons use monopolar cautery and cutting devices, which require an earthing plate to be attached to the patient. It is important to ensure that the earthing plate has a good contact. Don't forget to check whether the patient has any internal metalwork, in the form of hip or knee replacements, as earthing pads must not be placed on or near them. You also need to confirm whether the patient has a pacemaker, as some monopolar devices can interfere with these (especially defibrillating types).

With pacemakers, it is important to check what type, model and when it was last serviced. It may be necessary to have a cardiac technician present to monitor the pacemaker and/or apply a magnet to shield the pacemaker from the effects of the interference caused by the cautery.

Post-operative care

Depending upon the reconstruction technique used, the patient may need to be warned about particular aspects, such as having to care for a split-thickness graft donor site or having an eye temporarily closed for a period. Very occasionally, a patient may have an open wound – for example, in delayed reconstruction (see below). This will be dressed, but it may nonetheless be painful or irritating to the eye or it may bleed. It is therefore essential to educate the patient to enable them to understand what is happening under the dressing in relation to the surgery. They must also be given the means to contact someone if they have any concerns after the surgery.

There may be some post-operative pain and this will need to be controlled with appropriate analgesia. Remember, most patients will be day cases and will need to take medication home, so it is important to go over their medication requirements carefully. Bear in mind that they may be bandaged up and only have use of one eye. Spend some time explaining the potential frustrations and difficulties of being one-eyed, including clumsiness and the risk of banging into things.

Excision of the lesion and histopathological clearance

Once the biopsy has been undertaken and the diagnosis has been confirmed, the patient may need the reminder of the lesion to be removed (from a histological basis). There are several ways in which this can be done.

Excision and immediate reconstruction

If the surgeon is convinced that they can guarantee complete excision, they may excise the affected tissue and immediately go on to reconstruct. However, this is very rarely the case and may only be associated with direct closure of the wound.

Mohs micrographic excision

This is a specialist technique offered in some centres, which is seen as the gold standard for the removal of BCCs (and other tumours as well). The recurrence rate is very low with Mohs excision, and the success rate is as much as 98–99% (Platts *et al.* 2014).

A dermatologist who has undertaken specialist training to complete the technique usually carries out the procedure. The patient will attend a clinic to have the presenting lesion assessed and will then undergo a pre-operative assessment. Once the appropriate arrangements have been made, the patient will have the lesion excised under Mohs micrographic control and then, on the same day (or the day after), will be transferred to the appropriate tertiary oculoplastic unit to have the defect reconstructed.

Mohs excision of the lesion aims to remove the lesion in its entirety whilst also ensuring that the minimum of healthy tissue is removed. In order to do this, the lesion is excised in a certain fashion and the histopathology is undertaken at the same time by the Mohs surgeon.

Initially, the visibly obvious lesion is divided into sections and 'mapped'. Then, section by section, the tissue is removed and examined microscopically. If there is any evidence of cancerous cells in the specimens examined, the dermatologist marks their location on the 'map' and excises more tissue from that specific area. This procedure may be undertaken several times to ensure complete excision.

Excision under frozen section

Where Mohs excision cannot be accessed or specific types of tissue are being excised, excision under frozen section is a viable and accurate alternative. In this case, the patient attends theatre and has the appropriate tissue removed with a degree of margin, and this is immediately sent to the pathology lab. The tissue is prepared in the lab, frozen in a Cryostat machine between -20°C and -30°C, and cut in sections to be examined under the microscope.

Meanwhile the patient will have the open wound dressed and they will return to the day unit or ward. Very occasionally the patient and team may wait for the result in theatre or start to reconstruct. Usually within a short period (typically within an hour or two), there will be a result. Once clearance has been confirmed, the patient can come back to theatre to be reconstructed.

There are some technical limitations to this approach as regards the processing of the specimen and particular tissue types, which has led to it achieving arguably slightly less accurate results. However, the process is nonetheless well regarded and precise enough to warrant good outcomes.

Excision and delayed reconstruction

Alternatively, an excision and subsequent delayed reconstruction is a more accurate approach than frozen section. Permanent sections and better preparation of the specimens allows for a more accurate result.

With this approach, the patient attends theatre and has the appropriate tissue removed. The specimen is then formalin-fixed and sent to the pathology lab. Meanwhile the patient has the open wound dressed and returns for reconstruction several days later, once a result is made available and clearance has been obtained.

Reconstructive surgery

Once histopathological confirmation of tumour clearance has been established, reconstructive surgery can be considered. Each individual case is different and offers particular challenges when deciding on the most appropriate surgical approach to reconstruction. There are a number of recognised reconstruction approaches that can be used (or a combination of approaches), depending upon the nature of the defect. Some of the more common approaches are outlined below.

Laissez-faire

Some small defects can effectively be left to close through normal healing and granulation of tissue. If the appropriate patients are carefully selected, the outcomes can be good, with less scarring.

This approach requires appropriate wound care input and management. Essentially the appropriate dressings (if required) need to be chosen and careful wound hygiene applied. A non-stick dressing may be useful or Jelonet (Smith & Nephew) is applied initially, with a supporting secondary dressing (such as a foam dressing).

Wound care would certainly involve aseptic non-touch technique (ANTT), to protect key parts and sites from colonisation by micro-organisms. Further specific information regarding ANTT guidelines can be found at www.antt.org

The patient may have several visits to the outpatients' department for dressing changes or can be educated in how to manage themselves. The wound will need to be kept clean, using sterile water and topical antibiotics.

The wound should be monitored and its progression recorded with legible handwriting in the medical notes. It may also be necessary to get clinical photographs. The wound should also be observed for signs of infection, including redness, erythema, discharge and smell.

Intrinsic to appropriate wound care would be general care considerations, including stopping smoking, a good well-balanced diet, temperature control and good hygiene. The patient may well need support with some of these aspects and may require referral to the GP for additional help.

Primary closure

If there is enough redundant skin, the wound can be directly closed. However, the wound may need to be undermined to allow the skin to come together. Skin vectors and the direction of pull will need to be carefully considered when assessing the defect and the potential closure, to avoid a poor outcome. For example, direct closure of a lower eyelid wound in a horizontal (rather than the desirable vertical) vector could lead to an ectropion.

Eyelid re-approximation

Sometimes a full thickness lid defect, where a section of the eyelid has been removed, can be re-approximated, in a similar way to an eyelid wedge excision (as described on p. 19). Vicryl (5/0) sutures can be used bring the lid together and a horizontal lid margin suture Silk (6/0) is placed to create a slight eversion of the wound edge, with a modified mattress method (to reduce the likelihood of a lid notch).

(Lateral) Canthotomy and cantholysis

Releasing the lateral canthal attachments can allow the eyelid to be advanced horizontally to reduce a defect. This procedure is explained in more detail on p. 207, in relation to the emergency treatment needed to reduce pressure within the orbit.

Full thickness skin graft (FTSG)

Some small to moderately sized defects can be covered with a free skin graft harvested from an area elsewhere on the body that provides a good colour match and is not hair-bearing. A full thickness skin graft involves both the epidermis and dermis layers, as opposed to a split thickness graft which comprises only the epidermis and the uppermost dermis layers. Full thickness skin grafts anecdotally offer the best skin match, with the least contraction, compared to split thickness grafts. However, they also have poorer survival rates.

It will be necessary to ensure that there is a sufficiently good vascular bed for the graft to be placed on to enable it to survive. A full thickness skin graft can be harvested from various sites for use in oculoplastic reconstruction:

- Pre-auricular (in front of the ear)
- Post-auricular (behind the ear)
- Upper eyelid
- Supra-clavicular
- Inner upper arm.

If the defect is too deep, the skin graft will follow the contour of the defect and not look as cosmetically pleasing. To prevent this, it may be necessary to combine the FTSG with an underlying epicranial forehead flap or repositioning of the underlying orbicularis. An epicranial flap involves a vertical section of tissue being harvested (with a blood supply) from the forehead. The muscle tissue is then passed beneath the undermined skin to sit within the defect in order to bulk it out and create a vascular bed for the FTSG to be stitched onto.

Once the graft has been harvested, it is transferred into the defect and stitched (and/or glued) in place. The donor site is then undermined and closed. An outline of the surgery and competency can be found in Chapter 15 (see p. 314).

The sutures in the donor site can be removed at or around the tenth day post-op. The wound will need to be kept clean and should be protected from coarse clothing, which may rub and cause irritation.

In order to remove the sutures, ANTT protocol will need to be adhered to. Initially, wash hands and don gloves, then use toothed forceps (e.g. Adsons) and Westcott or suture scissors to remove the sutures. As the sutures used in the donor site are typically nylon/prolene, a non-toothed forceps probably wouldn't grip the sutures and might slip. Before starting, ensure that the patient is comfortable and the area is easily assessable. Use a magnifier lamp in order to gain better visibility.

Removing sutures can be painful, especially if they are difficult to access or are buried. Consider the use of topical or subcutaneous local anaesthetic in order to make the procedure more comfortable.

The graft donor site will require wound hygiene post-operatively, with regular cleaning with sterile normal saline or alternatively cooled boiled water and cotton balls/gauze. It is important to assess the patient's (or relative's) cleaning technique. Application of antibiotic ointment will be necessary in the first week following surgery. The sutures in the graft site will drop out if they are Vicryl, but it will be better to remove them early so as to reduce inflammation.

Post-operative graft site massage will be necessary for several months following the procedure in order to reduce scarring and contracture. The massage technique is outlined on pp. 15–16.

Rhomboid flap

This technique uses the basis of a rhomboid shape to create a flap that will be rotated into the wound (see Figure 5.9). The flap is stitched into place.

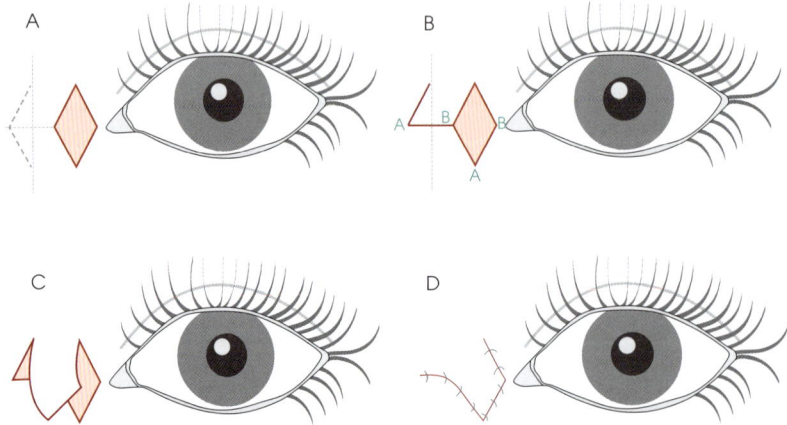

Figure 5.9: Rhomboid flap

The rhomboid flap is very versatile and can be used in various ways to correct numerous defects. There is usually a good skin match and blood supply and it heals very well.

In a similar way to the rhomboid flap, Zitelli (1989) outlined the modified 'bi-lobed' flap which can be created and rotated into a lower eyelid defect.

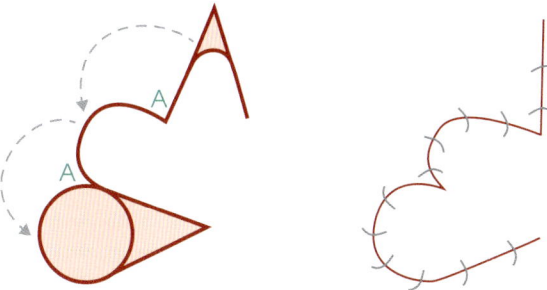

Figure 5.10: Bi-lobed flap

Hughes procedure

We can think of the eyelid as made of two layers sandwiched together, an anterior layer of skin/muscle and a posterior layer of tarsal plate/conjunctiva. In some full-thickness lower eyelid defects the reconstruction has, if possible, to be undertaken so as to recreate a posterior and anterior lamella to give the lid some form and stabilisation. In order to create a posterior lamella, a conjunctival/tarsal flap is created from the upper eyelid and bridged (transconjunctivally) over the eye and into the defect and stitched in place. This is called a Hughes flap. The flap is still attached to the upper eyelid in order to guarantee a blood supply. Then a full thickness graft is harvested and stitched over the abridging Hughes flap to recreate the anterior lamella.

The eye is closed for several weeks (the flap can actually be divided after 2 weeks in many cases) while the grafted element heals in place. This may cause some issues if the vision is poor in the non-operated eye, which may mean that the patient isn't suitable for this type of reconstruction. When appropriate, the patient comes back to theatre and has the flap opened.

Cutler-Beard reconstruction

In some ways, this is a similar procedure to a Hughes but to correct upper eyelid defects instead. A horizontal lower eyelid incision is made below the tarsus and a section of lower eyelid skin is released and advanced under the incision and bridged over the eye and stitched into the upper eyelid defect. This creates an anterior lamella. An auricular cartilage graft is harvested from behind the ear and is used to create a posterior lamella.

Tenzel and Mustarde flap

These are both moderate to large lateral rotational flaps that can be harvested to cover extensive lower eyelid defects. The Tenzel flap is the smaller of the two approaches and is a semi-circular flap harvested from the lateral canthus, curving temporally and superiorly just under the brow towards the ear. The flap is undermined so it is free and then advanced into the lower eyelid defect.

A Mustarde flap is a much larger myocutaneous flap and the incision goes from the lateral canthus all the way to the pinna of the ear – essentially it is an extended Tenzel flap. It is rarely used, but with sizable lower eyelid defects (75% of lid lost) this approach can be utilised. Great care has to be taken to protect the facial nerve. Nevertheless, post-operatively there can still be nerve paralysis, scarring, numbness, necrosis of the flap and haematoma.

At the time of surgery, a suction drain is placed (see p.240) in order to reduce the risk of post-operative haematoma. A compression dressing and bandage is applied as well at the end of procedure and this should stay in place for several days after surgery.

General wound care will be required post-operatively after the Tenzel/Mustarde flap reconstruction, including hygiene and application of antibiotic ointment. The sutures are usually nylon/prolene and will need to be removed at approximately 10 days.

References

Changing Faces (2019). https://www.changingfaces.org.uk (last accessed 31.10.2019).

Lee, Y. & Hwang, K. (2002). Skin thickness of Korean adults. *Surgical and Radiologic Anatomy.* **24**(3–4), 183–9. Epub 2002 July 12.

Nerve Tumours UK (2019). https://nervetumours.org.uk/ (last accessed 31.10.2019).

NICE (2015). Meibomian Cyst (Chalazion) Clinical Knowledge Summary. *https://cks.nice.org.uk/meibomian-cyst-chalazion* (last accessed 1.11.2019).

Platts, M., Danial, S., Cook, A. & Cooper, J. (2014). A review of the management options for periorbital basal cell carcinomas. *International Journal of Ophthalmic Practice.* **5**(1), 6–11.

Telfer, N., Colver, G. & Morton, C. (2008). Guidelines for the management of basal cell carcinoma. *British Journal of Dermatology.* **159**(1), 35–48.

Zitelli, J. (1989). The bilobed flap for nasal reconstruction. *Archives of Dermatology.* **125**, 957–59.

6

The eyelashes and trichiasis

Introduction

Probably one of the most overlooked aspects of the eye and its surrounding anatomy are the humble eyelashes. Interestingly, though, diagnosing and treating conditions related to eyelashes can actually represent an important part of the oculoplastic role, particularly if the lashes become malpositioned. It is therefore worth considering their role and physiology, and also appreciating their importance, not only anatomically but also cosmetically and psychologically.

Eyelashes can exemplify beauty, and sexuality, and they play an important part in a multi-million-pound cosmetics industry. They affect how we look and express ourselves, especially in relation to femininity. From a psychological perspective, eyelashes are a focus in non-verbal communication, particularly if they are long and lush. Beautiful eyelashes may suggest that the individual is healthy and free from conditions that might lead to them falling out. Long eyelashes may provide the illusion that the eye is wider, and this may be intensified with make-up such as eyeliner and mascara. Darkened eyelids, and eyelashes contrasting with the white of the eye, may further accentuate the impression of youth and beauty. In the same way as lipstick can highlight the lips, eye make-up can emphasise the eyes.

Clearly, eyelashes play a significant role in the human psyche and the psychosocial aspects of interaction. They reflect health and vitality and thus influence physical attraction between individuals. If there is any disruption in the natural presentation of the eyelashes, it can therefore have a powerful psychological effect on the individual.

Eyelash anatomy

The eyelid can be split into two halves. The outward portion is skin and muscle (orbicularis oculi) and is known as the anterior lamella; and the inner half is made up of the tarsal plate, meibomian glands and palpebral conjunctiva, and is called the posterior lamella. This division is observable at the lid edge and is visibly separated by a demarcation known as the 'grey-line'. This is important, particularly as a surgical landmark, and needs to be remembered as it is often referred to in various texts and medical notes.

The eyelashes originate from the anterior lamella and, depending upon the individual, there can be one or more rows. There are anywhere from 90 to 120 lashes in the upper eyelid and slightly fewer in the lower (around 70 to 80) but this number may vary between individuals.

The main function of eyelashes is to provide protection from injury and stop debris entering the eye. However, there are theories that eyelashes may also play a part in disrupting airflow near the eye and thus reducing the drying effect of air upon the cornea.

The morphology of the eyelash is similar to that of scalp hair but lashes are significantly stunted in length, compared to hair elsewhere on the body. Typically, the eyelashes on the upper eyelid grow to 8–12mm, and on the lower 6–8mm.

When eyelashes fall out or are removed, they take 6–8 weeks to regrow. There are five recognised phases to eyelash growth:

- Anagen – this is the growth phase where the lash is actively growing; it stops when it reaches a certain length (30–45 days)
- Catagen – at this stage the lash stops growing and its follicle shrinks (14–21 days)
- Telogen – this is the static or resting phase and lasts for approximately 100 days
- Exogen – in this stage, the lash falls out and a new lash starts to grow in its place.
- Kenogen – this is a phase when the follicle is empty and then the formation of a new lash begins.

Within the follicle of the eyelash, there are associated glands of Moll and Zeis. The gland of Moll is an apocrine gland and secretes a sterile, odourless, oily substance onto the eyelash, near the margin of the eyelid. This substance is thought to provide an immunological defence mechanism, as it contains molecules including IgA, MUC1 and lysozyme, which all have roles in protecting the surrounding lash and ocular surface from infection.

Similarly, the glands of Zeis are sebaceous glands and produce sebum, which helps maintain and condition the lashes. The follicle itself helps control growth of the lashes by means of a complex interaction of factors including hormones and neuropeptides. The base of the follicle is made up of connective tissue and is called the pupilla. The bulbous root sheath originates from where the lash is generated. The main body of the lash is known as the shaft, and the base is called the root.

Growth rates and the length of lashes can be affected by a particular glaucoma medication (Bimatoprost, which is a prostaglandin), which leads to excessive lusher growth of lashes. This product is also now available on the market as a beauty treatment to enhance and darken eyelash growth – under the name Latisse (marketed as Lumigan or Allergan). When taking a history, it is good to find out whether the patient is using this product and make a note of it. This product may also cause orbital fat atrophy and is not recommended.

Assessment of the eyelashes

From our perspective as practitioners, it is important to assess the eyelashes and consider the following questions.

Is there any loss of lashes (madarosis)?

- If there is an associated lesion on the eyelid, this could represent an aggressive aspect that can be related to a tumour and cause loss of lashes.
- Certain conditions can lead to loss of lashes, such as syphilis or psoriasis. Alopecia areata is a moderately common genetic condition, which essentially involves loss of patches of hair, including eyelashes.
- Taking various drugs, including anti-thyroids and anti-coagulants, can lead to lash loss.
- May be associated with hair being pulled out by the individual – trichotillomania. This can be related to anxiety, stress and mental health issues.
- Metabolic causes such as malnutrition, chronic zinc deficiency.
- Infection – specifically staphylococcal blepharitis and Demodex (parasitic).

Are there any colour changes (poliosis)?

This may involve premature and sometimes localised whitening of the lashes, which is secondary to several genetic syndromes, but can be associated with inflammation.

Are the lashes malpositioned in any way?

The inward turning of lashes that touch the eye is known as trichiasis and will be discussed further below.

Are there more than one/two rows of lashes?

Normally there are one or two rows of lashes anterior to the grey-line, but congenitally there can be multiple rows (often in the posterior lamella) that can cause issues. This condition is known as distichiasis.

What is the condition of the lashes?

If there is underlying skin disease (most notably blepharitis), there can be quite severe crusting around the lashes. Similarly, in a Demodex infestation (and with the benefit of a slit lamp), you might observe cylindrical crusting around the base of the lashes.

When observing the eyelashes through a slit lamp, it is important to take note of the condition of the lash, the position of the lash and any other associated issues. Is there any redness or swelling at the base of the lashes? Or are they misdirected or malpositioned?

You should also take note of whether the patient uses false eyelashes or stick-on lashes which may be used to enhance cosmesis. These can harbour infection and irritation of the eyelid margin, especially if the glue that is used to secure them is not completely removed.

Trichiasis

This is a common abnormality whereby the eyelashes turn inwards towards the eye (see Figure 6.1). There are various reasons for trichiasis, including blepharitis, Herpes Zoster, trauma, trachoma, Steven-Johnson syndrome, cicatricial pemphigoid, previous eyelid surgery, epiblepharon (more commonly in children) and mechanical rubbing of the eye.

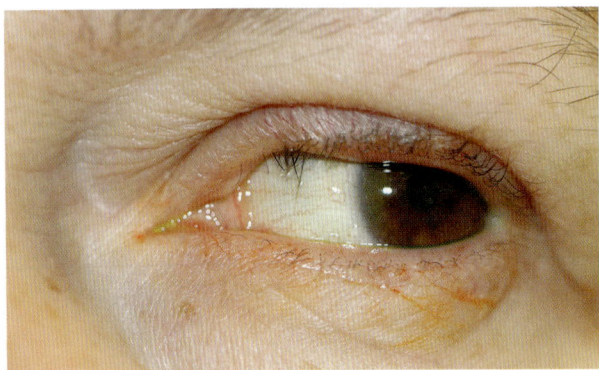

Figure 6.1: Trichiasis

The individual with trichiasis may experience a 'foreign body sensation' or really be quite irritated by the continual abrasion associated with the lashes touching the eye. If left untreated in patients with prolonged symptoms, trichiasis can cause epiphora, redness, photophobia, pain, corneal abrasion, corneal ulcers and reduction of vision. Trichiasis can involve anything from a single lash to more or less the entire eyelid. Using a slit lamp, and under a blue light with a drop of fluorescein, it may be possible to assess the amount of damage being caused by the eyelashes. If the problem is excessive, temporary relief may be gained by using a bandage contact on the cornea to protect it. However, be mindful of the potential infection risk of using a bandage contact lens for a prolonged amount of time.

Eyelash removal and treatment for trichiasis

The treatment for trichiasis includes initial removal of the offending lashes by actively pulling them out. This is known as epilation. Usually this needs to be undertaken with the use of a slit lamp or magnifying loupes (if a slit lamp is not available). It requires the practitioner to be quite dexterous and takes practice to refine the technique. Some patients may get frustrated and attempt self-epilation, but this should be discouraged as there is an obvious risk that they could cause harm to themselves.

Some lashes can be particularly thick and may require quite a significant tug to pull them out and this can hurt the patient. Conversely, some of the lashes can be quite fine and difficult to pick up. Occasionally, if the lid is malpositioned or there is a significant overhang of lid skin, you can find actual skin hairs or even brow hairs (if they are exceptionally long) abrading onto the eye that will require removal.

I use fine-tipped forceps (such as Birks) to undertake lash removal. Alternatively, actual epilation forceps can be used – although I find these somewhat cumbersome. Prior to starting the procedure, the patient will need to be prepared and the practitioner should explain what they are about to do. Usually verbal consent is sufficient for this procedure, but some practitioners may find it necessary to gain written consent.

When undertaking epilation, I prefer to rest my active epilation hand and fingers on the patient's forehead for upper lid lashes, and either the nose or temporal region for the lower eyelid.

Personally, I have found the best technique is to get hold of the lash literally a millimetre from its base at the lid margin and then pull swiftly and firmly in the direction the lash is pointing. If you take hold of the lash any further up the shaft it is more likely to break and this makes epilation trickier. When operating on the upper eyelid, I get the patient to look down . When operating on the lower eyelid, I ask them to look up . You may have to support the eyelid and provide counter-traction to get a cleaner pull – otherwise you will pull the lid as well as the lash. Epilation may require prolonged periods when the eye has to remain open. This can cause discomfort for the patient, so remember to stop or allow the patient to blink in between pulls.

After epilation the eye should be more comfortable, but of course after a few weeks the lashes will return. Epilation of lashes suits some patients and they will be willing to attend a regular clinic to have this done. However, there are other more permanent treatment options available.

Cryotherapy applied to the offending eyelids is one treatment option for trichiasis. This involves applying a cryo-probe onto the lashes and freezing the area. Whilst this can remove the lashes effectively, it can also be quite destructive to the surrounding skin and may cause tissue necrosis. It is therefore not the safest treatment option.

Similarly, argon laser treatment has also been suggested as a treatment for trichiasis, but again the success rates are anywhere between 60% and 80% and the complication rates are significantly high, at 20%. These complications can include lid hypopigmentation (colour changes) and notching of the lid.

The other relatively safe option for trichiasis treatment is electrolysis. This involves passing a hand-held fine-tipped wire down each individual lash to the follicle, approximately 2.5mm, and applying a monopolar electrical or radiofrequency current to burn and destroy the lash follicle. This can be a slightly laborious approach, particularly if there are a lot of lashes to treat. The success rates are also quite variable, approximately 50–60%. I therefore warn patients that repeat treatments are likely. The patient also has to have a local anaesthetic injection into the eyelid, which may put some individuals off. In order to visualise the lashes during the procedure, the treatment requires an operating microscope. The surgical competency for electrolysis can be found in Chapter 15 (see p. 276).

The equipment required for electrolysis is as follows:
- Radiofrequency electrosurgical diathermy machine
- Electrolysis needles and handpiece
- Epilation forceps
- Prep tray
- Local anaesthetic.

The process for electrolysis is as follows:
- Identify aberrant lashes prior to surgery, gain written consent and mark the appropriate site/side for surgery using the correct consent form
- Instill local anaesthetic drops into the affected eye
- Some practitioners use a protective eye shield
- Administer subcutaneous local anaesthetic to the area that requires surgery
- Check and prepare the equipment for use and check that the patient has a pad on to return the current back to the machine; if the patient has a pacemaker, be aware that this can be affected by the machine
- Wash hands and don sterile gloves
- Using the theatre operating microscope, identify the lashes requiring treatment
- Check with the patient the level of anaesthesia
- Pass the electrolysis needle down the side of the shaft of the eyelash requiring removal
- The electrical current is applied for 2–10 seconds. The appearance of blanching or bubbles at the eyelid indicates that sufficient current has been supplied
- The eyelash may well fall out when the electrolysis needle is removed, or it can be removed using epilation forceps – it should be easy to remove

- This will be repeated as necessary
- Apply topical antibiotics to the eyelids for one week post-operatively
- Care must be taken to protect the globe from accidental injury by not advancing the electrolysis needle too far into the follicle.

Following surgery, the practitioner will record the surgical episode in the patient's medical notes, including:

- Date of surgery
- Nature of the surgery and the reason for it
- The name of the practitioner
- The local anaesthetic used
- A detailed diagram showing the treatment areas
- An outline of the surgery performed
- Post-operative treatment and follow-up
- Signature.

The patient will require follow-up in clinic 6–8 weeks later to assess the outcome after the surgery.

Alternatively, the lashes can be removed surgically, using a specialised cannula (lacrimal trephine or Sisler cannula – BD Visitec). Essentially, this enables the practitioner to 'apple-core' the individual lashes out under a local anaesthetic. However, this is tricky and quite tedious to perform, especially if there are multiple misdirected lashes.

Occasionally the patient may require actual surgery to correct the issues associated with trichiasis, possibly including removal of the lash-bearing skin in its entirety. This is usually undertaken under a local anaesthetic. Using a super-sharp blade, a sliver of the marginal anterior lamella is removed with the eyelashes, leaving a raw area of marginal skin. Once healed, the lashes will hopefully not return as the follicles have been removed altogether.

If there is a small cluster of lashes causing a problem, that section of the eyelid can be removed. A wedge excision can be undertaken to remove them completely. However, this assumes that there is enough laxity in the eyelid to allow the wedge to be performed and that the eyelid will come back together safely. There are risks of wound dehiscence and scarring associated with the procedure.

The formation of new rows of lashes, arising from the eyelid margin, is known as dischiasis. These accessory lashes cause irritation and disruption. Removing them can be difficult and it requires more extensive surgery, which may include an anterior lamellar repositioning procedure. This involves splitting the anterior and posterior lamella and then repositioning the posterior portion 2mm anteriorly to the overlying anterior portion, which is sutured into place. However, this can cause eventual loss of eyelashes and the patient would need to be counselled prior to the procedure.

Eyelash hygiene

It is important to educate the patient on how to keep their lashes clean and there are a multitude of products on the market to help with this. Handy cleaning wipes are convenient and accessible. Some of these wipes have a tea-tree oil component, which can also help to combat a Demodex infestation. There are combined products which come as a cleaning foam and additional wipes. The old recipe of diluted baby shampoo is still commonly recommended for eyelid/lash cleanliness, but this is somewhat dated now, with so many specifically manufactured products available, and it's best to steer the patient away from this method.

I sometimes also suggest that the patient uses a brand new, clean mascara brush to help encourage the lashes to be swept in a more natural direction. I often notice on the slit lamp that not all the lashes are touching the eye and some may be lying horizontally along the lid margin, offering the potential to cause an issue. These are the sort of lashes that might benefit from a gentle brushing with a mascara brush.

If the patient uses false eyelashes, it is particularly important to clean/remove all the residual glue off the eyelashes. Similarly, if the patient has eyelash extensions it will be important to keep them as clean as possible, as this can trigger blepharitis. Likewise, make-up can build up on the lashes and cause further potential irritation. The key is to encourage regular lid and eyelash cleaning. This comes at a price and many products are not cheap but the alternatives (i.e. water or doing nothing) will potentially be more detrimental.

More recently the introduction of electromechanical eyelid margin debridement can be a useful adjunctive therapy – although it is not commonly available within the NHS. BlephEx™ (Scope Ophthalmics) incorporates a hand-held device that has a soft disposable rotational head. When used in conjunction with a cleaning foam, it can be gently applied to the lid and eyelashes to clean them.

In conclusion, there is clear evidence that misdirected lashes can have a significant impact on patients' wellbeing and their ability to carry out the activities of daily living. I have a dedicated clinic to manage these patients and many end up on my minor-op theatre list for electrolysis. Talking to these patients, I get a real sense of how much trichiasis affects their lives. Careful assessment and discussion of how to manage the problem are necessary, and people want the oculoplastic practitioner to provide an accessible and flexible service.

7

Blepharitis, meibomian gland disease and dry eye disease

Introduction

It might seem slightly odd that blepharitis and dry eye should warrant their own chapter in this book. However, it is justified by my experience as a practitioner. I spend a considerable amount of time talking to patients about these conditions so it seems worth devoting a chapter to a disease process that has such a profound effect on so many people.

Blepharitis and meibomian gland dysfunction (MGD) significantly affect the quality of tears – and the health of the ocular surface relies upon good-quality tears. If tear quality isn't maintained, there can be a reduction in visual acuity, and an increase in irritation and discomfort, which can all lead to a reduced quality of life. These problems are also becoming more prevalent (especially in women), with a notable increase in individuals presenting with related symptoms.

A considerable amount of research has been carried out in relation to dry eye disease (DED) and the ocular surface, and it has been summarised in the *TFO DEWS II Report Executive Summary* (Craig, J.P., Nelson, J.D., Dimitri, T.A. *et al.* 2017). In this report, the Tear Film and Ocular Society (TFOS) has drawn together research by the leading lights in this field. The 10-chapter report (of which a summary can be downloaded) has superseded the original Dry Eye Workshop (DEWS) report produced in 2007.

We will explore the composition of tears in more detail in Chapter 8. In this chapter, we will consider how blepharitis and meibomian disease affect the quality of tears and in turn the ocular surface. The symptoms that then manifest have to be controlled and reduced by means of patient education, and this can only be done if the practitioner has an insight into the mechanisms of these diseases.

A definition of DED

The DEWS II report defines dry eye disease as 'a multifactorial disease of the ocular surface characterised by a loss of homeostasis of the tear film'.

DED is complex and is affected by several elements, including tear film instability, hyperosmolarity, inflammation, neurosensory abnormalities and homeostasis disruption. Essentially there is a vicious circle of interacting processes and aetiology that ultimately causes dry eyes. Some of these effects are associated with environmental factors, or altered lacrimal function, but essentially are associated with tear evaporation.

We commonly recognise the term 'homeostasis' as a principle of equilibrium, but in DED the ocular surface is in a state of disruption and unbalance. As an oculoplastic practitioner, I am interested in the way eyelid-related conditions, such as blepharitis and MGD, play a part in affecting this delicate equilibrium.

DED risk factors

There are a number of consistent risk factors associated with DED, not just blepharitis or MGD. These include:

- Age – tear quality reduces as we get older
- Gender – more women are associated with dry eyes as they are firstly more likely to seek medical help and may have dryer eyes due to hormone-related associated changes and the menopause and also autoimmune conditions (which tend to be more common in women) (DEWS 2007)
- Ethnicity – dry eyes may be more common in Asian and Hispanic patients (DEWS 2007)
- Computer users – prolonged eye opening and reduced blinking, due to staring at the screen
- Contact lens wearers
- Hormone replacement therapy
- Medications – antidepressants, antihistamines
- Diseases – Sjogren's syndrome, connective tissue disease, diabetes, rosacea, thyroid disease
- Inconclusive risks – smoking, alcohol, Demodex infestation.

Dry eye disease (DED)

There are two recognised forms of dry eye disease:

- Aqueous deficient dry eye (ADDE) – a consequence of reduced lacrimal secretion, the osmolarity of the tears increases (hyperosmolarity) in normal evaporative circumstances
- Evaporative dry eye (EDE) – due to the increase in evaporation in tears from the surface of the eye, leading to hyperosmolarity, in the presence of a normal functioning lacrimal gland.

Whichever form is considered, the main pathophysiological cause of DED is the evaporation of tears from the ocular surface. This evaporation causes damage to the surface epithelium and increased hyperosmolarity, which in turn leads to inflammation.

Osmotic pressure is the tendency of a solvent to move in the direction of a lower solvent activity and is primarily determined by the solute concentration. If the concentration of the solute is changed, the osmolarity will be affected. In the context of DED, the relevant solute is the 'saltiness' of the tears – hyperosmolarity can therefore be seen as increased salinity in the tears.

Hyperosmolarity causes a cascade of events leading to the increased production of inflammatory mediators, which are thought to damage goblet cells within the corneal epithelium. This can be seen with a slit lamp, fluorescein and a blue light as punctate epithelial erosions (PEEs) and tear film instability. This in turn exacerbates the hyperosmolarity and so completes the vicious circle.

Meibomian gland dysfunction (MGD)

The major cause of EDE is MGD, due to the poor production of meibum, and the causes of MGD can be further subdivided into either cicatricial (scarring) or non-cicatricial. In addition, as people get older, the number of functioning meibomian glands reduces and this also contributes to MGD.

Cicatricial MGD is caused by inflammatory mechanisms related to certain cicatricial conjunctival diseases such as trachoma, pemphigoid and erythema multiforme. As a consequence of these diseases, the submucosal scarring closes the meibomian duct openings and drags them into the tarsal plate. The affected glands are displaced and/or narrowed and therefore cannot deliver meibum effectively. The reduced oil production leads to tear film instability and quicker evaporation, resulting in EDE.

Similarly, in non-cicatricial MGD, several underlying conditions are associated with the process, including acne rosacea, atopic dermatitis, psoriasis and seborrheic dermatitis. The usual outcome in non-cicatricial MGD is hyperkeratinisation of the meibomian duct openings, causing duct obstruction and dilation. Thickening of the meibum, due to changes in its composition, can exacerbate the problem. Plugging of the duct openings leads to reduced delivery of meibum and again contributes to tear film instability and faster evaporation, also resulting in EDE.

Blepharitis

Due to factors such as increased inflammatory mediators, and underlying issues such as skin conditions, the eyelids can become irritated and inflamed, leading to the condition known as blepharitis.

Blepharitis is one of the most commonly encountered problems in an oculoplastic clinic and is partly responsible for the increase in dry eye, as outlined above. It is associated with MGD and keratoconjunctivitis sicca (dryness of the conjunctiva and cornea), and other conditions such as rosacea.

Types of blepharitis

Blepharitis is subdivided into acute and secondary types. In the acute condition, underlying staphyloccal (or occasionally streptococcal) toxins contribute to the blepharitis, but it is essentially associated with rosacea, seborrhea and hypersensitivity. There can be an allergic component driving the inflammation rather than an infective process. Seborrhea is a papulosquamous skin disorder which causes scaling of the skin, greasy eyelid margins and itching that particularly targets the glands of Zeis.

Secondary blepharitis is caused by an infectious contributory process driven by bacteria/virus or Demodex infestation.

Due to the considerable overlap of classification, when an individual presents with symptoms of blepharitis it can be difficult to discern whether it is acute or secondary.

Blepharitis can also be seen as either anterior, affecting the lid margin (usually staphylococcal or seborrheic) or posterior (meibomianitis), involving the meibomian gland. MGD affects the meibomian gland and is therefore categorised as posterior blepharitis.

Symptoms of blepharitis

Symptoms of anterior blepharitis include:

- Discomfort – a burning, gritty 'foreign body' sensation
- Preseptal cellulitic presentation
- Mild photophobia
- Lash debris
- Collarettes (collar of debris around the base of a lash)
- Hyperaemia (increased blood vessels)
- Madarosis (loss of eyelashes, usually associated with seborrheic changes)
- Lid ulceration (beware of basal cell carcinoma!)
- Trichiasis.

Patients will often suggest that their symptoms are worse in the morning. On waking, their eyelids may be closed and congested with discharge and crusting.

Demodex are tiny mites that live around the eyelashes, causing irritation and secondary blepharitis and MGD. The mites are 0.3–0.4mm long, with segmented legs and body scales that allow them to attach themselves to the lashes. Demodex feast on skin cells and sebum. They are usually not directly identifiable, but the characteristic collarettes of debris around eyelash bases are indicative of a Demodex infestation.

Diagnosing blepharitis and MGD

A good history and careful questioning will initially help provide the clues required to diagnose blepharitis. There are a lot of potential differential diagnoses to rule out before arriving at the conclusion that the patient has blepharitis (acute or otherwise). Some of these differential diagnoses are potentially very serious, so beware. Particular consideration should be given to lid margin tumours (such as basal, sebaceous or squamous cell carcinomas), which can readily masquerade as blepharitis and be overlooked. Ulceration, lid obliteration and madarosis should set alarm bells ringing.

There are particular questions that can be asked, and even some dedicated questionnaires and assessment tools that can be used to gain the information needed to diagnose and grade the severity of the disease. The two outlined by the *TFOS DEWS II Report* (Craig, Nelson, Dimitri, *et al.* 2017) are the Ocular Surface Disease Index (OSDI) and the Dry Eye Questionnaire (DEQ-5).

A slit lamp examination should enable you to observe the condition of the eyelids and margins, and assess:

- Hypaeremia – increased vascular engorgement
- Tyelosis – hyperkeratosis
- Telangiectasia
- Margin serration
- Eyelashes – position and loss
- Lash debris – position, type and extent
- Corneal dryness – fluorescein and blue light (PEEs and staining)
- Tear break-up time (TBUT), see p. 122
- Blink coverage – lagophthalmos
- Lid margin meniscus height.

Then the meibomian gland openings should be assessed for:

- Orifice capping
- Distended orifices
- Opacified orifices
- Secretion quality – clear/fluid, yellow and thickened or toothpaste-like.

Applying firm but consistent digital pressure to the lid margin should enable discharge of meibum from the gland orifices. Observing the viscosity of the meibum will provide an indication of the secretion quality. If it easily presents as a clear fluid, this might be deemed normal. However, if the product is yellowish and harder to excrete, this may suggest MGD. In the worse cases, the secretion may be very thick and toothpaste-like or the glands may be completely blocked.

The upper eyelid should be everted to check for any underlying issues that might be contributing to the problem, such as papillae, which might suggest an allergic component.

Some ophthalmic companies have devised mechanisms to directly measure osmolarity, but unfortunately this isn't always readily available on the NHS. Alternatively, specific specialised imaging of the meibomian glands (using infrared or optical coherence tomography meibography) has been described as a safe and convenient way of assessing the quality of the glands, but there may be limited access to these types of scanning.

Treating DED, MGD and blepharitis
Treating DED

The treatment of DED, much like its diagnosis, can be complex and multifaceted. A combination of conservative actions and treatment options may be needed to get the condition under control. However, it is important to emphasise to the patient that blepharitis, once it manifests, is often a long-term, even life-long, condition that requires continual management.

The TFOS DEWS II Report (Craig, Nelson, Dimitri, *et al.* 2017) outlines a stepwise approach to treating DED.

Step 1:
- Patient education
- Dietary modifications
- Consider medication contraindications and modification of polypharmacy
- Ocular lubricants
- Lid hygiene regime.

Step 2 (if initial steps have not been successful):
- Preservative-free lubricants
- Demodex treatment – tea-tree oil
- Tear conservation (punctal plugs – see p. 125)

- Moisture chamber glasses
- Antibiotics/steroid treatment
- Cyclosporine
- Oral tetracycline.

Step 3:
- Oral secretagogues
- Autologous serum eye drops
- Therapeutic contact lens.

Step 4 (extreme requirements):
- Long-term corticosteroids
- Amniotic membrane grafts
- Surgical punctal occlusion
- Tarsorrhaphy.

Further treatment modalities for MGD and blepharitis

Patient education is paramount, and the practitioner needs to start by explaining the mechanism by which lid problems arise. Individuals need to understand the connection between their symptoms and the underlying aetiology. If they appreciate this, they are more likely to comply with the recommended treatment. The practitioner must therefore spend time outlining why the eyes are dry, and why the lids are inflamed and itchy. Once patients understand the relationship between the various problems, and the links between the individual causes of their irritation, they are more likely to understand that lid hygiene is just as important as eye lubrication.

Conservative treatment starts with eyelid hygiene. Traditional approaches with baby shampoo (diluted) are still sometimes advocated but have been largely superseded by scientifically proven formulas that are arguably more effective. Products such as Blephroclean (Thea) or Ocusoft Plus (OCuSOFT) are available in the form of easy-to-use and convenient wipes that can be used to clean the lid margin and eyelashes and remove debris.

For specialised lid-margin cleaning, known as microblepharoexfoliation, a hand-held device with a rotating soft-tip micro sponge is used to clean the lid margin. The device is BlephEx™ (Scope Ophthalmics). Unfortunately, it is not available within the NHS, but may be available in the UK from some private healthcare providers.

Heat treatment (hyper-thermic) once or twice a day is also very important in softening the meibum within the glands. Special 'eye-bags' have been produced by several companies for this purpose. They are reusable, microwavable and easy to clean. The eye-bag is placed over the closed eyes for several minutes and the heat is allowed to disperse within the eyelids. Many patients still use, or have been encouraged to use, flannels or face-cloths warmed by using hot water. But this is an inconsistent (and unhygienic approach) and the heat quickly dissipates and is largely ineffective. 'Eye-bags' are now available via prescription on the NHS in the UK or can be bought from pharmacists.

There is an order and methodology to undertaking eyelid hygiene. Firstly, the patient should apply heat treatment to soften the meibum and then apply firm massage at the lid margin to express the meibum. The patient has to take care not to poke themselves in the eye and should wash their hands before and after massage. Following this, they should carry out a thorough eyelid cleaning process using the products outlined above and being careful to include the lashes.

It is important to stress that this level of eyelid hygiene comes at a cost, both in time and money. It may be that not all patients can afford so much time and expense. For this reason, a cheaper, simpler (and more pragmatic) approach may have to be considered for some individuals.

Diet is another important aspect. Increasing omega-3 fatty acid intake or taking supplements can be advocated, as these have been noted to have an anti-inflammatory effect. Foods commonly associated with omega-3 oils include fish (salmon, mackerel, oysters, tuna, cod liver oil and herring), nuts/seeds (flax seed, chia, walnuts) and plant oils (flax seed oil, soybean oil and canola oil).

In acute infective blepharitis, topical antibiotics, such as fusidic acid, bacitracin or chloramphenicol, may be required to clear the infection (along with eyelid hygiene). In more seborrheic or dermatological presentations, the underlying cause may need to be treated simultaneously and this may have to be coordinated with the patient's GP.

Corticosteroids may help to reduce the inflammation (Fluorometholone/Maxitrol), but caution should be exercised due to the various side-effects associated with their use, particularly raised intra-ocular pressure. It is important to check that the patient does not have a history of glaucoma. A short reducing course over two weeks should be sufficient. In MGD, longer-term treatment may be required in the form of tetracyclines, but beware of their side-effects such as photosensitisation and hypersensivity. Also, 0.05% cyclosporine has been shown to be effective in the treatment of MGD (Nemet, Vinker & Kaiserman 2011).

Specific treatment of Demodex infestation is available in the form of tea-tree oil wipes – Optase (Scope Ophthalmics) and also BlephEx™ lid margin cleansing.

The eyes need to be kept lubricated and the patient needs to be assessed to ascertain the type and dose of drops required. A day-time lubricant can be used as often as is advocated and a more viscous night-time ointment can also be applied.

In summary, blepharitis and associated MGD is a complex and difficult condition to manage and treat. This chapter merely scrapes the surface. As a practitioner, it is therefore essential to appreciate the underlying mechanisms of these diseases and remember that patient education is as important as physical treatment.

References

Craig, J.P., Nelson, J.D., Dimitri, T.A. *et al.* (2017). *TFOS DEWS II Report Executive Summary.* The Ocular Surface. http://dx.doi.org/10.1016/j.jtos.2017.08.003 (last accessed 6.11.2019).

DEWS Epidemiology (2007). The epidemiology of Dry Eye Disease: Report of the epidemiology Subcommittee of the International Dry Eye Workshop. *The Ocular Surface.* **5**(2), 93–107.

Maher, T.N. (2018). The use of tea tree oil in treating blepharitis and meibomian gland dysfunction. *Oman Journal of Ophthalmology.* **11**, 11–15.

Nemet, A.Y., Vinker, S. & Kaiserman, I. (2011). Associated morbidity of blepharitis. *Ophthalmology.* **118**(6), 1060–68.

Putnam, C. (2016). Diagnosis and management of blepharitis: an optometrist's perspective. *Clinical Optometery.* 8, 71–78.

8

The lacrimal system and dacryocystorhinostomy

Introduction

In order to maintain the eye as a viable working organ, its external membranes require a continual flow of moisture to preserve and nourish it. The conjunctiva and cornea both need a sustained level of tears to ensure that they function and do not dry out.

Accordingly, the lacrimal system and the associated accessory glands, through their production of tears, provide a mechanism that protects the eye. The two systems combine to produce enough tears, in an even spread, to keep the eye in optimum condition. The accessory glands of Wolfring and Krause are situated within the fornices of the eyelid and are more medial to the lacrimal ductules.

The tear system essentially comprises the lacrimal gland, accessory glands, puncta, canaliculi, lacrimal sac and nasolacrimal duct into the nose. The lacrimal system includes several structures that normally produce and drain away tears. Initially the lacrimal gland manufactures tears, which then sweep across the eye through blinking. Eventually the tears drain away through tiny holes called puncta at the medial edge of the upper and lower eyelids, continuing through channels into the lacrimal sac and eventually out into the nasal passage.

Any malfunction or interruption to this system can be detrimental to the eye, causing dryness, irritation, discomfort, and in extreme cases infection, scarring and even lasting damage. Many patients who come to the clinic complain of excessive watering (epiphora) or dry, gritty, painful eyes. Both these situations (eyes that are too dry or too wet) can lead to very real frustration for the patient, affecting their lifestyle and in extreme cases leading to depression and despair. Excessive tearing can also cause maceration of the skin, causing it to become sore and irritated.

As a practitioner, it is important to appreciate the many aspects of epiphora and understand the related anatomy. Let us first consider the lacrimal system (see Figure 8.1).

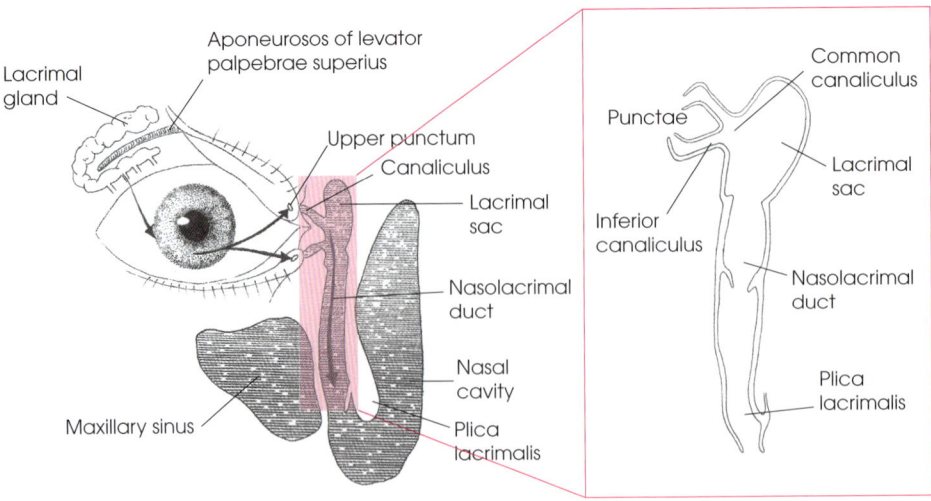

Figure 8.1: The lacrimal system

The lacrimal gland

A gland is a group of cells that collectively produce a substance or molecule that can either go into the bloodstream (endocrine) or into some external surfaces or cavities (exocrine). The lacrimal gland is an exocrine gland because its cells produce tears that help to protect and nourish the eye and overlying mucous membranes (conjunctiva).

The lacrimal gland is located just under the orbital rim supero-temporally in a concavity within the bone of the orbital roof known as the lacrimal gland fossa. The almond-shaped lacrimal gland is approximately 17mm in length and 15mm wide. It has two distinct lobes. The smaller palpebral lobe is the more anterior aspect and can just be seen as a small pinkish mass under the conjunctiva, resting on the eye (if you lift the upper eyelid and ask the patient to look down and medially). More posteriorly, there is the orbital lobe. Both lobes are separated by the fibrous septum, giving them the appearance of separate lobes. Small secretory ducts from both lobes transport tears to the surface of the eye via a row of openings within the palpebral conjunctiva.

The lacrimal gland itself is lobular and contains many acini (clusters of cells that resemble a group of minute berries). These cells produce the aqueous fluid that is tears. The tears are produced at a constant rate – about 0.2ml every 24 hours.

The lacrimal gland is innervated by the lacrimal nerve (a sensory nerve derived from the ophthalmic nerve) and greater petrosal nerve (an extension of the facial nerve) which provides the autonomic parasympathetic component of tear production. Blood supply to the lacrimal gland is from the lacrimal artery and the venous outflow is from the superior ophthalmic vein.

Tears

Tear production

The production of tears is known as lacrimation and is associated with the lacrimal gland and the accessory glands. Tears are essentially the interface between the eye and the environment. The tears:

- Lubricate the surface of the eye
- Clear the vision (along with blinking)
- Deliver and excrete nutrients
- Deliver metabolic products
- Protect against infection.

Under normal circumstances an adult produces approximately 1g of tears every day. The tears contain several products, including:

- Over 60 metabolites
- Proteins
- Water
- Lipids.

Tear layers

The tear film over the eye has three distinct layers: lipid, aqueous and mucous. It is important to consider all these layers as any disruption to these closely associated strata can directly affect the quality of the tears.

The lipid layer

The most superficial layer of the tears is the lipid layer. This thin layer (approximately 0.015 to 0.160µm thick) is made up of oils that have several functions. Some of the compounds found in the lipid layer include cholesterol, wax esters, fatty acids and phospholipids.

The hydrophobic element in the lipid layer ensures that the tears stay on the eye and reduces the risk of tears migrating away and essentially pouring down the cheek, providing a cohesive binding function. Secondly, the lipid layer prevents the tears from evaporating. Thirdly, the lipid layer provides a smooth surface for the lids to pass over when opening, closing and blinking. However, the main function of the lipid layer is to reduce surface tension and thus stabilise the tear film.

After each blink, the lipid layer is disrupted and moves over the aqueous layer. It is re-spread, but quickly re-exerts the surface tension deficit caused by the blink, thereby stabilising the tear film.

In the moments after the blink, the lipid layer will start to break up and destabilise, causing dots and streaks on the corneal surface. This can be observed on a slit lamp, with fluorescein, and is known as the 'tear break-up'. This is a measurable phenomenon and is recorded in seconds as the 'tear break-up time' (TBUT). In an individual with dry eyes the TBUT may be only 2 or 3 seconds, whereas in more usual circumstances it may be 10 or more seconds. TBUT measurement is a useful subjective measure of tear film stability and you may find reference to it in the patient's medical notes.

The lipid layer is supplied via sebaceous glands in the eyelids – the meibomian glands and the glands of Zeis. If any of these glands become damaged or inflamed, the amount and quality of lipid production may be significantly reduced – for instance, in blepharitis. Blepharitis is an inflammatory condition that affects a significant proportion of the population and is associated with redness, itchiness, crusting and blocking of the meibomian glands (see Chapter 7).

The aqueous layer

The middle layer of the tears, the aqueous layer, forms the largest component of the tear film. It is approximately 4μm thick and is made up of various electrolytes, proteins, metabolites and peptides. The two most common proteins found in the aqueous layer are lipocalin (which is thought to help tear film spreading) and lysozyme (which acts as an antimicrobial). But there are at least 60 other molecules and components within the aqueous, making it a rather more complex fluid than you might expect. Exploring the molecular level of the aqueous is beyond the scope of this book, but it is important not to underestimate the complexity of the tear film and to bear in mind that dry eye disease is multifactorial.

The aqueous layer also acts as a conduit for oxygen and nutrients, enabling them to reach the avascular underlying corneal surface. This continual flow helps to remove debris and pathogens with each blink.

The mucin layer

At the surface of the conjunctival membranes and cornea is the mucin layer, which is primarily composed of proteins that are anchored to the epithelium. Again, the main purpose of the mucin layer is tear stabilisation. However, it also has an antimicrobial element.

Tear types

When considering tear production, it is important to recognise that three distinct types of tears can be produced (each with its own composition): basal tears, reflex tears and psychic tears.

Basal tears
These are the fundamental tears that we produce that provide nutrition and protection for the eye.

Reflex tears
These are produced copiously in response to stimulation – for example, bright light, onions, vomiting or strong smells or odours. Reflex tears are produced to help wash away these irritants.

Psychic tears (Crying)
Uniquely, as humans, we produce tears in response to emotions such as sadness, happiness or stress. The limbic system in the brain is thought to be associated with the production of these tears, which have a different molecular make-up to other tears as they contain more protein-based hormones. A parasympathetic control of the autonomic nervous system is linked to the production of emotional tears.

Finally, there is another type of tearing known as 'crocodile tears', whereby the individual lacrimates when eating. This phenomenon is due to a 'mis-wiring' of the facial nerve and is often linked to facial palsy or recovery from facial palsy (see Chapter 13).

Schirmer's test

In order to determine whether the lacrimal gland produces enough tears to keep the eye sufficiently moist, a Schirmer's test can be performed. This is also known as the 'dry eye test' or 'basal secretion test'. There are many possible causes of dry eyes and poor tear production, including diabetes, leukaemia, rheumatoid arthritis, Sjogren's syndrome and vitamin A deficiency, to name only a few.

The test involves inserting a test paper/strip partially over the inferior eyelid margin, to measure how much moisture is captured on the paper a certain time after insertion. There is still some confusion as to whether or not local anaesthesia should be used with the test. If you perform the test without topical local anaesthetic drops, you are measuring basal and reflex tear production. This is because the 'foreign body' sensation created by having a paper inserted into the eye *will* cause the eye to tear more. Alternatively, the test can be carried out with topical local anaesthesia such as proxymetacaine, which measures basal tear production only.

The test strip typically has a folding point at which the paper is meant to rest over the eyelid margin, and the practitioner needs to make sure the paper is introduced at this point. The paper should be inserted laterally so as not to interfere with, or damage, the cornea. The patient should also be encouraged to keep their eyes gently closed. Time the test carefully and accurately for 5 minutes, whilst simultaneously reassuring the patient.

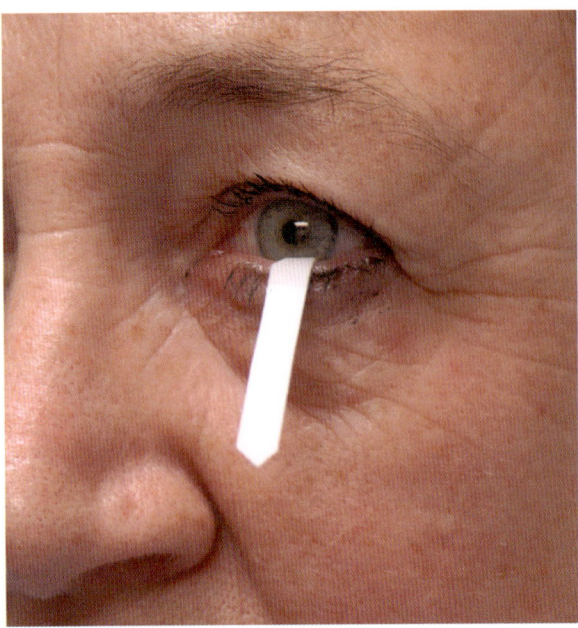

Figure 8.2: Schirmer's test

Once the time period is over, remove the test strip. Measure the extent of the lacrimation on the paper in millimetres and record the result in the patient's notes.

The test is not as commonly undertaken as it once was, and this is partly due to the lack of accuracy and reproducibility of the results. Research has shown that there can be significant fluctuation of results and suggests that there may be only a limited requirement for the test (Holland *et al.* 2013).

Blink mechanism

Blinking assists in the movement of tears across the eye and towards the puncta at the medial corner of the eye. There is also an associated 'pump' mechanism that contributes to the drainage of tears. When the eyelid closes, the orbicularis muscle (pretarsal) contracts and essentially squeezes and simultaneously closes the puncta and canaliculi, at the same time as the lacrimal sac is pulled open. The associated negative pressure helps draw the tears into the lacrimal sac.

The eyelid's blinking mechanism clearly contributes to the efficient flow of tears across the eye. Therefore, if the eyelids are malpositioned, this can contribute to the poor drainage of tears. Often a patient will present with a lower eyelid that is lax, but the signs can sometimes be more subtle – for example, a medial ectropion causing the puncta to be slightly out of position. Close examination of the eyelids, particularly with the use of a slit lamp, may reveal such issues.

An unusual phenomenon, known as Centurion syndrome, can be associated with poor lacrimal drainage. In this syndrome, which is associated with a prominent nasal bridge, there is an anterior displacement of the medial canthal tendon and its insertion to the bone, causing the puncta to be malpositioned away from the eye.

Puncta

The puncta are the small openings at the medial corners of the eyelid margins of both upper and lower eyelids. The inferior puncta are slightly inverted and in apposition with the tear meniscus against the eye. Both the puncta are located on a slight elevation in the eyelid margin known as the papilla.

When assessing the inferior puncta, they should not be visible unless physically everted. The size of the opening of the puncta varies a little between individuals, but measures about 0.6mm in diameter on average.

When assessing the patient on the slit lamp, it is important to observe the size, position and nature of the puncta. The opening size varies between patients. If it is very narrow or even absent, this may help explain why the patient is struggling with epiphora. Therefore, it is important to make note of the size of the puncta.

The position of the puncta is also crucial: commonly the puncta and medial lower lid position may have altered and fallen away from the eye, resulting in a punctal ectropion. This (sometimes subtle) malposition of the puncta can be enough to significantly affect tear drainage. The nature of the puncta also needs to be considered. For example, have the puncta been subjected to surgery to alter their size or shape?

Occasionally, patients who have had repeated infections or trauma may lose the puncta or it may be occluded due to scarring. In rare cases, infants are born with a congenital absence of the puncta known as 'punctal agenesis'. This can be associated with a membranous occlusion which can be overcome with probing, or the puncta may be completely absent.

Alternatively, there may be a plug or similar device in position in the puncta and this should be recorded in the medical notes.

It is important to gain an insight into the size of the opening of the puncta when assessing the patient. Punctal stenosis (narrowing) can have a significant impact in relation to tear drainage. Surgical opening of the puncta (punctaplasty) can help with drainage, but more conservative approaches to opening can often include the insertion of perforated punctal plugs to help open the orifice. Essentially these are tiny silicone devices that can be inserted into the puncta with an insertion device (usually included with the plugs). They are often placed in theatre and are removed several months later. They have a lumen running through them to allow some tear drainage.

Beyond the visible opening of the puncta, the punctal orifice narrows and becomes part of the canaliculus or drainage canal. The initial part, the ampulla, is approximately 2mm in length. It descends vertically in the lower eyelid and ascends in similar opposing fashion in the upper eyelid, before transecting 8mm medially toward the nose and the lacrimal sac. In the majority of patients, just prior to the lacrimal sac, the two canaliculi converge and join together to form the common canaliculus. It is important to note the relationship between the common canaliculus and the medial canthal tendon, as it lies between the anterior and posterior arms of the tendon as they attach to the nasal bone.

The lacrimal sac and the nasolacrimal duct

In a small deviation or groove in the bone (lacrimal fossa) of the inferior medial orbital rim, there is a collection bag known as the lacrimal sac. It is approximately 10–15mm long and acts as a conduit for tears to pass into the nasal cavity. The narrower posterior end of the sac is known as the nasolacrimal duct. There are valves within the tract of the duct which help prevent retrograde flow of tears, and these include the valves of Hasner and Rosenmüller.

Eventually the lacrimal and nasolacrimal sac pass through the bony nasolacrimal canal and into the inferior meatus of the nose, underneath the interior turbinate.

Sometimes, if there is a build-up of material in the lacrimal sac, this can lead to it swelling. It may then become infected and erythematous, causing a sore red lump to form in the inner corner of the lower eyelid. This is dacryocystitis and requires antibiotic treatment. Very rarely the infection can be so acute as to require lancing to express the infectious material.

Repeated infections associated with dacryocystitis are often related to blockage or narrowing (stenosis) of the nasolacrimal duct. Similarly, issues related to the lacrimal sac may cause collection of mucous material, eventually leading to infection. The patient may get repeated bouts of infection which can be distressing. The swelling can be painful and cause profound epiphora (excessive watering and tearing).

Whilst antibiotics will help in reducing the immediate symptoms, eventually the repeated infections will cause scarring and possibly exacerbation of the symptoms of epiphora.

Likewise, a blockage or stenosis anywhere along the length of the canaliculus prior to the lacrimal sac will also cause epiphora. The traditional way to investigate this is with a sac washout test.

The sac washout test (SWO) and probing

It would be easy to underestimate the importance of the sac washout test (SWO) as a simple means to pass some fluid through the lacrimal system to evaluate the patency of the system. But the SWO test should really be seen as a vital supplementary investigation in the practitioner's diagnostic toolkit. Traditionally the SWO test has been carried out by medical and nursing practitioners alike. No matter who undertakes the test, there needs to be an understanding of its importance in providing information related to the patency of the canaliculus and the lacrimal sac. With just feel, the practitioner can elicit subtle nuances within the system but this takes practice, initial supervision and learning.

To undertake a SWO test, the practitioner requires:

- 2–3ml syringe (must be Luer-lock)
- Disposable lacrimal cannula – curved, typically 26 gauge (see Figure 8.3)
- Normal saline 0.9% (sachet)
- Swab/tissue
- Oxybuprocaine or proxymetacaine
- Possibly – lacrimal dilator/Bowman's probe.

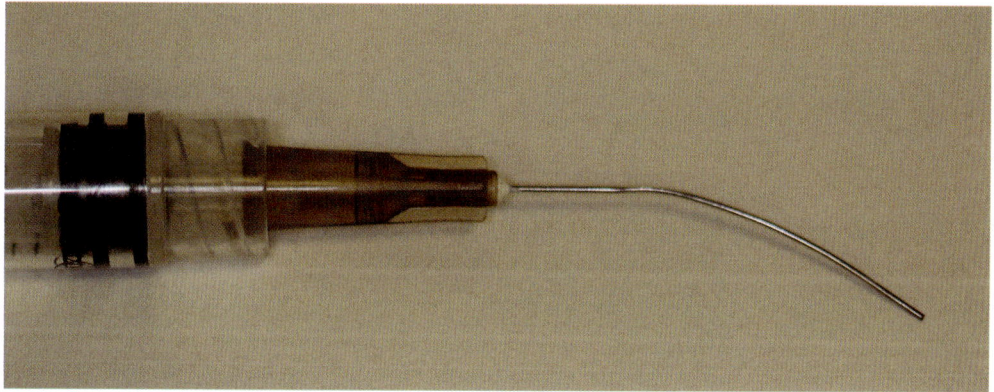

Figure 8.3: Lacrimal cannula

Initially, the patient needs to be prepared for the procedure. Ideally, a reclining bed or recumbent chair will provide comfort and head support. A run-through of the procedure will enable the patient to understand the nature of the test and what to expect. Verbal consent is all that is usually required but some individuals may still insist on written consent.

Once the patient is prepared, instil anaesthetic drops into the eye/s. It might be useful to place a protective hand towel or drape over the patient's clothes near the neck/shoulder to catch any overspill. Even though this test is not strictly sterile, a high level of cleanliness should still be maintained where possible, following local guidelines.

The practitioner will need to draw up some normal saline into the 2ml syringe and attach a lacrimal cannula. Remember the syringe should be Luer-lock (screw-fix). Sometimes reasonable pressure is required to pass the fluid through the system and this could cause the cannula to be displaced if any other type of syringe is used. It is always worth checking that the cannula is firmly fixed onto the syringe, even if it is a Luer-lock.

Presuming that the practitioner is right-handed and that the inferior punctum is to be syringed, they should stand to the side of the patient, obviously at the head end, with the patient laying semi-prone, and the patient's head at a 45° angle. The room requires good illumination and, if available, a head-light or spotlight can provide additional brightness. It may also be easier to use a magnifier or, for some practitioners, a pair of magnifying loups. Remember, the puncta can be remarkably small and difficult to identify.

Once the patient has been positioned and prepared for the procedure, use one hand to gently pull the lower eyelid down and also slightly horizontally laterally away from the nose to expose the punctum. This action puts the canaliculus in a more accessible position and reduces the risk of the tube becoming compressed like a concertina, once the cannula is passed.

If the punctum is especially small, it may need to be opened using a lacrimal dilator. Whilst holding the lower eyelid as described, use the tip of the probe to locate the opening if possible and gently allow the weight of the probe to exert minimal pressure into the punctal orifice. Do not to be tempted to apply undue additional pressure as this could damage the punctum. Now rotate the probe in order to open the punctum. If it is still difficult to find the punctum, a punctal seeker may be used to locate it, but medical assistance and some local anaesthetic may be needed, as this procedure can be uncomfortable.

Assuming the punctum is accessible, place the tip of the cannula gently into the punctal orifice, merely using the weight of the syringe to provide initial inward pressure. Once the cannula has entered the punctum, the patient can find it uncomfortable, so make sure you reassure them and anticipate their reaction. If the discomfort is intolerable as you advance, you may need to stop. Also, remember the ampulla is in a downward trajectory – not medial – so head downward initially and then turn to move toward the nose along the canaliculus.

If the patient continues to tolerate it, carefully advance the cannula. Remember the cannula should advance freely, not under duress, and the lower eyelid should be kept under horizontal traction. However, it may become apparent that it isn't possible to advance the cannula and there is a restriction or even a complete blockage. In this case, don't force the cannula, as this could create a false passage or damage the canaliculus

Sometimes there may be an initial restriction, which gives way as a loss of resistance and then you may be able to continue to advance the cannula. Experience and practice over time will enable you to adopt the best course of action, but if you have any doubt, you should always seek help. Keep feeling your way along, consciously assessing resistance, restriction and observing how the cannula progresses along the system.

As you advance the cannula, be mindful that the total length of the canaliculus into the lacrimal sac is only 10mm and that is not far. If you have advanced further than this, you are likely to be in the sac. Occasionally, the action of advancing the cannula 'rucks' up the canaliculus (concertina) and this in turn prevents you from advancing any further. The feeling as you do this is bouncy/spongy and is described as a 'soft stop', often caused by a canalicular blockage. If you were to retract back and inject saline, most of the fluid would probably regurgitate through the upper canaliculus and punctum.

Alternatively, you may freely advance and then come across a firm termination. This will probably be the cannula pressing up against the bony posterior wall of the lacrimal sac and is said to be a 'hard stop'.

When you think you have advanced sufficiently, you may want to see how freely the saline passes along the system and in many cases it will do so unabated. Alternatively, you may get little or no saline to pass and it will be necessary to anecdotally provide an estimate as to how much saline has either freely passed into the nasolacrimal duct or similarly how much has regurgitated back. This will need to be recorded in the medical notes. You may also get discharge of mucus, pus, blood and other foreign materials, and these should be noted as well.

Clearly, there is a lot more to the 'simple' act of undertaking a SWO test than many people assume, and don't let anyone convince you otherwise. This test is really important when assessing the patency of the lacrimal system. The results will influence decisions made on clinical management and ongoing treatment, so the test must be performed carefully and accurately. If you are in any doubt about the results, get a colleague to double-check.

Reflex Epiphora

Despite what appears to be a 100% patent nasolacrimal system, the patient may still get epiphora. This may be reflex tearing, whereby the patient is parasympathetically over-lacrimating as a direct response to dry eyes. This condition may be exacerbated by particular conditions, such as windy days, air conditioning or staring at computer screens. Reflex epiphora is probably the most common cause of excessive tearing, so it needs to be assessed, using fluorescein and blue light on the slit lamp, to distinguish how much dryness may be contributing to the problem (see Chapter 7). Whilst on the slit lamp, don't forget to check the size, position and nature of the puncta as well.

Lacrimal scintillography

Alternatively, despite a patent system, there may be a functional flow issue within the lacrimal system. Rose and Verity (2011) define a functional nasolacrimal duct obstruction as a 'clinical diagnosis often given to patients presenting with epiphora, but in whom there is no clinically apparent abnormality of the eyelid and lacrimal apparatus'. The SWO test will not readily help you to assess this. Further, more specialised investigations may be required. Lacrimal (dacryo) scintillography (DSG) may be useful in these circumstances, whereby a radioactive tracer is dropped into the medial tear lake and its progress recorded with a gamma camera. A series of x-ray images are produced that provides a pictorial representation of the flow of fluid through the lacrimal system. However, there is some controversy as to the relevance of this test in certain circumstances and it may have 'severe' limitations due to its lack of correlation with symptoms and clinical picture (Vonica, Obi, Sipkova et al. 2017).

Ultimately, if there is a blockage of the nasolacrimal system and this cannot be overcome by any conservative means, an operation to create a new passageway will be required. In infants and children, the blockage may be a mucus plug which can very often be overcome by syringing alone. However, this is much less commonly the case in adults. The most common procedure to overcome epiphora from a blocked nasolacrimal duct is a dacryocystorhinostomy or DCR.

Further examination and assessment of the lacrimal system

There are some other elements of the examination that the practitioner needs to consider when assessing someone with epiphora, or which they might see written in the medical notes. Externally you have to check for any lid deformities, trichiasis (eyelashes turning in and irritating the eye), incomplete blink, eyelid lesions, punctal eversion and ectropion/entropion. All these can impede the flow of tears towards the puncta and should be noted.

Two other important observations/tests include a fluorescein dye disappearance test (FDDT) and assessment of the 'tear lake'. After considering the relative position of the eyelids, insert a drop of fluorescein (2%) – then observe how long it takes for it to disappear and how it disappears. Normally the fluorescein should be completely gone from the eye within 5 minutes through natural drainage – assuming the patient hasn't wiped it away with a tissue (make sure you tell the patient not to dab). It is important to specify in the notes how long it took for the dye to disappear and how efficiently it disappeared. Some practitioners may summarise this by describing the FDDT result as 'brisk', 'moderate' or 'slow'. However, these terms are somewhat subjective and it is better to record the actual time it took to disperse in minutes. Any delay may indicate an obstruction to the drainage of the dye and necessitate further investigation

Whilst the fluorescein is in the patient's eye, you can also observe the height of the meniscus of the tears at the lower lid margin and against the eye – known as the 'tear lake'. Usually it is less than 1mm, but in patients with drainage issues it could be double that. Additionally, in conjunction with a SWO and probing, it may be prudent to examine the nasal cavity with an endoscope. The nose can be prepared before examination by using lidocaine spray to anaesthetise the cavity. The endoscopic examination enables the practitioner to look for any abnormal nasal anatomy, such as polyps, tumours or gross deviations of the nasal septum.

It may also be necessary to use a nasal decongestant in order to view the anatomy and make more space within the nose. This usually comes as a spray for adults and in drop form for children (and may be combined with a local anaesthetic).

No matter which decongestant spray is used, you need to prepare the patient, as it won't taste very nice and inevitably some of the spray contents will be swallowed. If a local anaesthetic is used, it will numb the patient's throat, and this can be a little disconcerting. Warn the patient not to eat or drink anything hot whilst the spray is active in the oral-pharyngeal cavity – typically 2 hours.

The nasal cavity is separated by the nasal septum. In many individuals there is a small degree of septum deviation and this doesn't cause any concern. However, it is important to assess this using a nasal endoscope. A significant degree of septal deviation may well remove the option of having an endonasal DCR.

A septoplasty (removal of the septum) can be performed at the time of surgery to create the necessary space for the endoscopic DCR surgery to take place. However, it is important to assess this in outpatients or at pre-assessment. A septoplasty also presents other risks and considerations for the patient (and surgeon) and these need to be discussed prior to consent being sought. Specifically, there are further risks of bleeding, pain or discomfort. And because the nasal septum is essentially weakened, there is a small risk of it breaking down and creating a hole between both sides of the nasal cavity, sometimes causing an audible whistle when breathing.

When undertaking a nasal endoscopy, it is also important to look at the nasal turbinates (middle and inferior). Normally, tears drain through the nasolacrimal duct into the nose, under the inferior nasal turbinate, in the space known as the inferior meatus. This isn't really accessible without manipulation of the turbinate. However, with the endoscope you might see the fluorescein that was previously injected if a SWO has been undertaken.

Stenting of the lacrimal apparatus

If a nasolacrimal duct narrowing (stenosis) is suspected, the initial treatment option may be to stent the lacrimal system. This generally involves using a length of silicone tubing which has a metal intubation stylet at each end. One end of the tubing and stylet will be used to intubate the upper puncta, the other the lower puncta. The stent is tied in the nose. Only a very short length of the stent will be visible between the upper and lower puncta.

In principle, the stent is used to dilate the canaliculus and it is eventually removed after several months. This may be effective and prevent the patient having to undergo any more protracted surgical options. However, for some patients, stenting may be ineffective or shortly after removal the canaliculus may become stenosed again.

From a nursing perspective, anyone who has a canalicular stent will need to be informed of the potential risk that the stent could migrate. Normally only a small portion of the stent is visible between the upper and lower puncta (see Figure 8.4), but if it migrates out a whole length of tubing may be in view. If this is the suspicion but the patient hasn't arrived on the Eye Ward or EED, it is advisable to encourage them to tape the prolapsed stent to the side of their nose – but certainly not to cut it. Then advise the patient to attend the outpatients' department in order to assess and reposition (or occasionally remove) the stent. The stent can migrate for several reasons but it is commonly associated with sneezing, coughing or accidentally rubbing the eye (see below).

Ballooning of the lacrimal apparatus (dacryoplasty)

An alternative to nasolacrimal duct stenting is to use a balloon intubation (dacryoplasty). Its use is usually restricted to congenital stenosis but it can be used in adults. This is a similar process to the one described above but the tube used to intubate has a tiny balloon on the end, not unlike a urinary catherter (but obviously on a much smaller scale). Once cannulated and in the appropriate position (i.e. the point of the stenosis), the balloon is inflated for a specified time, e.g. 60–90 seconds, and then deflated. This process may be repeated several times (especially in adults) and in several different points in the lacrimal system. The pressure is measured at the time of the intubation with a momometer dial/gauge somewhere in the region of 8 atmospheres (8atm) of pressure.

Dacryocystorhinostomy (DCR)

If there is a nasolacrimal blockage it may be necessary to perform corrective surgery, known as a dacryocystorhinostomy or DCR. This procedure can either be carried out externally or endoscopically, but the outcome is largely the same. The external DCR is the most common approach, but many surgeons perform endo-DCRs as a viable and equally (or slightly less) successful procedure. The main advantage of the endoscopic approach is that no skin incision is required and there is therefore no scarring.

The indication for DCR is essentially chronic inflammation and recurrent/chronic dacryocystitis. However, DCR surgery should be avoided in acute dacryocystitis and if there is any suspicion of a lacrimal sac tumour.

Both the external and endoscopic procedures are usually carried out under general anaesthetic (GA) but can also be done under a local anaesthetic with sedation (LA Sed). General anaesthetic is the preferred option, as the patient's airway is protected (usually with an endotracheal airway or laryngeal mask). Without this protection, fluid, blood and bone fragments could drop into the airway and could potentially cause irritation and coughing, especially if swallowing is hindered by heavy sedation.

External DCR

This procedure involves the following steps:

- Identifying the correct side
- Marking the incision site with an imaginary line halfway between the bridge of the nose and the medial canthus, then marking downward for 15mm
- Administering local anaesthetic (whether GA or not)
- Some surgeons may use a nasal pack to decongest the nose to reduce nasal bleeding (the nasal mucosal lining is quite vascular) within the nostril of the side being operated on
- Making an incision with a bard-parker blade through skin
- Reflecting back the underlying periosteum and exposing the nasal bone
- Identifying the lacrimal crest (anterior lacrimal sulcus bone)
- The lacrimal sac is then reflected out of the sulcus and to one side
- Using bone punches, a hole is made in the bone of the lacrimal crest
- Creating a small opening through the nasal bone, exposing the underlying nasal mucosa
- Once a sufficient opening has been created in the bone, the inferior and superior puncta are cannulated with a Bowman's probe
- The probe should be seen to press against the lateral wall of the lacrimal sac; using the probe to tent up the sac, an H-shaped incision is made into the sac using a crescent knife (or similar)
- The tip of the probe will now be visible, having passed completely through the lacrimal system and the new opening made in the sac lining

- Often at this stage any mucus/pus collection is likely to pour out – this may require swabbing for culture and sensitivity
- The nasal lining is now opened in a similar manner to the lacrimal sac, in an H-shape
- The posterior flap of the lacrimal sac is then anastomosed to the posterior flap of the nasal mucosa, and then similarly to the anterior flaps. There is now a direct new channel straight through the lacrimal sac into the nasal cavity.
- This new channel can be intubated with a bi-canalicular silicone stent.
- The stent is passed through the puncta and through the new channel and is tied in the nasal cavity
- The external wound is then closed with Vicryl sutures
- A simple dressing is usually applied.

Pre-operative DCR care considerations

At pre-assessment, it is important that the patient is prepared for a general anaesthetic and that they are safe to proceed. A full medical history (including medications, allergies and social history) should be taken. If there are issues related to the airway or that might affect the anaesthetic, the patient should be seen in the anaesthetic clinic before surgery.

When assessing patients due for DCR surgery, the key issue is to ascertain whether there is any suggestion of a bleeding risk. If there is any indication that the patient is on anti-coagulant or anti-platelet therapy, this should be identified and managed prior to surgery. It is also important for the patient to avoid aspirin (if possible) and anti-inflammatory medications.

In addition, the practitioner should investigate any possibility of the patient being a poorly controlled hypertensive. This may need further input from the GP and the patient's blood pressure needs to be optimised prior to surgery.

This procedure can be treated as a day-case, but it is important to warn the patient that if there are any issues during the operation, they will have to stay in overnight. Again, the most likely issue is usually associated with epistaxis (nose bleed). It is always good practice to have a 'DCR tray' in the unit, which contains local anaesthetic spray, nasal speculum, nasal tampons, scissors, torch, lubricating gel, gloves and swabs. It is useful to have these items close at hand. If the patient has a significant nose bleed post-operatively, for instance, it may be necessary to insert a nasal tampon in order to stop the flow of blood. If this doesn't curtail the nose bleed, the patient may have to return to theatre to have the troublesome blood vessel cauterised.

It is also important to counsel the patient pre-operatively about issues that may arise after the surgery so they know what to expect. After a DCR, the key issues include epistaxis and pain/discomfort. The patient should also be advised that there will probably be a bi-canalicular stent in situ and this is likely to remain in place for 2 months.

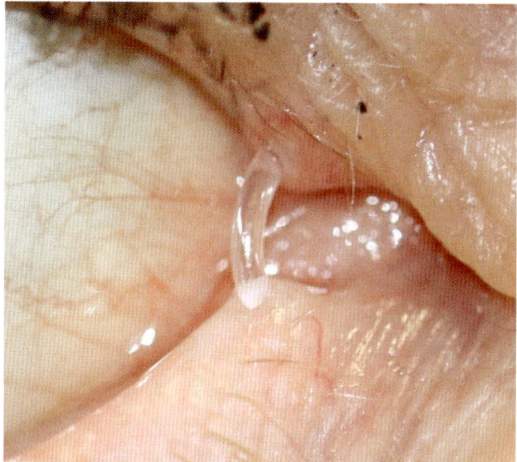

Figure 8.4: Bi-canalicular stent

During surgery the stent is passed in through the puncta and into the new system. The stent is tied within the nasal cavity, but a small section can be seen bisecting the eyelids between the puncta (see Figure 8.4). This type of stent acts as a stabilising scaffolding that allows everything to heal in an appropriate manner. The patient shouldn't be aware of the stent, but occasionally it can cause irritation either in the nose or in the medial corner of the eye where it can be seen bridging between the upper and lower puncta. It is important to inform the patient that whilst the stent is place it will partially or even completely occlude the tear drainage passageway. Their symptoms of epiphora may therefore continue after the surgery and until such time as the stents are removed. It is also important to encourage the patient to support the tube and prevent migration in circumstances such as sneezing by placing a finger over the medial canthus.

There are other types of stent, including a mono-canalicular type and mini-monoka, both of which are single-ended and therefore are only used to cannulate one of the puncta/canaliculi. The mini-monoka stent passes through the system in the same way and can be trimmed to the required size. The distal end of the mini-monoka stent has a footplate that allows it to rest against the punctal opening, preventing it from being pulled down the canaliculi. These types of stent are easier to remove as they can simply be pulled out via the puncta with fine forceps. They are typically used in trauma cases, or if one or other of the canaliculi are blocked and therefore cannot accommodate a bi-canalicular stent.

Post-operative DCR care

The main potential problem post-operatively is a nose bleed. A small amount of blood may be noted from the nasal cavity post-op and this shouldn't be too disconcerting. However, a continual and persistent nose bleed that doesn't naturally stop with some simple first-aid measures will require further intervention. Initially the patient should be encouraged to sit with their head forward and to pinch their nose firmly at the junction of the bony and soft part of the nose. Sometimes a cool pack over the bridge of the nose may also help slow bleeding.

If these simple measures do not work, insertion of a nasal tampon may help stop the bleeding. These usually come individually packed and with a string attached. They may need to be trimmed to fit some noses, bearing in mind that everyone's anatomy is different, so make sure you have some scissors to hand. Also, to help insertion, a layer of lubrication (such as Vaseline or Lacrilube) should be applied. In order to insert the tampon correctly and safely, it should be passed horizontally into the nose and should move unrestricted. If there is any resistance, it should be taken out and reinserted in a slightly different trajectory. The assistance of an oculoplastic medical practitioner may be required to ensure that the tampon is inserted correctly.

If bleeding persists, the patient may need to go back to theatre. For several days after the procedure the patient may notice some intermittent bleeding; it is important to reassure them that this is normal – as long as it stops naturally and isn't persistent. It will be necessary to encourage the patient to avoid hot drinks and food for the first 24–48 hours after surgery to reduce the risk of bleeding. Getting the patient to sleep in a more upright position may also help with this.

The patient will probably get some pain and discomfort for a few days and should be encouraged to take simple analgesia. The patient will also need to apply antibiotic ointment to the wound (if they have had an external DCR) and may need to be prescribed oral antibiotics if the surgery is associated with a history of infection (dacryocystitis).

Otherwise, it is important to advise the patient not to blow their nose for at least 1 month following the procedure. This can be annoying for the patient but doing so could cause problems, especially if there is a risk of dislodging the canalicular stents or causing a nose bleed. Similarly, the patient should be advised not to rub their eyes, as this too may dislodge the stent.

Inevitably, and despite the best intentions of the patient (and possibly through no fault of their own), the stents can still prolapse forward and out of the puncta. I occasionally get contacted by patients concerned by a 'piece of thread' sticking out of their eye. It is important to tell them about this potential risk before they go home after surgery or preferably at the pre-operative assessment. The temptation for some individuals to cut the 'thread' or attempt to pull it out may be too great, and of course this could be detrimental to the success of the surgery – so it is really important to educate them about the stent. I usually suggest that if they see the stent, or are aware of it having become dislodged, they should immediately contact the practitioner and then it can be explored in clinic. The patient should be encouraged to tape the stent to the side of their nose and to contact the hospital. Ensure that you give the patient contact details for the relevant staff member/s so it is easy for them to get into contact with someone if they have issues.

With some careful manipulation, it may be possible to reposition the stent but occasionally it may have to be entirely removed.

Endo-nasal DCR

As has already been mentioned, DCR surgery can also be approached endo-nasally, meaning that the whole procedure is carried out from within the nasal cavity. Not all patients are suitable for this approach, as their nasal cavity may not be wide enough or may be restricted due to an abnormality or variation in the anatomy. This needs to be explored in clinic, at the stage of listing and consent.

Assuming the nasal space is appropriate and the surgery can safely be undertaken, the outcome is essentially the same – we are just approaching it from the opposite direction. Endoscopic DCR is especially advantageous if external scarring is to be avoided, especially in those who might scar excessively such as those with a tendency to keloid or hypertrophic scarring.

The pre-operative care considerations are largely the same as with the external approach. But an emphasis on peri-operative bleeding and its management is important. The practitioner needs to investigate any potential risks associated with potential bleeding very carefully. Bear in mind that eliciting this information can be difficult, especially if the patient isn't entirely clear who their cardiologist is or who deals with their regular anti-coagulant therapy.

The procedure involves the use of various endoscopic instruments to undertake the surgery and the steps may include the following:

- Preparing the nose by applying local anaesthesia and decongesting it
- Once the local anaesthesia and decongestant have been allowed to work, a flap incision is made into the nasal mucosa adjacent to the middle turbinate
- The mucosa flap is then deflected back
- An opening in the underlying bone is made using either a combination of rongeurs or a drill. A motorised drill with a specific burr (usually diamond-tipped)

can be used. The diamond tip provides good removal of bone without damage to soft tissue or mucosal linings. The hole created in the bone is called an osteotomy
- Once the bone is removed, the lacrimal sac is revealed, and its presenting posterior wall is then opened using a blade; the sac is then deflected open
- Silicone stents are then passed, in a similar way to the external approach.

Post-operative care

Most of the post-operative care is similar to that used with the external approach. The main issues are: bleeding risks, stent prolapse and avoidance of hot food/drinks and blowing the nose.

Additionally, however, irrigation of the nasal cavity to remove blood clots is encouraged at least once a day with saline solution. Saline solution can be purchased via local chemists or may be prescribed in some circumstances. The use of topical steroid nasal drops may also be encouraged to reduce inflammation.

Some surgeons pack the nose (with a nasal tampon) initially (for the first 24 hours) if this is warranted, especially if there has been significant bleeding during the procedure.

Remember to advise the patient to take it easy for the first few days after the procedure, so as to not trigger any bleeding. When there is no external wound, patients often underestimate the extent of the work that has been undertaken. So it is important to spend time emphasising the need to relax and avoid strenuous activity immediately after the operation.

Lester Jones tubes

Occasionally, in patients with a complete blockage of the upper/lower eyelid canaliculi through scarring or who have an absence of canaliculi, a variation to the traditional surgical approach to alleviate symptomatic epiphora is required. This procedure is called a conjunctivo-dacryocystorhinostomy or CDCR.

This particular approach, which is similar to a traditional DCR, can be performed both externally and endo-nasally. However, a stent cannot be used because it simply can't be passed down the canaliculi as they are blocked. An alternative mechanism is therefore required to allow the tears to pass into the nasal cavity through a conduit known as a Lester Jones tube (LJT).

The LJT is a pyrex glass tube that varies in length and width. At its superior end it has a flange and the inferior end is often tapered. The tube is placed at the medial canthus, passing through the bony osteotomy that has been created and straight into the nasal cavity. Essentially it acts like a small drainpipe, providing a direct channel for tears to drain from the eye into the nasal cavity.

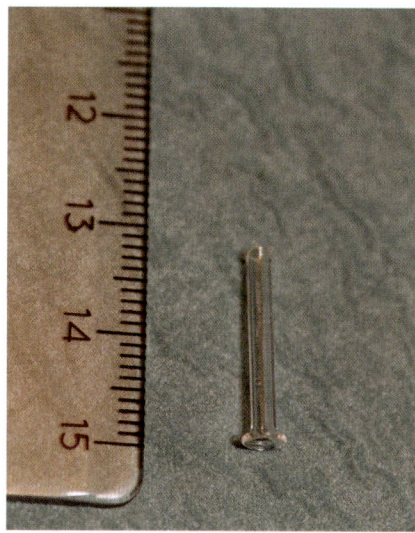

Figure 8.5: Lester Jones tube

The LJT will need to be ordered in advance and sterilised prior to surgery and particular adjunctive surgical instruments will be required in order to position the tube. The length and width of tube varies in each case and needs to be anticipated prior to surgery. The width of the tube is between 3 and 5mm and the length ranges from 10 to 24mm. Any longer than this makes the tube unstable and more likely to break. Typically, the length is around 14mm.

There are also several alternative LJTs available for particular circumstances, including:

- Angled – this tube has a deliberate kink approximately a third of the way along it. In certain patients, this may allow the tube to sit better, particularly in the nose if a straight tube abuts the middle turbinate.
- Frosted – in order to reduce migration, the outer part of the tube is frosted and rough, ensuring that it will be kept in position due to the friction against the tissues.
- Putterman-Gladstone – again in order to prevent migration the tube has a bulbous section in the upper third of its length.
- Baylis – this is a 60-degree curved tube, not unlike the angled tube, to overcome difficult corners.
- Suture Holed – some LJTs come with a hole in the flange to allow for a suture to initially help keep it in place.

Lester Jones tubes offer an effective way to overcome the difficulties of epiphora in this specific group of patients, where there are no alternatives. However, their use also raises a lot of considerations in relation to patient education and tube care.

Firstly, patient selection is important. The practitioner needs to ensure that they appreciate the pros and cons of LJTs. Once inserted, the tubes require care and attention and for life. Therefore, it is important to ascertain that the patient is willing to care for the tube and that their epiphora is severe enough to warrant the attention and input that will be required to maintain an LJT.

To keep them patent and open, LJTs require regular flushing with topical drops. Hypromellose drops are inserted into the eye and at the same time the opposite nostril is occluded, and then the drop is sniffed through the tube. This forceful passage of fluid through the tube is important to remove debris and mucus that can collect within the tube and cause it to block. This may be especially true if the patient has a heavy cold.

Unfortunately, the tube can migrate and shift position, either by moving undesirably into the nose or becoming more prominent at the medial canthus. This may mean that it needs to be adjusted, either in clinic or (more likely) in theatre. It is therefore important for the patient to understand that they may require a further visit to theatre after the initial surgery for fine adjustment.

In rare cases, the tube can fall out altogether. This is problematic as the soft-tissue passage created for the tube can quickly occlude, making reinsertion difficult, particularly if it is left for too long. In this case, a new passage will have to be created (in theatre). At pre-assessment it would be pertinent to tell the patient that up to one-third of people who receive a Lester Jones tube will require an extra visit to theatre to adjust the tube and a further one-third of cases may require several such trips.

Post-operatively, if the patient coughs or sneezes there is a risk that the force generated will blow the tube out. This may be prevented by teaching the patient to quickly cover the flange of the tube with a free finger when they realise they are about to sneeze.

The patient may be aware of the passage of air through the tube and this can be a little unsettling at first. Some patients describe a cold sensation (or, very rarely, even a sound) associated with breathing.

Damage to the lacrimal system

In some circumstances, the tear drainage system can be damaged through trauma or occasionally as a consequence of treatment (such as radiotherapy) or surgery. It is important to elicit this information as part of the history-taking process.

Not uncommonly, patients will present in emergency centres with trauma or lacerations to the face involving the lacrimal system. Typically, medial canthal lacerations can directly sever the canaliculi. It may be possible to salvage this using bi-canalicular or mono-canalicular stents to cannulate the system. The stents may then act as scaffolding and also help to bring the rest of the lacerated skin together. In this case, if they are tolerated well, the stents may stay in place for up to a year.

When using an endoscope to visualise stents within the nose, remember that those stents placed at the time of DCR surgery will be more apparent near the middle turbinate, but stents inserted for canaliculus repair will be under the inferior turbinate and typically harder to see and remove.

Conclusion

I hope you can now recognise and appreciate the complex dynamics of the lacrimal system and apparatus. Clearly, there are several inter-related anatomical aspects to the system and its overall efficiency.

Caring for patients who suffer the frustration of epiphora is difficult and we need to help them understand the broader problems associated with the underlying causative factors. I therefore spend a lot of time explaining why they need to use drops when they have reflex epiphora (dry eyes causing excessive lacrimation). I also emphasise the importance of eyelid hygiene and care in order to reduce the likelihood of blepharitis. Guarding against blepharitis and related problems can improve tear quality, which can in turn reduce dryness and therefore improve tear production. If we spend more time explaining the reasons for all these protective measures, patients are likely to be more compliant and meticulous in caring for the eye – time well spent, I think.

References

Holland, E., Marris, M. & Barry Lee, W. (2013). *Ocular surface disease: Cornea, conjunctiva and tear film*. (Chapter 7). Elsevier.

Rose, G. & Verity, H. (2011), Concepts in lacrimal dynamics and a practical course of treatment. *Expert Review of Ophthalmology.* **6**(6), 603–10.

Vonica, O., Obi, E., Sipkova, Z., Soare, C. & Pearson, A. (2017). The value of lacrimal scintillography in the assessment of patients with epiphora. *Eye* (London). **31**(7), 1020–24.

9

Thyroid eye disease

Introduction

First described in 1835 by Robert J. Graves, thyroid eye disease (or Graves' orbitopathy) is a complex and occasionally clinically challenging condition to manage. From a nursing perspective, thyroid eye disease (TED) can be an emotionally debilitating and physically demanding disease for the patient. The cause of Graves' disease continues to be uncertain and is associated with various extraneous factors. Clinically, thyroid eye disease is associated with swelling of the extra-ocular muscles, causing the eyes to bulge out (known as proptosis). The outward proptosis can in turn cause eyelid retraction and eye exposure, leading to possible corneal damage (see Figure 9.1).

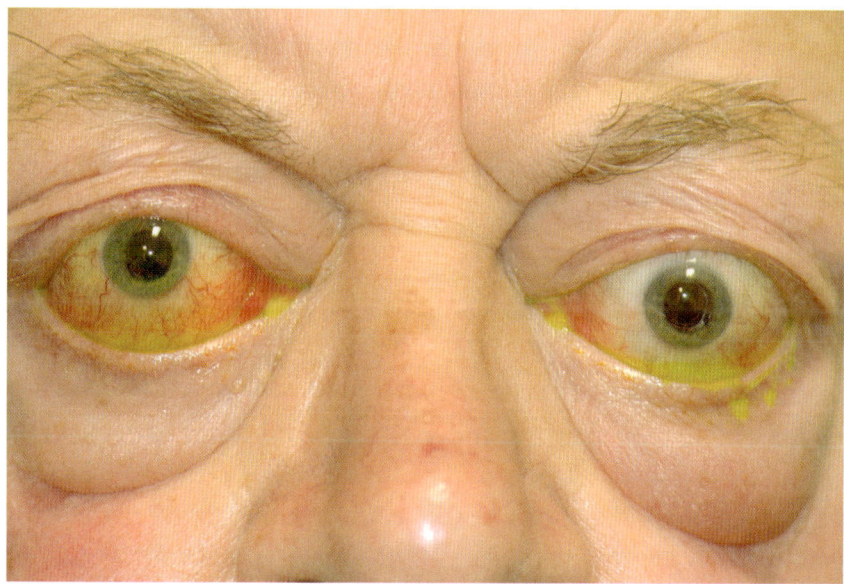

Figure 9.1: Thyroid eye disease

In order to appreciate the natural history of thyroid eye disease, it is important to understand how the thyroid gland manufactures and regulates thyroxine production within the body.

The pathology of thyroid eye disease

The production of thyroxine is regulated by a feedback system and by the level of iodine in the thyroid gland. The thyroid gland is an endocrine gland located in the neck, just below the larynx. It is said to be butterfly-shaped and is bi-lobed, lying on either side of the trachea. Within the thyroid gland, there are follicles which produce thyroxine. On a cellular level, thyroxine is synthesised by several processes that take place within the thyroid follicles. This involves iodide and the amino acids tyrosine and thyroglobulin. As part of the synthesising process, the attachment of tyrosine to iodine and further coupling of these molecules creates T4 and T3 within the colloid of the follicle. These molecules diffuse through the cell membrane and into the blood supply. Generally, more T4 is secreted than T3. However, T3 is several times more potent than T4, and most T4 circulating in the blood will eventually be converted to T3. A negative feedback system controls the level of thyroxine within the body, involving the hypothalamus in the brain and the anterior pituitary gland, and several hormones. So, for example, if there were a high blood concentration of thyroxine, its production would be suppressed. Alternatively, if the serum concentration of thyroxine were too low, the hypothalamus would be stimulated to increase thyroxine levels.

If you imagine a low blood level of T3 and T4, the negative feedback system will:

- Stimulate the hypothalamus to secrete the thyrotropin-releasing hormone (TRH), which then travels to the pituitary gland.
- Release TRH from within the interior pituitary gland to stimulate secretion of the thyroid-stimulating hormone (TSH). The TSH then stimulates the production of T3 and T4 within the follicles of the thyroid gland.
- Increase the levels of T3 and T4 entering the blood supply, which in turn inhibits the release of TRH and TSH.

Thyroid hormones regulate many actions within the body, including oxygen use, metabolic rate, cellular metabolism, growth and development. Hypothyroidism is associated with myxedema, the symptoms of which include: brachycardia, sensitivity to cold, muscle weakness, general lethargy and weight gain. Adversely, hyperthyroidism is associated with increased metabolic rate, heat intolerance, increased sweating, weight loss, insomnia, tremor and nervousness.

Graves' disease is associated with a genetic predisposition and environmental factors. Activation of an immune response is thought to be facilitated by cleavage of the thyroid-stimulating hormone receptor binding site in the cell membrane, leading to the over-production of T3 and T4. This in turn leads to increased metabolic response, including tachycardia, enlargement of the thyroid gland (known as a goitre) and enlargement of the extra-ocular muscles within the orbit. Auto-antibodies specifically target the fibroblasts in the eye muscles and adipose tissue in the orbit, leading to swelling and inflammation. The inferior and medial rectus muscles are most commonly affected, but it is not unusual for all the extra-ocular muscles to be targeted. The muscles degenerate with the formation of collagen and infiltration of fat.

Clinical ophthalmic manifestations of the disease are associated with eyelid swelling, proptosis, conjunctival injection, caruncular swelling, pain and discomfort, chemosis and reduced visual acuity. There are many outward symptoms of thyroid eye disease, including:

- Diplopia
- Ache/Pain both at rest and on eye movement
- Epiphora
- Dry eyes
- Eyelid swelling
- Proptosis
- Eyelid retraction
- Photophobia
- Foreign-body sensation
- Blurred or reduced vision
- Infection/discharge
- Lagophthalmos
- Restriction of eye movement
- Conjunctival injection and chemosis.

Graves' disease is also known as thyroid-associated orbitopathy. As it affects the orbital and peri-orbital tissue, the terms are often used interchangeably. Graves' disease is up to five times more common in women than men, and is more prevalent in patients over the age of 60. This disease is self-limiting and often becomes inactive after a period of approximately two years.

Rundle's curve

The natural history of Graves' orbitopathy was originally described and depicted by Rundle and Wilson in 1945. They found that, from diagnosis, there is a steep prominence of the disease during a 'dynamic' initial phase, during which it reaches its maximum severity. Then, over a period varying in length (but typically 12–18 months), the disease process appears to stabilise and this is referred to as the 'plateau' phase.

Subsequently, the disease may reduce and ebb to a point. This process was plotted on a graph (see below). Known as 'Rundle's curve', it is still seen today as important in portraying the disease process. Bartley (2011) described Rundle's curve being used 'as shorthand in the lexicon of Graves' ophthalmopathy as a descriptor of the disease's putative natural history' and Rundle's curve has been referenced in many articles and books ever since its conception.

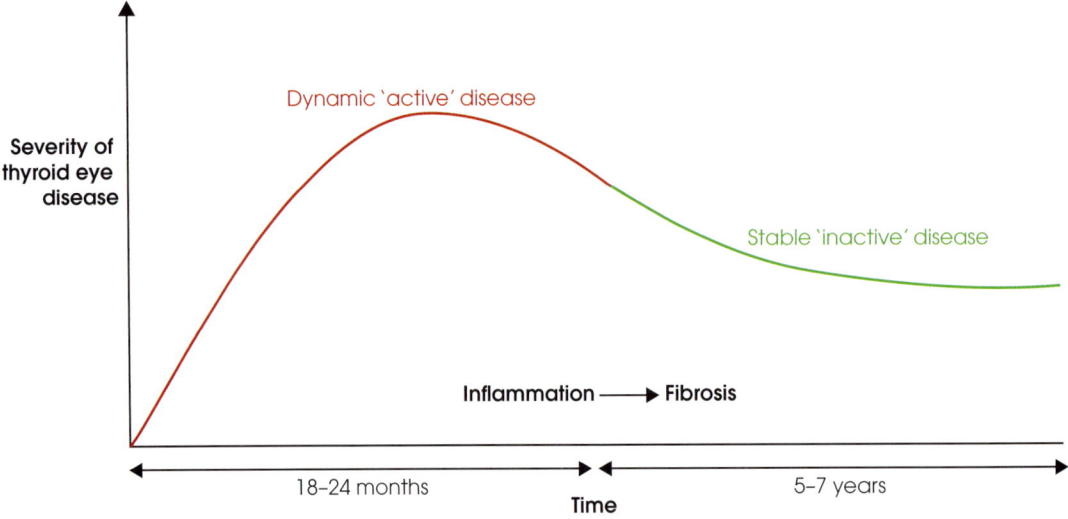

Figure 9.2: Rundle's curve

Smoking and thyroid eye disease

Smoking is one of the most common contributory factors in thyroid disease, and evidence suggests that smoking can make the effects of the disease process up to seven times worse (Thornton *et al.* 2006). Smoking cessation is therefore an essential part of the treatment for these patients. However, this is not always easy as many patients with thyroid disease suffer from low mood and find comfort in continuing to smoke.

Nevertheless, once the facts about smoking have been stressed to the patient, they often become more motivated to stop. 'Vaping' arguably provides a safer alternative to smoking, though the evidence on the effects of vaping on TED is still inconclusive, so stopping completely is the preferred option where possible. From a nursing perspective, supporting the patient to stop smoking is extremely important. There are various support groups and organisations that the patient can be guided towards, including Freedom from Smoking (2016) and NHS Smokefree. NHS Smokefree also provide an app for use on a smartphone that can provide guidance and a personal help plan.

There are smoking cessation support courses for nurses that provide the knowledge and information needed to help patients quit. The patient's GP can also provide a lot of help and support by referring them to stop-smoking courses and prescribing nicotine replacement therapy or stop-smoking medication such as Champix (Varenicline) ®Pfizer Ltd.

Selenium treatment for thyroid eye disease

Selenium (Se) is an essential mineral which has many uses, including in the glassmaking process, pigments, photocopying, photo-cells and importantly in many intercellular processes. It is found naturally in the soil, tuna, grass-fed beef, turkey and Brazil nuts. The recommended daily dose of selenium can be gained by eating one or two Brazil nuts.

Selenium is involved in the regulation and metabolism of thyroid hormones and is known to reduce thyroid peroxidase antibodies by as much as 20%. It also has an anti-oxidant property. Amounts of selenium found naturally within foodstuffs can vary and can also differ in abundance and availability from country to country.

Selenium can be purchased in many healthfood stores and may play an important part in helping to reduce some of the symptoms of thyroid disease. It is therefore helpful for the nurse to provide information about selenium and to encourage the patient to buy it as part of a treatment regime. The recommended dose of selenium in thyroid eye disease is 200 micrograms per day, but the specific dose for individual patients should be regulated in consultation with the GP and the endocrinology team.

Initial assessment for thyroid eye disease

Patients with Graves' disease will require formal assessment in the outpatients' clinic. The European Group on Graves' Orbitopathy (EUGOGO) guidelines (2008) suggest that this should be undertaken where possible within a multidisciplinary team (MDT) setting. The team should include an oculoplastic consultant, an endocrinologist and nursing support. In order to treat and manage the disease effectively, it is necessary to have a holistic approach and this can only be successfully achieved with access to information about the patient, appropriate assessment of the patient and the application of a consistent MDT approach.

In the first instance, a full clinical history is required. Apart from the usual demographics, other essential information includes:

- Past medical and ophthalmic history
- Medications
- Family and social history
- When the disease was diagnosed

- Whether the patient's thyroid disease is being monitored by an endocrinologist
- Whether or not they should be on any prescribed medication (such as Carbimazole or PTU) to control thyroxine production
- Results of any recent blood tests, especially including TSH, T3, T4, TPO
- Whether the patient smokes and how many 'pack years'
- Does the patient have any other outward signs of thyroid disease including dermopathy, myxedema or acropathy?
- Does the patient have any other co-morbidities, such as diabetes, other auto-immune diseases or malignancy?

Ophthalmic assessment for thyroid eye disease

In order to gain a complete understanding of the extent of the patient's thyroid eye disease, the practitioner needs to undertake a complete ophthalmic assessment, including all the following aspects.

Visual acuity (VA)

This probably goes without saying, but a LogMar visual acuity result is important when ascertaining baseline distance vision. Visual acuity remains a crucial tool when assessing subtle changes in sight but it is easy to underestimate the importance of this test because it is used so frequently. The practitioner must always take time to check the visual acuity and make sure it is competently undertaken, to the best of the patient's ability.

Along with visual acuity, it may be necessary to undertake a refraction and Humphrey field test, so it is important to align appointments with orthoptic colleagues.

Colour vision (Ishihara)

Checking the patient's colour vision can highlight subtle deficiencies in colour perception. Certain degenerative diseases, including age-related macular degeneration and retinal damage due to diabetes, may cause a reduction in colour perception. However, the main cause of a reduction in colour vision may be nerve compression at the apices of the orbit, as a direct consequence of extra-ocular muscle/orbital fat swelling.

Eyelids

It is important to carry out a careful appraisal of the amount of eyelid swelling caused by similar inflammation processes. Patients often find eyelid swelling quite distressing, especially if it is associated with proptosis. The swelling may be a consequence of underlying fat hypertrophy bulging anteriorly, and it is important to distinguish between eyelid swelling and fat hypertrophy. Simple eyelid swelling is likely to be fluid-like oedema, whereas fat hypertrophy is firmer to palpation. The eyelid swelling may be angry and hot, suggesting erythema.

Eyelid measurements
The practitioner also needs to complete a set of basic eyelid measurements including pupillary aperture, marginal reflex distance and levator function (see Chapter 3, p. 46).

Eyelid retraction
Similarly, it is necessary to ascertain the level of eyelid retraction and whether this involves either the upper or lower eyelids. It is often more readily seen inferiorly and can be quite marked.

Proptosis
One of the most commonly associated signs of thyroid eye disease is proptosis, due to the underlying rectus muscle swelling. Ascertaining the degree to which the eyes are proptosed is an important part of the assessment (exophthalmometery). To measure the proptosis, the practitioner will need to use an exothamometer (see below).

Bell's phenomenon (palpebral oculogyric reflex)
This is a defensive/protective mechanism whereby the eye rotates both upward and outward when an attempt is made to open closed eyes. It is important to understand the degree of a patient's Bell's phenomenon, especially if there is poor eyelid function to protect the eye. This is relatively easy to ascertain. The patient can be asked to close their eye while the practitioner simultaneously tries to firmly open the eyelids (without hurting the patient).

Eye assessment
Using a slit lamp, the practitioner should carry out a complete assessment of the eye, observing for conjunctival chemosis and injection (including the caruncle), clarity of the cornea and punctate epithelial erosions (PEES), and checking the intra-ocular pressure (IOP) and fundoscopy.

Other investigations
Further to a comprehensive medical and ophthalmic history of the patient, other important investigations may be required to gain a complete picture of the extent of the disease process.

Blood tests
Firstly, it may be necessary to repeat serum blood tests, especially TFT, thyroid peroxidase antibodies (TPOAb), T3 and T4, as well as full blood count and U&Es.

Normal ranges for thyroid blood test results for men and non-pregnant women may

vary widely. Typical thyroid blood test results in relation to thyroid function are:
- TSH 0.4–4.0 mU/l
- FT4 9.0–25.0 pmol/l
- FT3 3.5–7.8 pmol/l

To help understand thyroid function in conjunction with blood test results:
- If the TSH is high and (free) T4 is low, the patient has hypothyroidism
- If the TSH is low and (free) T4 is high, the patient has hyperthyroidism
- If the TSH is slightly elevated but free T4 is within normal limits, the patient has subclinical hypothyroidism (test TPOAb to help determine risk of subclinical disease converting to clinical hypothyroidism)
- If the TSH is low and (free) T4 is also low, this may indicate a failure of the pituitary gland.

Scanning

A computerised tomography (CT) scan of the head and orbits will show the degree of muscle swelling within the orbit and especially any apical congestion. Equally, magnetic resonance imaging (MRI) can play an important role in the diagnosis and management of thyroid eye disease. Computerised tomography uses computer-processed x-ray measurements taken from various angles to produce an image. Various body structures can be identified, based on their ability to absorb x-ray beams. The resulting image is very useful for identifying soft-tissue changes and details such as blood vessels and other small structures. However, the patient is subjected to a large dose of radiation which may increase their risk of cancer. MRI scanning can be used as an alternative to CT scanning. This process is longer and more expensive but has the advantage of not subjecting the patient to any radiation.

Classification of stage and activity of Graves' orbitopathy

It can be difficult to distinguish the factors and symptoms associated with Graves' orbitopathy and attempts have been made to create methods of classification by assessing variables associated with the most common symptoms of Graves' disease. A couple of assessment tools have been created, each with their own merits and disadvantages, including NO SPECS (Werner 1969) and VISA (Dolman & Rootman 2006). The main tool I am familiar with, and which is commonly used, is the Clinical Activity Score (CAS), developed by Mourits, Koornneef, Wiersinga, et al. (1989) and later amended by EUGOGO (1997).

The CAS is based on the assessment of seven key factors, each of which scores a point if apparent (scoring between 0 and 7). They include:

- Spontaneous pain (orbital)
- Gaze-evoked orbital pain (on movement)
- Eyelid swelling attributed to active GO
- Eyelid erythema
- Conjunctival redness (also due to GO)
- Chemosis
- Inflammation of caruncle/plica

A further three criteria are assessed in follow-up patients: an increase in proptosis, decrease in ocular excursion (deviation) and decrease in visual acuity.

A CAS of 0–3 is deemed 'mild' and wouldn't necessarily require any treatment apart from routine adjuncts such as analgesia and lubrication. However, a CAS over 3 may trigger the need for treatment, including corticosteroids.

The CAS system is widely used but it is subjective and open to a degree of interpretation, and it may also not be particularly sensitive to small changes in the symptoms. However, the EUGOGO (2008) committee have produced quite robust guidelines to aid the clinician to minimise potential subjectivity. Certainly, if the practitioner has a particular interest in this area I would guide them to the EUGOGO website (http://www.eugogo.eu).

Anti-thyroid management of thyroid eye disease

The drugs used to control thyroid production are known as anti-thyroid agents. In the UK, two main medications are used to manage thyroid eye disease – namely carbimazole and propylthiouracil (PTU).

Carbimazole is the first-line drug used in order to reduce the production of thyroxine. This drug acts by disrupting the molecular manufacture of thyroxine. Often, a patient known to be showing signs of hyperthyroidism will be commenced on a titrated course of carbimazole. This may need to be adjusted to the lowest dose required to maintain a more normal thyroid function. Once the disease process has run its course, it may be possible to reduce the dose of carbimazole and then stop completely. Alternatively, a 'block and replace' approach can be used, whereby the dose of carbimazole completely stops thyroid production and the patient takes a daily dose of levothyroxine to replace the thyroxine. This may require close monitoring at first to titrate the dose of levothyroxine. The side effects of carbimazole most commonly cause a rash, but more seriously bone marrow suppression, which in turn causes a reduction in white blood cell production – agranulocytosis and neutropenia. This only occurs in rare cases but any patient who describes the sudden onset of a sore throat, fever or mouth ulcers should seek medical advice urgently. Recent advice from the Medicines and Healthcare Products Regulatory Agency (2019a, 2019b) suggests that carbimazole has also been associated with acute pancreatitis and congenital malformations.

Propylthiouracil (PTU) is used as an alternative to carbimazole, particularly if the patient cannot tolerate carbimazole or is in the early stages of pregnancy. PTU works in a similar way to carbimazole but is slower in its initial action. It is also a slightly more onerous form of medication, as more tablets have to be taken on a daily basis, which may be confusing for some patient groups.

PTU has been associated with serious liver injury and it is therefore prudent to monitor the patient's liver function while they are taking the drug. Warn the patient to be aware of signs of liver injury – particularly yellowing of the sclera, which is a common sign of jaundice.

While the patient is taking these medications, they must be closely monitored by an endocrinologist, and patients with thyroid-related eye disease should preferably be cared for by a multidisciplinary team approach.

Radioactive iodine treatment for hyperthyroidism

As has already been mentioned, iodine is crucial for the production of thyroxine. Patients who have hyperthyroidism which is difficult to control may also have an enlarged thyroid gland (goitre). In this instance, it may be necessary to use radioactive iodine to stop the thyroid gland from over-producing thyroxine. The form of radioactive iodine used is called I-131. The radioactive iodine I-131 is given by mouth, usually as a drink or a tablet. It is not typically associated with many side-effects, though it may sometimes cause mild pain in the neck which can be controlled with over-the-counter analgesics. The patient also needs to be informed of their potential low-grade radioactivity and the associated risks of exposure to others.

The following precautions are advisable (timings may vary depending on dosage and local guidelines):

- Sleeping in a separate bed from your partner (10 days)
- Keeping away from children and pregnant women (5 days)
- Delaying a return to work (5 days)
- Not travelling on public transport (3 days)
- Not preparing food for others (2–3 days)
- Not sharing utensils with others (2–3 days)
- Flushing the toilet two or three times after use.

Note that doses of radioactive iodine can be detected, for example, by scanners used in airports, so it may be prudent to have a supporting letter from a medical practitioner if the patient needs to travel during the initial period of treatment.

Note also that it can take several months for the thyroid to become completely functionless, during which thyroid function may fluctuate.

Orbital radiotherapy treatment for thyroid eye disease

Until quite recently, orbital radiotherapy was used as a treatment for several aspects of thyroid eye disease. Typically, it was given as an external beam approach, with 20Gy over 10 days to each orbit.

The indications for this included:

- Optic neuropathy and relief of distension at the orbital apex
- Inflammation and congestion within the orbit
- Improvement of strabismus and ocular motility.

The use of low-dose orbital radiotherapy remains controversial, with recent trials suggesting that for patients on oral corticosteroids there was no additional benefit for them to also have orbital radiotherapy (Rajendram, R., Taylor, P.N., Wilson, V.J. *et al.* 2018). Nonetheless, as a practitioner caring for these patients, you may come across individuals who have had this treatment for the reasons outlined above.

Corticosteroid treatment for orbital inflammation

The most common treatment for orbit inflammation is steroids. Patients with moderate to severe orbital inflammation may require intravenous methylprednisolone. Initially, intravenous (IV) steroids are commenced with a test dose (250mg), and thereafter doses of 500mg to 1g are given per treatment. Prior to treatment, it is necessary to check the patient's liver function. Most importantly the maximum amount that can be provided in one year is 8 grams. There are many side effects and contraindications for the use of IV steroids and this may affect a patient's ability to receive them. Some common side effects include:

- Tachycardia (rapid heartbeat)
- Stomach irritation/ulcer
- Feeling hot or cold
- Flushing of the face or upper torso
- Poor sleep

- Headaches
- Agitation
- Liver-related issues
- Weight gain.

Prior to the steroid treatment, the patient needs to be informed about the potential side effects. Although intravenous steroids can be very effective in reducing orbital inflammation, they may not work in every case. In this instance, a last resort would be immunosuppressant treatment in the form of azathioprine.

Azathioprine treatment

This drug can be used for many purposes, including the prevention of rejection following organ transplant and to treat a range of autoimmune diseases. It has a number of potential side effects, including nausea and vomiting, hypersensitivity, dizziness, fatigue and rashes. It is also known to suppress bone marrow and patients can therefore develop anaemia and be more susceptible to infection. Azathioprine can be a viable alternative to steroids but again the patient will require particular support and guidance with regard to using this drug.

Orbital decompression

Once the disease has run its course, some patients (approximately 20%) may be left with a residual proptosis, causing physical issues related to eye exposure and eyelid retraction. This may cause them some distress and embarrassment. In this case, the only way to reduce the proptosis is to intervene surgically with a procedure known as orbital decompression.

Essentially this surgery creates openings in the bony orbital walls to allow the soft tissue to fall back into the spaces created. Alternatively a decompression (with just orbital fat removal) may be sufficient in some patients with mild proptosis. The relative severity of the proptosis will dictate how many orbital walls have to be decompressed. In some cases, a lateral wall decompression (with orbital fat removal) may be enough to gain an optimal decompression. In other, more severe cases, it may be necessary to decompress the lateral and medial walls (and even occasionally some of the orbital floor).

Surgery to alleviate proptosis is usually elective. However, in very rare cases, it is undertaken for urgent compressive optic neuropathy This is when the extra-ocular muscles swell so much that they compress the optic nerve at the apex of the orbit, causing sudden deterioration of vision.

Pre-operative preparation

Pre-operative preparation is necessary, as this surgery often takes 2 to 3 hours to perform and is usually undertaken with a general anaesthetic. The practitioner therefore needs to ensure that the patient is haematologically as stable as possible. It is also important to ascertain whether the patient is on any anti-coagulant therapy and manage it appropriately.

Other considerations before surgery include ensuring that the CT scans are available, as there can be individual variations in muscle and bone thickness. The relationship, position and proximity of the cribriform plate are also important, as this plate could be breached during surgery, and lead to a cerebrospinal fluid leak.

As mentioned earlier, the degree of proptosis will determine the extent of decompression required, i.e. how many orbital walls will be involved. Most commonly, the medial and lateral walls are decompressed, but occasionally the orbital floor may also be involved. Therefore, prior to surgery, the practitioner will have to undertake a full examination, including ocular morbidity, intra-ocular pressure, anterior segment exam, dilative fundus exam, and measurement of ophthalmometry for proptosis.

Surgical approaches for orbital decompression

Surgically, the procedure I am most familiar with is the swinging eyelid approach, which is undertaken as follows:

- Incision – swinging lower eyelid approach to the lateral wall and floor, releasing of the lateral canthal tendon, also caruncular approach to the medial wall
- Progress is made to bony orbital rim
- The periosteum is lifted off the bone
- Openings are then made into the orbital bones and some of the surrounding bone may be burred down
- Once sufficient bone has been removed, openings are then made in the periorbita and orbital fat is removed or is usually allowed to herniate into the space created
- Finally the wounds are closed
- Other lower eyelid surgical techniques include a transconjunctival or subciliary/skin crease approach, and these methods are adopted by many surgeons.

This procedure may also be undertaken endoscopically via the nose to access the medial orbital wall/orbital floor. This approach is particularly useful for orbital apical congestion and of course it means that there is no external surgical excision or scarring.

Post-operative care following decompression

Remarkably, very few patients have significant post-operative pain following this procedure. However, it may still be necessary to provide oral analgesia for the first week after surgery. Some patients are likely to stay in hospital for one night after the procedure where the pain can be monitored closely.

The most significant risk after surgery is a post-operative peri-orbital bleed. However, given that the surgery has provided an outlet for this by opening the sinuses, the chance of post-operative bleeding causing a significant problem is very rare (unless only the lateral wall has been decompressed or if a fat-only decompression has been performed). Any potential bleed is likely to amass within the maxillary sinus. This is not to say that the practitioner caring for the patient should not still be vigilant and monitor the patient for signs of bleeding, including sudden increased pain, loss of vision and tension within the orbit.

Immediately after the surgery the patient should not have a compressive dressing in place for longer than 24 hours. During this time the patient's visual acuity should be carefully monitored. Initially this will mean that the dressings will need to be removed and replaced in the first 24 hours. Using aseptic technique will be important when removing or reapplying the dressings. The patient may find it difficult to focus on the vision chart, as they may be blurred with ointment etc. It may also be painful. To focus the vision, make sure the patient uses their glasses (if they normally use them) or an occluder with a pinhole will likely improve the visual potential. Record the outcomes in the medical and nursing notes.

Importantly, if there is any discernible deterioration in the vision, you should report it immediately. This may indicate an orbital bleed, which could lead to blindness.

Topical lubricants should be encouraged in the initial weeks after surgery and it will be important to monitor the patient's instillation technique. After approximately a week, the patient should be encouraged to start gentle lower eyelid upward massage to reduce the risk of retraction.

The patient should not blow their nose for at least 6 weeks post-operatively as this may forcibly blow air into the orbit.

Other post-operative effects may include:

- Swelling and bruising for some days after the procedure but this should settle, with little further effect.
- Some patients describe having numbness in the maxillary region (infra-orbital anaesthesia) – again, this should recover over time but can take several months to do so.

- The patient may have double vision (diplopia) after the surgery. Again, this may settle with time and reduction in swelling but it also may require surgical input at a later stage to correct. In the short term, the use of prisms on the glasses may sometimes be useful.
- Having undergone decompressive surgery, further surgical input may be required to deal with under- or over-correction of the proptosis.
- Extremely rarely, there is a risk of a leakage of brain fluid (cerebral sinus fluid), with a potential associated risk of meningitis.
- Orbital cellulitis.
- Hypoglobus (inferior displacement of the globe).
- Enophthalmos (excessive decompression).
- Blindness is a very rare and devastating outcome from decompression surgery but the risk needs to be outlined at consent.

Initially there may be some notable post-operative improvement of the proptosis. However, only after further time has elapsed (up to 12 months) will the patient appreciate the full outcome of the surgery. It is important to prepare the patient for this – so that they realise it will take time for the decompression to be completely healed. Only then can any other corrective surgery be considered – for example, eyelid retraction correction and/or potential squint surgery for diplopia.

This recovery time can be frustrating for the patient and it is important to support them fully throughout this period. Psychologically, it can be deflating for them to wait for corrective surgery to be performed while still suffering from the effects of thyroid eye disease.

References

Bartalena, L., Baldeschi, L., Dickinson, A. *et al.* (2008). Consensus statement of the European group on Graves' orbitopathy (EUGOGO) on management of Graves' orbitopathy. *European Journal of Endocrinology.* **158**(3), 273–85.

Bartley, B. (2011). Rundle and his curve. *Archives of Ophthalmology.* **129**(3), 356–58.

Dolman, J. & Rootman, J. (2006). VISA classification for Graves orbitopathy. *Ophthalmic Plastic & Reconstructive Surgery.* **22**(5), 319–24.

European group on Graves' orbitopathy (EUGOGO). http://www.eugogo.eu (last accessed 5.12.2019).

Freedom from Smoking (2016). www.freedomfromsmoking.org (last accessed 5.12.2019).

Leatherbarrow, B. (2019). *Oculoplastic Surgery.* 537–61. USA: Thieme.

Medical and Healthcare Products Regulatory Agency (MHRA) (2019a). *Carbimazole: risk of acute pancreatitis.* https://www.gov.uk/drug-safety-update/carbimazole-risk-of-acute-pancreatitis (last accessed 12.11.2019).

Medical and Healthcare Products Regulatory Agency (MHRA) (2019b). *Carbimazole: increased risk of congenital malformations; strengthened advice on contraception*. https://www.gov.uk/drug-safety-update/carbimazole-increased-risk-of-congenital-malformations-strengthened-advice-on-contraception (last accessed 12.11.2019).

Mourits, M., Koornneef, L., Wiersinga, W., Prummel, M., Berghout, A. & Gaag, R. (1989). Clinical criteria for the assessment of the disease activity in Grave's ophthalmopathy: a novel approach. *British Journal of Ophthalmology*. **73**, 639–44.

Mourits, M., Prummel, M., Wiersinga, W. & Koornneef, L. (1997). Clinical activity score as a guide in the management of patients with Graves' ophthalmopathy. *Clinical Endocrinology*. **47**(1), 9–14.

NHS Smokefree (2019). https://www.nhs.uk/smokefree (last accessed 5.12.2019).

Rajendram, R., Taylor, P.N., Wilson, V.J. et al. (2018). Combined immunosuppression and radiotherapy in thyroid eye disease (CIRTED); a multicentre, 2 x 2 factorial, double-blind, randomized controlled trial. *The Lancet Diabetes & Endocrinology*. **6**(4), 299–309.

Rundle, F. & Wilson, C. (1945). Development and course of exophthalmos and ophthalmoplegia in Graves' disease with special reference to the effect of thyroidectomy. *Clinical Science*. **5**(3–4), 177–94.

Thornton, J., Kelly, S., Harrison, R. & Edwards, R. (2006). Cigarette smoking and thyroid eye disease: a systematic review. *Eye*. 21(9), 1135–45.

Werner, S. (1969). Classification of the eye changes of Grave's disease. *The American Journal of Ophthalmology*. **68**(4), 646–48.

10
Enucleation and evisceration

Introduction
The end goal for all ophthalmic practitioners and ophthalmologists is essentially to preserve sight wherever possible. However, despite our best endeavours, some individuals are forced to have an eye removed, for various reasons. As one might imagine, this has a profound effect on the patient and their well-being. Therefore, it is important for practitioners to understand the impact of this procedure on the patient and their family.

The term 'enucleation' refers to the surgical removal of a mass without cutting into it. Obviously in this context it means the removal of an eye. In practical terms, this means surgically removing the eye as a whole unit, with the extra-ocular muscles and the optic nerve detached. This is in contrast to 'evisceration' which essentially means to 'disembowel' or 'take the contents out'. In ophthalmological terms, this means removing the contents of the eye but leaving the sclera behind. Both procedures will be discussed in more detail later in this chapter.

Previously known as 'extirpation', removal of the eye by surgical means has been performed for many years and has been refined to an efficient technique that is carried out across the world.

Indications for eye removal
There are various indications for eye removal, including:
- Intra-ocular tumour/malignancy
- Trauma
- Severe infection
- Blind painful eye/Phthisical eye
- Sympathetic ophthalmia.

I have always considered patients who require eye removal in two distinct groups: the acute group and the chronic group. Each of these groups come to the procedure with differing perspectives and different psychological backgrounds and outlooks. A patient with a long-term chronic eye condition that has slowly got worse, resulting in a visionless, painful eye, is more likely to have come to terms with the need for removal than a patient who suddenly loses an eye through trauma.

For many patients with a long-term chronic painful eye, the situation can be likened to having a painful tooth that requires removal. The removal may actually represent a new chapter in that particular patient's life, and an opportunity to move on. Many of these patients have a cosmetically unsightly eye that causes them constant pain and discomfort. The eye may even shrink in size and become what is known as a phthisical eye. Of course, it would be wrong to assume that this is how *all* patients feel but I have found it to be the case for a significant number, after many years of caring for such patients.

Alternatively, there is the patient who suddenly loses their eye through trauma or cancer. Eye removal in this situation often has a more profound effect. Whilst many patients will put on a brave face, their unfortunate situation may well lead to underlying feelings of angst, disappointment and anger. Certainly, with a traumatised eye, enucleation should be left for a few days until there is opportunity to discuss the surgery and gain the patient's consent – to give the individual a chance to absorb the situation, at least in the very short term.

Given that trauma is the most common reason for enucleation surgery, it could be argued that more should be done to increase social awareness and knowledge in order to reduce traumatic events. How do we address the continued apathy concerning the risks involved in using metal grinders and other heavy machinery, for example? At the same time, we need to acknowledge that there has been progress in some areas. For instance, the legal requirement to wear seat belts has had a profound effect, significantly changing road accident outcomes and reducing the number of associated enucleation procedures.

Psychological impact

Many patients will, understandably, have feelings of anger due to blaming themselves or others for the avoidable 'moment in time' when a split-second decision led to a traumatic event. There is also the pain of having to lose what might have been a perfectly seeing eye. However, most traumatic events actually involve several factors that combine to create a life-changing accident. Even in such a devastating situation, time can eventually heal and, when appropriate, it may be possible to make the point that adapting to the new situation can lead to a new set of possible and positive outcomes.

The eye's vital position as a sensory organ, a means of communication and an essential cosmetic facial landmark, makes it a most important part of the human body. The dramatic change from stereo- to monocular vision has significant implications for most individuals. Losing an eye can affect relationships and emotions, as well as having an impact on financial and work-related issues and social interaction. Some patients experience a process of loss and grief following enucleation. Disappointingly, there is often little time immediately after the trauma to prepare the patient for potential eye removal, so much of the support has to come after the event. There is no doubt that some individuals suffer from depression and anxiety following eye removal surgery for trauma.

The other issue to contend with, within the UK's NHS service, is that referral for such patients for psychological support can be lengthy. Certainly, there is little time to formally assess the patient's psychological well-being pre-operatively. Unfortunately, very few eye hospital units have such clinical psychology services.

There may also be a possible lack of understanding from the patient's perspective about life with one eye. Assuming that the remaining eye is healthy and has good visual acuity, there is nothing to say that the patient cannot, for example, drive, undertake sports, work and carry on with a relatively normal life.

As I have said, time is definitely the best healer and for many patients, with a good cosmetic and practical result following eye removal surgery, the outlook can be very good. But in the beginning adapting to the loss of an eye, and changing from stereo to mono vision, can be disorientating. The loss of depth perception can create all sorts of issues. For instance, a simple act such as picking up a cup of tea from a table can initially be disorientating. Due to the slight alteration in depth perception, many individuals will at first knock the drink over. Similarly, individuals will bump into walls or other objects due to the slight change in spatial perception. This can add to the patient's overall frustration and annoyance. When coupled with possible anxiety about losing the eye, the patient may experience greater overall feelings of loss of control.

Apart from the environmental and practical aspects, we also have to consider many other variables that may affect the way a patient reacts to a traumatic event like this, including their personality, social status, culture, age and level of support from family and friends. Children with congenital conditions that require eye removal seem to cope rather better than adults in certain circumstances. But personality undoubtedly plays a massive part. Over the years, I have witnessed a whole host of personality traits in people who cope in a multitude of ways in such situations. As practitioners, we need to understand the individual personalities involved and use all our skills to help support the patient. It may be helpful to provide contact details for a support group where patients can meet other individuals who have undergone eye removal surgery or, where possible, to meet the oculo-prosthetists who fabricate cosmetic eyes.

An excellent book by Charles Slonium and Amy Martino, entitled *Eye Was There: A Patient's Guide to Coping with the Loss of an Eye* (Author House Publishing 2011), puts a really positive spin on how to cope with enucleation and provides real-life anecdotes as well. Another useful book is *A Singular View: The Art of Seeing with One Eye* by Frank Brady (1988), a pilot who lost an eye but resumed his career despite this setback. Another book which I can also recommend, offering similar advice, is by Jay Adkisson, entitled *Lost Eye* (2006). All patients should be directed towards these great resources, written by individuals who are well placed to comment on their experiences and coping strategies.

Perhaps unsurprisingly, little robust research has been undertaken to quantify the magnitude of the effects of eye removal. A piece by Kondo *et al.* (2013) offers some interesting findings. These researchers compared health-related quality of life in patients following surgical removal of one eye – and interestingly concluded that there was little difference between a normal (binocular) group and those who were monocular, having lost an eye.

Cosmetic impact

Cosmetically, the outcomes from eye removal surgery can be very good, with a reasonable level of eye movement associated with a fabricated prosthetic eye-piece that can barely be distinguished from the unaffected eye.

Most cosmetic eyes are manufactured in the UK via the National Artificial Eye Service based in Blackpool. A few eye units have their own prosthetic service but they are certainly in the minority.

The input of a dedicated ocular prosthetic department is fundamental in the post-operative rehabilitation of the patient.

Pre-operative considerations

Other specific pre-operative considerations include the usual general anaesthetic work-up, which involves checking haemolytic status, cardiac stability and the general well-being of the patient. As usual, there are particular concerns associated with patients on anti-coagulant therapy and this should be recognised and managed appropriately prior to surgery.

Sympathetic ophthalmia

It is also important to outline the risk of sympathetic ophthalmia (sometimes known as sympathetic uveitis) to the patient if the reason for surgery is associated with trauma or infection. This is a very rare condition in which the unaffected eye can have an inflammatory response, potentially leading to blindness. Certainly, in the initial days following trauma, it is prudent to observe the unaffected eye for any potential signs of sympathetic ophthalmia, which is essentially a delayed hypersensitivity reaction. Epidemiology of the condition is approximately 0.01% of penetrating wounds.

Early signs of sympathetic ophthalmia may include lots of accommodation and eye floaters. As the condition progresses, the symptoms may include severe uveitis, photophobia and pain.

Evisceration versus enucleation

Both these procedures are widely accepted as ways to surgically remove an eye. The approaches are different but the outcomes fairly similar. In both procedures an orbital implant can be used to replace the deficit created by removing the eye (bearing in mind that the volume of the eye is approximately 7.5ml). In the past, evisceration was associated with a greater risk of sympathetic ophthalmia but more recently this has been shown not to be the case.

The advantage of evisceration is that it is an easier surgical approach, making it quicker to perform, with fewer potential side effects. In its most basic form, this procedure can be undertaken by an experienced surgeon in approximately 30–45 minutes. It may be performed under a local (with sedation) or general anaesthetic. This is important, because some individuals who may be clinically unstable or unwell may not be able to tolerate the longer enucleation procedure, and evisceration may therefore offer a safer solution.

Evisceration may be indicated for endophthalmitis, phthisis bulbi (shrunken, non-functional eye), traumatic injury and painful blind eye.

In the case of intra-ocular malignant tumour, enucleation is the only option. (Performing an evisceration may not ensure complete removal of the tumour if there has been localised spread beyond the globe.) Enucleation is a lengthier procedure and involves removal of all the extra-ocular muscles from the globe and reattachment on the implant. It could therefore be seen as more expensive, given the longer surgical time, implant costs (usually the implant has to be covered with a Vicryl mesh to which the extra-ocular muscles are attached) and longer exposure to general anaesthetic for the patient. Given the financial pressures on the modern NHS, it may be that some physicians are choosing evisceration over enucleation because it is a cheaper procedure to perform.

Both surgical options can offer a degree of motility of the prosthesis once healed, but controversy exists as to which provides the best movement. Some practitioners also argue that the evisceration procedure is associated with less pain immediately post-operatively.

Types of orbital implants used in eye removal surgery

Several types of orbital implant are available to the surgeon when performing eye removal surgery. The main types are:

- Integrated
- Semi-integrated
- Non-integrated
- Dermis fat graft.

Integrated

These are implants which have a porous, bone-like structure which allows vessels and tissue to grow into the implant, becoming integrated with the body. The common types are:

- Hydroxyapatite – coral-like
- Bio-ceramic
- Medpor – polyethylene
- Alumininum oxide.

When they are inserted during surgery, these implants are often covered in a Vicryl mesh, which allows the extra-ocular muscles to be attached to the implant. Over time, this mesh will dissolve.

This type of implant has been associated with excellent mobility. Once integrated (6–12 months following insertion), hydroxyapatite implants could be drilled with a small central hole, which in turn could accommodate a prosthetic eyepiece with a peg on the back. This could provide even greater mobility. However, confidence in this system has waned, due to issues with infection and exposure (Fahim, Fruch, *et al.* 2007).

The main disadvantage of integrated implants is their cost, often amounting to several hundred pounds. They are also difficult to remove if the need arises and there can be issues with infection and exposure. To prevent exposure, some surgeons add a protective layer when closing the conjunctiva, in the form of an autologous scleral patch or temporal fascia patch graft.

Semi-integrated

These implants are not in any way porous but allow extra-ocular muscles to be attached directly onto the implant, so making it semi-integrated. These are much less commonly used these days, but they include the Allen implant and semi-hemispheric implants. They are relatively inexpensive implants which can provide good post-operative outcomes and movement.

Non-integrated
These are usually hard plastic spherical implants that do not in any way integrate with the body. They have to be wrapped in autologous sclera or Vicryl mesh during surgery. They are very cheap implants, often costing as little as forty pounds, and are not associated with a high risk of exposure. However, they can migrate within the orbit, which can create issues with the over-riding prosthetic eye-piece.

Dermis fat graft (DFG)
Occasionally the patient doesn't tolerate the orbital implant or has issues with discharge or infection. In these instances, the last resort is a dermis fat graft (DFG).

The DFG is usually harvested from the abdomen (iliac region) or from the outer superior aspect of the buttock. The procedure involves marking out a circle, usually with an approximate diameter of 1.5mm. Beyond, an ellipse is marked to allow for better skin closure. Local anaesthetic is infiltrated subcutaneously, creating a *peau d'orange* (dimpled) effect which essentially helps delineate the dermis from the epidermis. The epidermis is then removed, usually using a 15 blade. Following the original circle, the dermis is pierced and a pledget of underlying fat is removed, along with the dermis, to the required amount. This is then stitched into the orbit. Extra-ocular muscles can be attached but this offers little post-operative movement.

This is a relatively straightforward way of correcting an orbital deficit. However, given that there are two wounds, there is arguably a greater risk of infection in the initial post-operative phase.

As the graft is autologous, there is little risk of rejection. However, there can be problems with post-operative atrophy and physical shrinkage of the graft. This can in turn lead to issues with the prosthesis and superior sulcus formation.

The donor sites will require post-operative care. Initially they will be covered with a simple dressing which can be removed 3–4 days after surgery. The patient should be advised to keep the wound clean. The stitches in the wound are nylon and will need to be removed 10–14 days post-operatively.

Surgical approaches to evisceration and enucleation
The basic surgical steps in evisceration are as follows:
- Local anaesthetic is administered (peribulbar injection).
- A 360° peritomy at the limbus is performed and the conjunctiva is resected back.

- A stab incision is made at that limbus and then a circular cut is made all around the limbus to remove the cornea, ciliary body and lens.
- The remaining contents of the eye are scooped out and may be sent for histopathology.
- The inner surface of the sclera is then cleaned using absolute alcohol.
- Relieving incisions are made in the sclera.
- The amount of volume required is then measured, typically anything from 16 to 22mm (diameter).
- An orbital implant may then be positioned and the sclera wrapped over the implant.
- The Tenon's layer and conjunctiva layer are sutured over the sclera or implant.
- Some surgeons may then place a plastic conformer shell in the socket to help reduce post-operative swelling, along with a suture tarsorrhaphy.

The enucleation procedure is similar but has several additional elements, which obviously contribute to the complexity and length of the procedure:

- Local anaesthetic is administered (peribulbar injection).
- A 360° peritomy at the limbus is performed and the conjunctiva is released.
- Each extra-ocular muscle is identified, isolated and Vicryl stitch inserted. The muscle is cut away from its attachment to the globe.
- Once all the extra-ocular muscles have been removed from the globe, the eye itself is ready to be removed.
- A snare or enucleation scissors are used to remove the eye by cutting the optic nerve. Any bleeding is controlled using diathermy.
- The amount of volume required is then measured, typically anything from 16 to 22mm (diameter).
- An orbital implant may then be replaced and the sclera wrapped over the implant.
- Then all the extra-ocular muscles are reattached to the Vicryl mesh/implant.
- The Tenon's layer and conjunctiva layer are sutured over the sclera/implant.
- Some surgeons may then place a plastic conformer shell in the socket to help reduce post-operative swelling, along with a suture tarsorrhaphy.

Prior to commencing surgery, it is important to check the patient and perform a WHO check – especially clarifying which eye is to be removed (it may not be distinctly obvious). It is also important to make great efforts to protect the non-operating eye during surgery. Ensure the un-operating eyelids are closed and taped closed.

Protection also applies beyond surgery in that the patient will need to be educated to protect their remaining eye. Encourage the use of protective glasses, especially if work activities and/or social pastimes might pose a risk to the eye.

There are several points that need to be considered peri-operatively in relation to eye removal surgery. Firstly, the implant size is very important with regard to getting the correct fitting of the prosthetic post-operatively. Recently, the consensus has been that the bigger the orbital implant, the better (Custer 2008). This means a smaller and lighter ocular prosthetic, which can in turn mean fewer long-term issues such as lower eyelid ectropion and laxity. However, if it is too big it may be restrictive and the ocular prosthetist may find it more difficult to fit a prosthesis.

As a consequence of the manipulation and stimulation of extra-ocular muscles and ultimately the cutting of the optic nerve, there can be a significant vaso-vagal reaction, causing in some cases a complete cardiac asystole (known as the oculo-cardiac reflex or Aschner phenomenon). This is due to the stimulation of the ophthalmic branch of the trigeminal nerve, of which the efferent arm is the vagus nerve (Cranial Nerve X). If triggered, this nerve can diminish sinoatrial node impulses and then cause bradycardia. A similar response can be initiated with associated post-operative nausea/vomiting – known as the ocular-cardiac vomiting reflex. The anaesthetist, or theatre or scrub practitioner should be aware of this phenomenon, as it is not uncommon. In extreme circumstances, it can cause cardiac arrest (and notably children seem more sensitive to this). The use of a retrobulbar local anaesthetic injection prior to surgery will completely abolish the potential for an oculocardiac reflex.

At the end of the procedure, it is quite common for some surgeons to insert a surgical conformer into the socket. This is usually a clear convex acrylic structure that sits on top of the conjunctiva and behind the eyelids. The role of the conformer is two-fold. Firstly, it helps reduce oedema and inflammation. Secondly, it serves to maintain upper and lower eyelid fornices, which will be important later when the prosthesis is being fabricated. If the fornices are too shallow, it may be difficult to ensure that the prosthesis stays in position.

It is important to inform the patient that a conformer is in place, as they will be aware of something being in the socket and may be unsure what it is and what it is doing there. The conformer will also need to stay in situ for several weeks until such time as the prosthetic eye-piece has been fabricated and fitted.

The insertion of a suture tarsorrhaphy at the end of the procedure (which physically closes the eyelids) will help reduce conjunctival oedema and prevent a conjunctival prolapse. The lids are usually closed with a nylon stitch and plastic bolsters are used on the skin to reduce the chances of the stitch cheese-wiring through the eyelid. The tarsorrhaphy usually stays in position for a few days following the procedure and is taken out in clinic. As a practitioner, it is important to make the patient aware of this suture, as it will need to be cared for and cleaned, and also to ensure that the patient does not try to remove it themselves.

Post-operative care following eye removal

There are several key issues following eye removal surgery. Usually there are more issues related to enucleation than evisceration, but many of these issues can affect the patient no matter which procedure has been undertaken.

Immediately post-operatively, the main issues are likely to be pain and nausea/vomiting. Some patients will still experience the effects of the local anaesthetic immediately after the surgery and may not be affected by pain in the recovery room. However, when the local anaesthetic has worn off 2–3 hours later they may well be in some discomfort. Anecdotally, most of this discomfort seems to be associated with a combination of oedema/swelling, due to the manipulation of tissue and the compressive dressing exerting pressure on the orbit.

As most patients will have a pad and bandage on following surgery, it is important for the practitioner to ensure that this is not applied too tightly as this can contribute quite significantly to post-operative pain. In some cases, the practitioner may have to release some of the pressure of the bandage to allow the patient to gain some comfort. The bandage can be removed the following day after surgery.

Most often than not, simple analgesia will be sufficient to keep the pain under control but it has been shown that some patients do get quite significant pain following this surgery which can be persistent and long-term (Hegarty, Coakley & Dooley 2014). In these cases, it is important to ensure that the appropriate analgesics (such as opioids and non-steroidal anti-inflammatories) are available to be prescribed. Many of these patients will be discharged the following day and the practitioner needs to ensure that they have adequate pain relief to take home. For those patients who are kept hospitalised due to their pain, the input of the pain control nursing team may be required. In my experience, it is often left too late to request the assistance of the pain management team.

Similarly, with nausea/vomiting, early intervention and control are beneficial. Many anaesthetists provide some anti-emetic drugs peri-operatively and also prescribe them post-operatively. However, it is important to remember that there are various modalities associated with anti-emetic drugs and the way they work, and that it may be prudent to use anti-emetics with different modalities to control extreme forms of nausea/vomiting.

In the days following the procedure, patients should be instructed to be aware of signs of infection, including pyrexia, increased pain, swelling, discharge and erythema.

Many patients complain of difficulty in contacting anyone when there is a problem. Practitioners should therefore make the point of providing contact details so the patient can more readily make contact should the need arise. Pre-operatively the practitioner should also provide information and instructions pertaining to the tarsorrhaphy and conformer.

Another issue that some of my patients have complained about is how to deal with the bandage that is often applied at the end of the procedure. This can be reapplied in the immediate post-operative phase but can be left off after 24 hours.

Once the bandage is removed, and any other underlying dressings, the eyelids and surrounding area will need to be kept clean. Therefore it will again be important to show patients how to undertake this safely and with the least possible risk of infection. A basic form of aseptic technique should be shown to the patient, emphasising the need for vigilant handwashing.

There will possibly be inflammation and swelling in the surrounding eyelid tissues for a few days or even weeks following the procedure. This is usually non-infective oedema, but again the patient has to be aware of signs of infection. If the swelling becomes erythematous or hot to touch, with a possible discharge, the patient should seek medical attention as soon as possible.

The prosthesis should not be fitted for at least 8 weeks post-operatively to allow for complete healing of the socket. Once fitted with a prosthesis, the patient should be advised on how to care for it. It will be important to remove it and clean it with a mild, non-scented soap on a regular basis.

Instructing the patient on how to remove the artificial eye:
- Wash hands
- Use a mirror
- Place a towel in front of you – to allow a soft landing for the prosthesis (it can easily get chipped or damaged by falling onto hard surfaces)
- Gently pull the lower eyelid down, the lower edge of the prosthesis will present itself
- Pressure alone may then push the prosthesis out, or an extractor may be used to lever the prosthesis out over the lower eyelid
- There are specialised suction devises that can be used to help remove the prosthesis.

And to put it back in:
- Wash hands
- Use a mirror
- Lift the upper eyelid, slide the top edge of the prosthesis in and hold the position

- Then, with the other hand, pull down the lower eyelid and at the same time manipulate the prosthesis into the socket.

The patient should also use lubricant drops (especially if they have an incomplete blink). If there is an incomplete blink, the prosthesis will need more regular polishing and cleaning.

In the longer term, there may be one or two other issues, including implant exposure or extrusion. Whilst rare, continued friction and irritation of the conjunctiva by the overlying prosthesis can cause thinning and eventual exposure of the orbital implant. In these circumstances, further surgery may be required to cover the defect, possibly using a temporal fascia patch graft.

The same mechanical action can cause continued discharge of mucus and occasionally socket cysts. This may require treatment (for example, with steroids) or even surgical intervention. The patient should also be advised that the prosthetic eye-piece should be kept clean and have an annual polish to keep it in good condition.

References

Adkinsson, J. (2006). *Lost Eye*. iUniverse, USA.

Bailey, F. (1988). *A Singular View: The Art of Seeing with One Eye*. Bailey Publishers.

Custer, P. (2008). *The Choice of Enucleation Implant. American Academy of Ophthalmology.* https://www.aao.org/current-insight/choice-of-enucleation-implant (last accessed 5.12.2019).

Fahim, D., Fruch, B., Much, D. & Nelson, C. (2007). Complications of pegged and non-pegged Hydroxyapatite Implants. *Ophthalmic Plastic and Reconstructive Surgery.* **23**(3), 206–10.

Hegarty, D., Coakley, D. & Dooley, I. (2014). Psychological reactions and persistent facial pain following enucleation. *Pain Research and Treatment.* https://www.hindawi.com/journals/prt/2014/232989/abs/ (last accessed 5.12.2019).

Kondo, T., Tillman, W., Schwartz, T., Linberg, J. & Odon, V. (2013). Health related quality of life after surgical removal of an eye. *Ophthalmic and Plastic Reconstructive Surgery.* **29**(1), 51–56.

Slonium, C. & Martino, A. (2011). *Eye was there: A patient's guide to coping with the loss of an eye* Author House Publishing, USA.

11

Exenteration and socket wound management

Introduction

Very rarely, and for various reasons, it may be necessary to remove not only the eye but also the surrounding tissue, including the eyelids, orbital contents, lacrimal apparatus and even orbital bone. This is known as orbital exenteration surgery. This is life-changing and has a profound effect on the individual involved. Furthermore, the patient may have to endure the removal of a perfectly healthy seeing eye at the same time, and their distress may be compounded by having to undergo adjunctive treatments such as radiotherapy.

A lot of supportive care is necessary and several cosmetic and practical issues have to be addressed. This takes time and can have a big impact on the patient's morale. However, on a positive note, the long-term outcomes can be good, with the appropriate support and prosthetic input.

In this situation, the oculoplastic practitioner's main role is to provide support and wound care. However, any patient who may have to undergo orbital exenteration will need to be cared for by a multidisciplinary team.

Orbital exenteration surgery can be:

- Total
- Sub-total
- Extended.

A total exenteration involves the complete removal of the orbital contents, whereas a sub-total exenteration preserves the eyelids and these can be used to line the orbit (see Figure 11.1, p. 172). An extended exenteration obviously involves other surrounding adnexa.

Indications for exenteration

Orbital exenteration is most commonly associated with (potentially life-threatening) malignant tumours but it can also be undertaken for other disorders, including benign tumours, life-threatening infections, fungal infections, severe orbital deformity, orbital inflammatory disease associated with pain and end-stage socket contracture.

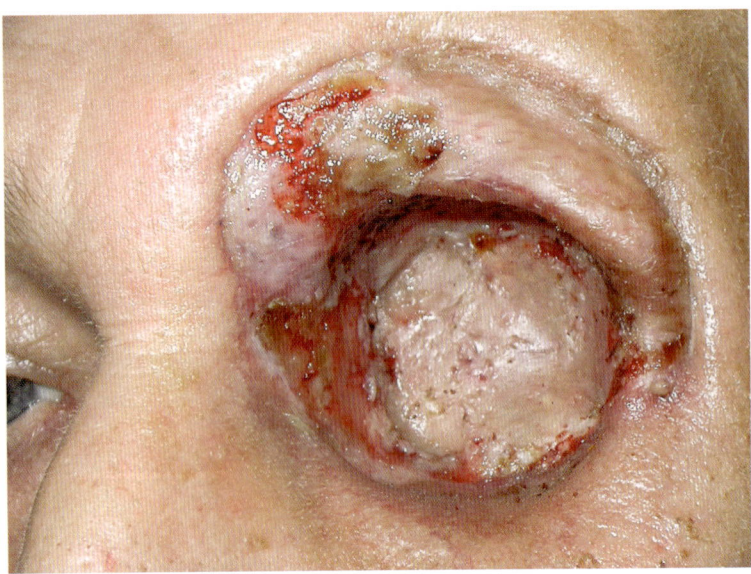

Figure 11.1: Total exenteration

There are several malignant tumours but the most commonly occurring include basal cell carcinoma, squamous cell carcinoma, sebaceous cell carcinoma and melanoma. These can be cutaneous, sinus, primary orbital or lacrimal gland tumours.

Orbital exenteration does not improve survival rates in all cases and this needs to be taken into account when balancing the type and extent of the tumour against the magnitude and likely impact and outcome of the surgery. In certain circumstances it can take up to twelve months to recover from orbital exenteration surgery, with many hospital visits and a great deal of care input. This needs to be borne in mind and may influence clinical decision-making and choice of treatment modalities.

Types of tumours commonly associated with orbital exenteration

Basal cell carcinoma (BCC)

This is the most common type of skin cancer and is sometimes referred to as a 'rodent ulcer'. The cause of BCC is usually related to ultraviolet sun damage (and sunbeds). BCCs are usually slow- growing tumours. They very rarely spread so significantly that orbital exenteration is required to excise them, as they are likely to be identified long before this happens. (For further discussion of BCCs in the eyelid, see Chapter 5.)

Squamous cell carcinoma (SCC)

Again, SCC is related to UV skin damage, which alters the underlying DNA of keratinocytes within the epidermis of the skin, causing an exponential growth of SCC. This type of tumour is more aggressive than BCC and it can metastasise to the lymph nodes (or other areas of the body).

Sebaceous cell carcinoma

This is a rare skin cancer which originates from sebaceous glands within the skin that produce lipids. This type of cancer is relatively slow growing but can again metastasise to other areas of the body. Sebaceous cell carcinoma is associated with other non-cancerous lesions such as benign adenomas, exposure to radiation or a genetic condition known as Muir Torré syndrome.

Melanoma

Cells (melanocytes) between the dermis and the epidermis of the skin help to protect the body from UV light and provide the skin with its natural colour. Over time, UV radiation can cause mutation of the DNA of the melanocytes, leading to cancer (melanoma). Sun damage and sunbeds are the most common cause, but individuals with a large number of moles on their skin have a greater propensity to aquire melanoma, and there is also a genetic link to the disease.

Patients with melanoma will present with various potential symptoms, including proptosis, ptosis, hypoglobus, red-eye, exposed eye, pain and discomfort, an obvious lesion that may discharge, crust over or have a tendency to bleed. It may be very obvious that there is a significant tumorous growth, but not always. Further investigations, including scanning, blood results and biopsy/histopathology, may be required to ascertain the extent of the disease.

Psychosocial considerations

In my experience some patients appear in clinic, having been urgently referred with a lesion, expecting that some surgery may be required to treat the problem, but not necessarily anticipating the potential extent of that treatment. They are often unprepared for the outcome, which may come as a considerable shock. Ideally the breaking of such bad news should be done sensitively and in a way that is as patient-centred as possible. Unfortunately, this isn't always possible in the confines of a busy clinic, and it is often felt that clinicians and nurses are ill prepared to deliver such news.

As oculoplastic practitioners, it is important to seek such training, and a course in breaking bad news or basic counselling skills may be helpful. However, if you are aware that you lack such skills, it may be better to ask someone who already has them to break the news to the patient, in order to avoid causing them any additional distress.

As a practitioner, it is important to be empathetic and give the patient an opportunity to discuss their fears and concerns. Simply offering a listening ear is a good place to start, but be cautious about taking an excessively emotional approach, as this may not be helpful and can end up making the patient feel even more negative and hopeless about their situation.

As oculoplastic practitioners, we are well placed to provide the time, availability and continuity of care required by the patient. And of course the family may well require support as well. I have occasionally heard the comment, 'I can cope, but I worry about my husband,' for instance. Discussing the issues with both the individual and their partner may be helpful, especially if the patient struggles to take in all the information.

Beyond patient- and family-centered requirements, we also need to consider broader cultural, religious and spiritual beliefs. Many individuals may seek solace in their faith in these difficult times and it is wise to have contact details of spiritual services the patient may wish to access within the local community or within the hospital.

The patient needs to fully understand the extent of the problem and, from the practitioner's perspective, it's important that the message is fully understood. You may need to start by finding out how much the patient knows about the condition or problem before bombarding them with new information. This will also help you understand how much the patient wants to know. It is important to give the patient all the information they need, while bearing in mind that they may *not* want to know about particular aspects of the treatment. Once you have found this balance, you can start to provide additional individualised information about specific aspects of the condition and the surgery they may undergo.

Everyone is different so attitudes towards orbital exenteration surgery vary widely. Patients may express anything from belligerent denial or avoidance to surprising acceptance ('there is always someone worse off than me'). Either way there is likely to be a process not dissimilar to grieving. The patient's reaction may be difficult to predict but it is essential that the discussion is undertaken in a structured and planned way. Here are some tips:

- Get it right first time – we have the chance to set the tone for a patient's journey, with careful consideration and planning.
- Get the setting right – make sure it's quiet, private and comfortable.
- Be prepared to spend time with no interruptions and turn the phone off.
- Allow the patient to be accompanied by family members or relatives if they wish.

- Find out what the patient knows – don't assume anything. Patients often know quite a lot, and many will have looked up their condition on the internet and may have insight into their diagnosis and treatment.
- It is essential to clarify poor or wrong information.
- Convey some hope but be clear when presenting the facts – any vagueness or conjecture may result in the patient getting the wrong message.
- Consider the language you are using to convey the message. Avoid jargon and keep it as simple as possible.
- You may not have all the answers to the patient's questions – don't be afraid to admit this and arrange to give them the information when you have found it out.
- It is all right to show some emotion – we are all human. However, there may be a fine balance. If the practitioner expresses too much emotion, it may make things harder for the patient. You may know the patient already or a strong professional relationship may have developed and feelings can spill over. Staff members may also require support so it may be prudent to consider how this can be arranged.
- We can't always judge what constitutes bad news. Remember, for some individuals, orbital exenteration may provide a sense of relief that they are getting rid of the problem.
- The process demands a lot of energy both from the patient and the carer. After the meeting, the practitioner may require an opportunity to reflect or talk about it.

Some practitioners may even follow a recognised protocol to approach such an issue. A commonly used methodology is the SPIKES template (Baile, Buckman, Lenzi *et al.* 2000). Although every situation is unique, it is useful to have a protocol to follow. The acronym SPIKES stands for:

Setting up – preparing as outlined above

Perception – ascertaining what the patient knows and what questions they have

Invitation – to share what the patient wishes to know

Knowledge – providing information about the issue, but initially warning the patient that there may be bad news

Emotions with empathy – addressing the patient's response

Strategy – creating a clear plan going forward.

This is a widely accepted and valued approach to conveying bad news and instigating a structured approach to the initial meetings with the patient. Most of the points outlined by the protocol have been discussed above, but the last element suggests that a strategy needs to be developed for the future, beyond in this case the surgical procedure. It may be that a specific time and place has to be arranged to have such a conversation, but nonetheless at the end of the discussion both the patient and the practitioner should have a clear plan for the next stage. Certainly, the patient is likely to require time to digest the diagnosis and treatment plan.

Post-operatively the socket may eventually be able to accept a prosthesis – usually a bespoke handmade unit fabricated from silicone. However, the fabrication process requires several stages and this will need to be planned and discussed with the patient. Consequently, there is something to aim for regarding recovery. Whilst it is by no means perfect, the prosthesis provides an end point and may allow the individual to get on with their life relatively normally.

Interestingly some patients aren't keen to have a prosthesis (given all the treatment required in order to have one and wear it on a regular basis) and they may opt to just wear eye pads.

Exenteration care requires a multi-disciplinary team approach, whenever possible. Good communication across the wider oculoplastic team is vital in streamlining care and the oculoplastic nurse practitioner is undoubtedly central to this process.

Pre-operative considerations

Apart from the psychological preparation, there are some other practical issues that need to be considered prior to surgery. Firstly, there is a reasonable prospect of blood loss during the procedure and if the patient is on anti-platelets or anti-coagulants this will of course contribute to this. Therefore, careful management of any blood thinning therapies is required before surgery.

Preparing the patient for the post-operative outcomes is very important. They need to know that there is likely to be some pain and discomfort, although (interestingly) not as much you might expect.

Nausea/vomiting is quite likely, given the nature of the surgery, and it may be necessary to administer anti-emetics both during the surgery and immediately post-operatively.

It is really important to warn the patient that there will be numbness in the maxillary and forehead regions and this is likely to be permanent. The infra and superior orbital nerves are often sacrificed during the surgery, which means that these areas will feel numb afterwards. This may be something that patients find difficult to cope with. I can recall a patient I looked after who struggled for many years after orbital exenteration surgery because he had numbness particularly in the cheek area, and found the sensation disturbing.

Again, it is equally important to outline the wound care regime following surgery and this ultimately depends on the type of exenteration performed and the subsequent reconstruction. I have developed a wound care assessment tool – The Manchester Orbital Exenteration Wound Assessment Tool (MOEWAT) (Cooper & Waterman 2011) to help provide a consistent and reliable mechanism to evaluate the socket post-operatively and this should be introduced pre-operatively.

Prior to surgery, it is necessary to get facial photographs (with the patient's permission). Additionally, the patient will require their scans to be available to review during the surgery. Make sure any pre-operative scans are available.

A full pre-assessment work-up should be undertaken, including up-to-date bloods, basic observations and an outline of the patient history including allergies. Ensure that contact details are available for relatives and friends.

Having considered a care plan based on the activities of daily living, certain issues may be highlighted that require further input and support. One particular area might be the significant loss of vision as a consequence of losing an eye. This might require the provision of further aids and support mechanisms around the home, although this might be difficult to arrange in the short time prior to surgery. Organisations such as Henshaws (www.henshaws.org.uk) can often provide such support.

Table 11.1: The Manchester Orbital Exenteration Wound Assessment Tool (MOEWAT)

1. BMI (↓↑)	No change = 0	BMI of 1 = 1	BMI of 2 = 2	More than 2 = 3	
2. Bone exposure	Nil/lid-sparing = 0	Small 0–25% = 1	Med 25–50% = 2	Large 50–75% = 3	Exten 75%↑ = 4
3. Wound appearance					
a. Necrotic	Nil = 0	Small 0–25% = 1	Med 25–50% = 2	Large 50–75% = 3	Exten 75%↑ = 4
b. Yellow slough	Nil = 0	Small 0–25% = 1	Med 25–50% = 2	Large 50–75% = 3	Exten 75%↑ = 4
c. Red granulation	Nil = 0	Small 0–25% = 1	Med 25–50% = 2	Large 50–75% = 3	Exten 75%↑ = 4
d. Epithelialisation	Nil = 0	Small 0–25% = 1	Med 25–50% = 2	Large 50–75% = 3	Exten 75%↑ = 4
e. Overgranulation	Nil = 0	Small 0–25% = 1	Med 25–50% = 2	Large 50–75% = 3	Exten 75%↑ = 4
4. Fistula/Sinus	Absent = 0	Present 0–1/3 = 1	Present >1/3 = 5		
5. Exudate					
a. Type	Nil = 0	Serous = 1	Haemoserous = 2	Purilent = 3	
b. Amount wound	Nil = 0	Low 0–30% = 1	Mod 30–60% = 2	High 60↑ = 3	
c. Amount dressing	Nil = 0	Low 0–30% = 1	Mod 30–60% = 2	High 60↑ = 3	

6. Wound margin				
a. Oedema	No = 0	Yes = 1		
b. Maceration	No = 0	Yes (0–50%) = 1	Yes (50–100%) = 2	
7. Pain Score (VNRS)				
a. General	Nil = 0	Low 0–3 = 1	Mod 4–7 = 2	Severe 8–10 = 3
b. Dressing	Nil = 0	Low 0–3 = 1	Mod 4–7 = 2	Severe 8–10 = 3
8. Therapy	No = 0	Yes = 3		

Orbital exenteration surgery

Prior to commencing surgery, it is important to check the patient and perform a WHO check – especially clarifying which eye is to be removed (it may not be distinctly obvious). It is also important to make great effort to protect the non-operating eye during surgery. Ensure the un-operating eyelids are closed and taped closed.

Protection also applies beyond surgery in that the patient will need to be educated to protect their remaining eye, encouraging the use of protective glasses especially if work and/or social pastimes might provide risk to the eye.

Most patients who undergo this surgery have a general anaesthetic, but it can also be undertaken under a local anaesthetic with sedation if the patient isn't deemed medically stable enough to have a general anaesthetic. Even patients who are having a general anaesthetic should also be given a local anaesthetic block with adrenaline. This will initiate some short-term analgesia in recovery and also provides vasoconstriction, reducing peri-operative bleeding.

Manipulating extra-ocular muscles, and eventually severing the optic nerve, can provoke the oculocardiac reflex (Aschner phenomenon) which can cause a significant bradycardia or even asystole. It is important that the anaesthetist and their support team are aware of this and that they take suitable precautions, usually by administering glycopyrrolate (a muscarinic anticholinergic medicine). Pre-operative peribulbar local anaesthetic injection will also reduce the oculocardiac reflex.

Total exenteration

This approach involves removing all orbital soft tissue including the eyelids and lacrimal apparatus. The area to be removed is marked and a blade or monopolar cutting diathermy device is used to dissect all the way around the orbital rim and down to the periosteum. The periosteum is then lifted and deflected off the bone of the socket using an elevator (commonly a Freer's elevator).

The periosteum is dissected off all the orbital plains: roof, floor, medially and laterally. All the major blood vessels are cauterised and the nerves severed along the way. Careful dissection along the orbital roof is required, as the roof can be quite thin and any break may cause a leak of cerebral spinal fluid (CSF). Continued dissection is taken all the way to the apex of the orbit dorsally, beyond the globe, depending on how much tissue has to be excised to remove the tumour.

Once the periosteum is completely freed, the remaining soft tissue, including the optic nerve, is cut (or a disposable snare can be used), freeing the final tissue at the apex of the orbit. The specimen is removed, checked and transferred to the histopathology container.

Subsequent reconstruction may involve:

- Spontaneous granulation, in which the socket is left to granulate from the orbital wound edges. This approach is rarely used and usually only if the procedure needs to be completed quickly due to the medical instability of the patient. Perhaps surprisingly, the outcomes can be quite good, but healing time can be very lengthy (taking 12 months or more).
- A split-thickness skin graft (STSG) into the socket. An STSG can be harvested, usually from the thigh, and used to line the socket. This can heal very well (within a couple of months) but there will be the co-morbidity of the donor site to manage as well as the socket.
- Temporalis muscle transposition flap or bi-lobed forehead flap/cheek advancement flap – a maxillofacial approach to filling and covering the socket. This often results in a shallower socket, which may make prosthetic rehabilitation difficult. There will also be either a temporalis or forehead defect which some patients may find unsatisfactory. However, there is less healing time, as the socket has been covered.

Sub-total orbital exenteration

This surgical approach is similar to a total exenteration but the eyelids are spared. Once the orbital contents have been removed, the lid skin is stitched together and used to line the socket. This makes for a much quicker recovery and fewer wound healing issues. Immediately post-surgery, the same regime described below, using Lyofoam® (Seton Healthcare) and Mepitel (Molnlycke), should be followed to prevent adhesion of the dressings. The Lyofoam is cut into circular pledgets, which are layered on top of each other until the socket is filled and Mepitel is placed over the top.

Occasionally, the lid wound can open and become dehisced, leading to leakage of fluid from behind the lids. This may be because there is a void or pocket behind the closed lids within which fluid can accumulate and cause issues. It may be advisable to warn the patient pre-operatively that this can happen in rare cases. Usually the wound heals well but it might require closer monitoring initially.

Split-thickness skin graft (STSG)

As previously mentioned, a split-thickness skin graft can be harvested (usually from the thigh) to line the socket. In theatre a dermatome is used to harvest the skin. This is a hand-held electric, battery- or sometimes air-driven device that slices a predetermined depth of skin, using a blade and cutting mechanism (5,000–6,000 cycles per minute). The depth and width of the graft are pre-selected. Once the skin has been harvested, there will be an exposed and raw area of dermis on the thigh. A non-stick foam dressing may be used to protect the wound and wick any serosanguinous fluid away.

Once harvested, the STSG can be passed through a meshing device (rather like a mangle) which puts little perforations into the harvested skin. This allows it to expand and potentially cover a wider space. Having placed the skin so that it lines the socket, a combination of glue and/or stitching is used pin the graft in. I then use Mepitel 8 x 10cm (Molnlycke) silicone dressing over the graft. In order to gently apply pressure onto the graft and pin it to the back of the orbit, a series of ever-larger circular pledgets of Lyofoam® (Seton Healthcare) can be layered into the socket. Alternatively, AquaCell® (Convatec) ribbon can be used.

Over the coming weeks and months, it may be necessary to repeat this dressing regime until such time as the graft has completely granulated. I have found that applying a non-stick/atraumatic membrane provides additional assurance that the foam will not stick. I use Mepitel 12 x 15cm® (Molnlycke) silicone dressing and then Allevyn non-adhesive 10 x 20cm foam dressing® (Smith & Nephew) and initially cover with a light bandage.

At the first dressing consultation, usually a week after surgery, take care when removing the dressing as it can be painful. I may continue to use this dressing regime until such time as the wound has granulated. For several months the patient may find it uncomfortable to wear trousers or especially jeans over the donor site wound as it is very sensitive. Once the dressings have stopped, the patient will be encouraged to keep the wound clean and apply Vaseline to soften the skin.

Post-operative care

There are some specific post-operative issues related to recovery following orbital exenteration and the practitioner therefore needs to:

1. Monitor and treat pain. Remarkably, in my experience, post-operative pain is mild to moderate in most patients so a simple analgesic regime (such as paracetamol/

codeine phosphate) may be sufficient to keep discomfort under control. Certainly, in the period immediately after surgery, it will be necessary to monitor the patient's pain. You should also ensure that the patient has appropriate analgesia on discharge.

2. Treat nausea and vomiting. Some patients complain of nausea after the procedure and this can be controlled with anti-emetics which can be instigated peri-operatively by the anaesthetist. Simple measures can also be undertaken by the patient, including drinking clear ice-cold drinks, eating small amounts of bland foods such as rice or plain crackers, and drinking ginger tea.

3. Monitor bleeding in case of haemorrhage. Occasionally there may be a small post-operative bleed that soils the dressing. This is usually minimal and ceases with gentle pressure or a compressive bandage and is nothing to worry about. However, a profuse bleed that soaks the dressing and doesn't appear to stop with simple first aid may require the patient to return to theatre for further cautery. Close monitoring is essential for the first 48–72 hours after the procedure. Ensure the patient takes plenty of rest and doesn't over-exert themselves, as this may trigger a bleed. It might be useful to consider constipation medication if required to reduce the possibility of over-straining.

4. Encourage the patient to mobilise in order to reduce the risk of deep vein thrombosis.

5. Check for infection. Over the course of the healing period following surgery there is a risk of infection which will warrant antibiotics. The wound care may need to be more frequent to keep control of any exudate, including dressing changes every 3–4 days. Topical antibiotics in the socket (such as chloramphenicol ointment) may only have limited effect. Alternative dressings can be considered in these circumstances. For example, Aquacell Ag® Ribbon (Convatec) is useful for controlling exudate and (due to its silver content) can help combat infection and colonisation.

6. Monitor for tissue necrosis. There can be some tissue loss or necrosis and quite often not all of the grafted material will survive. It may be necessary to remove any dead tissue with Westcott scissors.

7. Control overgranulation. Alternatively, during the healing phase, there can be overgranulation of tissue that can interfere with healing. Overgranulation can appear as a soft, shiny, oedematous tissue and may be associated with an increase of exudate. Outside the orbit, foam dressings can help to control overgranulation but this is difficult within the orbit. Topical steroids or silver nitrate can be applied to reduce overgranulation.

8. Monitor sinus formation into the nasal cavity. The ethmoid bones of the medial aspect of the orbit are very thin and can break down during the recovery period, creating a track into the nasal cavity. This will not heal over and can disrupt healing within the socket. However, a socket prosthesis can occlude this passage so it may not prevent rehabilitation continuing. Sinuses can present other practical problems, as anything can migrate from the nasal cavity into the socket, especially when the patient has a heavy cold or smokes! The important thing is to reassure the patient that this is a common occurrence and won't necessarily stop their recovery continuing.

9. Optimise wound healing. Several factors can affect wound healing and it is important to help the patient control these where possible. The relevant factors include smoking, obesity, poor nutrition, certain medical conditions such as diabetes, and temperature regulation. Conversely, during this difficult time, the patient may not be at their most willing to consider smoking cessation or modifying their diet. It may therefore be best to suggest small improvements at first (such as encouraging them to consider eating more fruit, for example) rather than major lifestyle changes.

10. Use a recognised wound assessment tool to monitor subtle changes in the wound healing process. For instance, the MOEWAT (Cooper & Waterman 2011), which has been specifically developed for orbital wound care, can be used to provide a regular and consistent monitoring tool.

11. Remember that many patients will require concurrent therapy. Some patients will commence radiotherapy soon after the surgery and this is likely to affect wound healing, so this needs to be anticipated. Extra clinic time and support may be required.

Choosing an orbital prosthesis

At the end of the healing journey, there is an opportunity to consider what options are available to disguise the socket. At present, a few centres have an oculoprosthetic department that can fabricate an orbital prosthesis. Otherwise, the maxillofacial services can make an orbital prosthesis, after the patient has been reviewed in one of their outreach clinics.

It will take several visits in order to create the final product and this may take many weeks to complete'. The orbital prosthesis is largely made of silicone and has to be glued into place within the socket and around the orbital rim. Wearing glasses over the prosthesis (even without a prescription) can help to disguise the edges of the prosthesis, making it less obvious.

Not everyone will relish the prospect of using a silicone prosthesis and some may experience frustration when positioning and wearing it. If it is not secured well, it can fall out, causing embarrassment and frustration. On the positive side, many patients would not be seen without their prosthetic orbital implant and can regain a lot of confidence by using it. The prosthesis serves several functions (essentially of course to provide cosmesis) but it obviously has its limitations – it can't move or blink, it won't change colour as normal skin might, some patients may have intolerance to the glues used, and it is often difficult to work with when getting it into position or gluing the edges. Society often expects physical perfection and symmetry, and we all feel the need to confirm to this. Consequently, some individuals are very keen to look 'normal' after exenteration and will therefore persevere with wearing the prosthesis. For instance, they may say, 'I wear my prosthesis for everyone else, not for me'. But some choose not to wear a prosthetic eye or even abandon their prosthesis, preferring to use a stick-on patch or a 'pirate' patch over the orbit.

A small number of individuals do not wear anything and are happy to go about their lives with the empty socket uncovered. No matter which option the patient adopts, we need to support their decision (as oculoplastic practitioners) and get them to where they want to be.

Titanium orbital implants

A minority of patients have had titanium orbital implants placed in the orbital rim and magnets inserted into their prosthesis in order to fix it in place better. In my experience, however, these often have mixed outcomes, with implants falling out or becoming unstable over time. However, as an oculoplastic practitioner, you may still come across this in your practice.

Conclusion

There is little doubt that orbital exenteration surgery has a profound effect upon those unfortunate individuals who have to endure it. As practitioners, we go to great lengths to provide that support. Patients need to know, from the start, that after surgery the journey is a long one, with many ups and downs. We should strive to guide the patient to the end goal as best we can, but it will be challenging for all concerned.

References

Baile, W., Buckman, R., Lenzi, R., Glober, G., Beale, E. & Kudelka, A. (2000). SPIKES – a six step protocol for delivering bad news: application to the patient with cancer. *Oncologist*. **5**(1), 302–11.

Cooper, J. & Waterman, H. (2011). The MOEWAT as a proposed method of evaluating orbital exenteration wounds. *British Journal of Woundcare*. **20**(10), 478–83.

Henshaws (2019). https://www.henshaws.org.uk/ (last accessed 19.11.2019).

12

Emergency oculoplastic care

Introduction

Many tertiary and some district hospitals will have a dedicated eye emergency centre or unit run by a mixture of nurse practitioners and ophthalmic medical colleagues. Apart from these specialist units, there are of course general Accident and Emergency (A&E) departments, which accommodate individuals who require urgent care, some ultimately involving ophthalmic issues. Within all these units an ophthalmic doctor may be called upon to review cases and treat patients accordingly.

Undoubtedly, some of the cases presenting at these units require some oculoplastic team involvement. These cases can involve anything from simple lacerations to complex multiple medical conditions, acute illness or life-threatening multi-organ/system injuries.

It is clearly impossible to cover all the potential eventualities that might present in an A&E department so this chapter focuses on the more common conditions and injuries that are likely to occur. Undeniably, different A&E units will have differing approaches, policies and procedures related to specific issues – for example, using different antibiotic regimes to treat a particular condition. It may therefore be advisable to check all treatment regimes discussed in this chapter against the protocol in your own hospital or unit.

There are certain organisations that are dedicated to providing consistency and best practice in emergency ophthalmic care. One such body is the British Emergency Eye Care Society (BEECS). Furthermore, there are some dedicated ophthalmic related emergency care texts that will offer greater depth and context for broader eye emergencies such as *Eye Emergencies: a practitioner's guide* (Field, Tillotson & Whittingham 2015) and the *Handbook of Emergency Ophthalmology* (Long & Koyfman 2018).

It is also worth noting that some of the more commonly occurring urgent issues outlined below may occasionally present in individuals who have several other related (or unrelated) modalities that require treatment. For example, a patient who is involved in a road traffic accident may have various other injuries. For ease of understanding, I have treated each of the specifically oculoplastic-related issues below as isolated presentations, but the practitioner should of course be aware of other aetiology and potential problems when carrying out their assessment.

When working in emergency care, there can be a tendency to focus solely on the presenting injury or medical problem. However, practitioners also need to consider other related complications such as psychosocial issues, mental health/wellbeing, learning disabilities and safeguarding problems. Many of these related and extremely important issues are covered in much greater depth in other publications.

The oculoplastic practitioner is unlikely to work within an A&E department, and therefore often only becomes involved in the care of such patients secondarily, maybe prior to surgery or subsequently in the outpatients' department. However, greater knowledge and understanding of the emergency care that has already been rendered will provide a foundation for the patient's subsequent care. At this point, it is crucial for the oculoplastic practitioner to fully appreciate and elicit the chronological history of the patient and the treatment provided to date. A vigilant and thorough practitioner will be able to formulate more structured care by means of good history-taking and attentive observation.

Key triage points

When the patient presents at the Eye Emergency Department (EED), the practitioner has to undertake a full and thorough assessment (bearing in mind that the patient may be unconscious). The triage stages are as follows.

1. The incident

Initially it is important to note the time, date and place where the incident or problem started to occur. It would be foolhardy always to assume that it happened within hours of the patient presenting – it may have ensued days or even weeks prior to arriving in the EED. Some individuals may quite innocently ignore or trivialise an injury or problem, thinking that it has had no further consequence, until it causes other issues.

It may be sensible to ascertain whether there were any witnesses to the incident, particularly in relation to children or if the individual lost consciousness. It is also prudent to get an independent account of what happened. Careful and diligent questioning will allow the practitioner to ascertain the facts and gather more understanding of the preceding circumstances as well as those following the event, whilst evaluating the evidence and rejecting anything that is irrelevant or incorrect. This is a skill in its own right, balancing considerable underpinning knowledge gained from years of experience with detective expertise in order to get a clear picture of events. Practitioners need to be able to listen to the patient and ask the appropriate open questions that will elicit the information required, whilst at the same time maintaining clarity and an understanding of the context in which events may have occurred. Remember, the patient may be upset, emotional, in pain and frightened, amongst many other emotions. It may therefore be difficult to gain a clear understanding and appreciation of the history.

Of course, it is extremely important to record in writing all the relevant information, whilst also reporting some of the less obviously significant facts. Some of the information you elicit may have wider use, beyond a medical context (in legal proceedings, for example), so remember to record the facts accurately and clearly.

The mechanism of the injury is important, especially if there has been a head injury and any associated loss of consciousness, fitting, nausea or vomiting. Again, it is useful to understand the relationship between each of these symptoms if there is one. It is equally important to ascertain if there have been any other injuries elsewhere on the body, recording their location and extent. It may be necessary, particularly if the patient is unconscious, to look for any other injuries by undertaking a full body/system assessment. This needs to be done carefully so as to not cause any further injury or discomfort, whilst being sensitive and empathetic.

If the problem is not trauma-related and is associated with a medical condition, it is equally necessary to ascertain date of onset, the nature of the symptoms and how they have manifested subsequently (i.e. whether they have got worse, whether there have there been additional issues, and what the patient has done to control the symptoms).

2. Ophthalmic symptoms

It is essential to ascertain the symptoms in relation to the eye. These may include pain, diplopia (double vision), floaters, flashes, loss of vision (whether sudden or gradual), blurring of vision, field defects, swelling (of lids). Ascertaining the duration, magnitude and severity of the symptoms is also important.

3. Visual acuity (VA)

The visual acuity test is vital as a simple way of assessing the distance vision potential and it should be carried out as early as possible. LogMar visual acuity is arguably more sensitive as a measurement of distance vision than the Snellen test, but any VA is better than none. Remember to ensure that the patient is wearing their glasses, or that they have their contact lenses in (if they wear them). If a chart is not readily available there are several downloadable apps that can be used on a mobile phone, but check their suitability and reliability before using them.

4. Past medical and ophthalmic history

Make sure you gain a picture of the past medical, surgical and ophthalmic history where possible, as the presenting complaint may turn out to be an exacerbation of a previously known condition (such as thyroid eye disease).

5. Social history

Gaining an understanding of the patient's social history will give the practitioner a broader understanding of the context within which the patient may be presenting, including, for example, smoking, alcohol intake, work, drug misuse and family support.

6. Medications

It is extremely important to understand what medications the patient is taking. If they are not able to tell you this, they may be carrying an up-to-date prescription. Looking at a prescription sheet may help you understand the underlying medical history, especially if the patient can't remember or is unconscious. Specifically, it is helpful to know what ophthalmic medications they are using.

Don't forget to ask about any herbal or homeopathic remedies or mineral supplements as well.

It may be necessary to clarify these details with the patient's GP or with a relative/partner.

7. Allergies

Ascertain whether the patient has had any reactions (especially to particular medications) or any intolerance of particular drugs.

8. Visual assessment

Apart from the VA (which is very important), it is necessary to undertake an assessment for a relative afferent pupillary defect (RAPD), using a torch and swinging-light test to observe for the pupils' reaction to light in both eyes. Usually when a bright light is shone into an eye, both the pupils will constrict equally and when the light is taken away they will both enlarge equally. However, if there is an afferent defect (signals not going from the eye to the brain), there is likely to be less (or absent) pupil constriction in the affected eye.

Colour vision (red-green defect) needs to be assessed using an Ishihara book. This test helps determine whether there is any colour desaturation between the eyes which may suggest optic nerve issues.

Also, a visual field test helps to elicit disruption or dysfunction in the patient's central and peripheral vision. Several conditions may affect the field of view, including stroke, pituitary lesion, glaucoma, brain tumour and neurological defects. A simple confrontational field test can be undertaken by the practitioner in the clinic, or a more formal test can be performed using a perimeter machine.

Check the eye movements if possible by getting the patient to follow a finger and pen tip, usually in an H-shape. Observe for any misalignment or if the patient complains of diplopia. Record your findings and if you have any uncertainty organise an orthoptic check.

9. Intra-ocular pressure (IOP)

The IOP needs to be assessed, ideally with an applanation tonometer (AP) but this may not be possible given the nature of the injury. Alternative approaches may include an

ICare tonometer machine to measure IOP, which is hand-held and less invasive than AP tonometry. The normal range is between 14 and 22mmHg, although this varies slightly during the day. Remember to record the method, time and outcome pressure in the notes.

Also, remember the eye may have a laceration (seen or otherwise) and be unstable. If checking pressure, bear this in mind so as not to cause any further damage inadvertently.

10. Assessment of the eyes

A structured approach should be adopted to assess the eyes, essentially working grossly from the outside, towards and then into the eye.

- Face: Look for symmetry (palsy), lacerations, lesions, fractures (nose). Test for loss of sensation – use the end of a rolled-up tissue or cotton ball to touch the skin of the face (with the patient's eyes closed) and ask them to comment if they feel the sensation (and if it varies from side to side) upon the forehead, cheek and jaw (essentially following the trigeminal nerve CNV – V1, V2 and V3).
- Orbit: Sensation, gently feel round the bony rims of the orbit to ensure they are intact.
- Lids: Look for lacerations, malposition, lesions, swelling, oedema, ptosis. Measure the degree of ptosis – marginal reflex distance MRD1 (see p. 46). Remember to evert the upper eyelid if possible.
- Globe: Look for hypo/hyperglobus (eye has moved down or up), proptosis (eye has moved forward), enophthalmos (recession of the eye into the orbit), rupture.
- Conjunctiva: Look for subconjunctival haemorrhage, chemosis, infection, discharge.
- Sclera: Look for jaundice, thinning, laceration, lesion.
- Cornea: Using a slit lamp, look for abrasion, laceration, opacity, infiltrate, limbitis.
- Anterior chamber (AC): Using a slit lamp, consider the depth of the AC, flare, cells, blood, infection.
- Iris: PEARL (Pupils Equal And Reactive to Light?), anisocoria, traumatic mydriasis (dilation), foreign body, iridodonesis (vibration of the iris).
- Lens: Opacity, dislodged (subluxation), foreign body, pseudophakic.
- Vitreous: Haemorrhage, foreign body.
- Fundus: Fundoscopy (retina detachment, oedema, haemorrhage, tear, optic nerve).

From an entirely oculoplastic perspective, the gross anatomy will be the focus of your attention, but it is important to check the eye for any potential issues, such as a globe rupture. Further investigation might involve a B scan (ultrasound) or computerised tomography (CT) scan (orbits/face) with 2mm slices (so as not to miss anything).

11. Lid eversion

As mentioned above, lid eversion is crucial to ascertain whether there are any issues related to the underside of the upper eyelid. Everting the lower eyelid is usually straightforward, while the upper is slightly trickier (see Chapter 3 for further details). The steps are as follows:

1. Get the patient to look down.

2. If you are right-handed, use your left hand to gently take hold of the patient's upper eyelid eyelashes with your thumb and forefinger, and gently pull down and away from the globe.

3. At the same time, using a cotton bud in the right hand to press down onto the upper eyelid just behind the superior edge of the tarsal plate, pull the lid upwards with your left hand.

4. Remove the cotton tip.

5. Gently hold the lid upwards with the thumb of the left hand. If executed correctly, the upper eyelid will fold at the junction of the superior edge of the tarsal plate, but it can be tricky in certain patients (especially if they have short or absent eyelashes). In this position, you may be able to observe the palpebral conjunctiva for lacerations, follicles, papillae and foreign bodies. It will also enable you to see the top of the globe and, to some extent, the anterior lacrimal gland, so any lesions or swelling may be observed.

Investigations

Blood tests

Various blood tests may be required, depending on the particular circumstances. These may include:

- Full blood count (FBC)
- Urea & Electrolytes (U&Es)
- Thyroid function test (TFT) and thyroperoxidase antibodies (TPO)
- Inflammatory markers – antinuclear antibodies (ANA), antineutrophil cytoplastic antibodies (ANCA), angiotensin converting enzyme (ACE), C-reactive protein (CRP), erythrocyte sedimentation rate (ESR)
- Immunoglobulins (IgA, IgG, IgM)

Computerised tomography scan (CT scan)

This uses x-rays from a multitude of angles, which are computerised to create a cross-sectional image. These images are particularly good for bone and tumours.

CT scans are cheaper and quicker than MRI scans but expose the patient to a significant dose of radiation and some patients may be allergic to the contrast mediums used. Some x-ray departments insist on an up-to-date renal function test prior to injecting contrast.

Magnetic resonance imaging (MRI) scan

This uses radio waves and magnets to create an image. The radio waves rebound off the water and fat within the tissue and are captured to create an image. An MRI full-body scanner can be claustrophobic for the patient and very noisy so patients have to wear ear protection. It is also contraindicated for patients who have pacemakers and various other metal implants. Generally, MRI scans are good at showing soft tissue and reveal excellent anatomical detail.

X-ray

This is rarely requested as x-rays have been largely superseded in orbital imaging by CT or MRI scanning. However, x-rays may show objects that are not radio-opaque, such as wood and glass.

Ophthalmic ultrasound B scan

Acoustic echoes present two-dimensional images that can be useful in identifying posterior segment pathology and intra-ocular masses. A hand-held transducer is placed over closed eyelids and, with lubrication gel, an image can be generated on a screen. This is a relatively quick, cheap and painless way of providing simple images of the globe to view particular pathology. It also has some uses within oculoplastics, and is especially useful in identifying intra-ocular tumours.

Exophthalmometry

This test is useful to measure the degree of bulging of the eye anteriorly (also known as proptosis). The exophthalmometer (see Figure 12.1, p. 192) is held in place by the practitioner, resting against the orbital rims. This device uses prisms (with a measurement scale) to discern the degree of proptosis in millimetres, allowing the observer to view and record the extent of proptosis. The measurement is the distance from the edge of the orbital rim to the anterior aspect of the cornea.

One has to be consistent, using the same type of exophthalmometer each time and recording findings, including the model used and the inter-pupillary distance, as this can vary between models. The normal range of globe position is 12 to 21mm. Anything greater than this would be deemed proptosis. Also, if the difference between each eye is more than 2mm, this might be significant. Be aware that there can be differences between races and there is also a degree of subjectivity in individual operators' assessments.

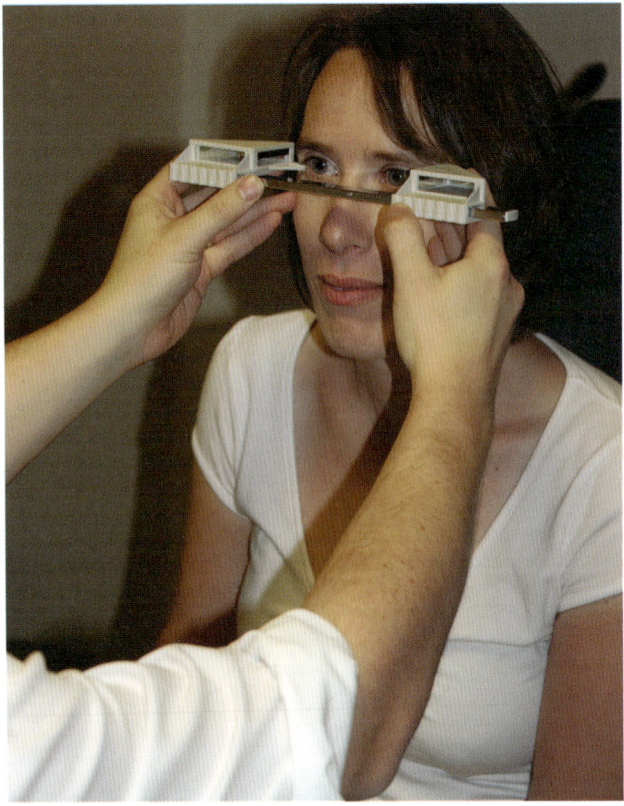

Figure 12.1: Exophthalmometer

Auscultation

Using a stethoscope bell placed on a closed eye can elicit a 'bruit'. This is an auditory sound generated by a flow (usually turbulent) of blood in an artery due to an obstruction or an unusually high rate of blood flow which is unrestricted. This may be associated with a carotid cavernous fistula (CCF), which is an abnormal communication between the arterial/venous system, causing venous blood flow to be hindered by the arterial pressure within the cavernous sinus. This creates an engorgement of the vessels in the eye, proptosis, loss of vision and a bruit.

Selected presentations that may occur in the EED

It would be impossible to consider all the clinical presentations that could potentially occur in any given eye emergency unit, but there are some relatively common oculoplastic pathologies that should be covered. Stabilising the patient systematically obviously takes priority over any eye considerations and any subsequent surgical reconstruction may have to be delayed until such time as it is safe to proceed. In the following section, I have assumed that the patient has already been stabilised.

Orbital cellulitis

There are very few real non-trauma eye emergencies but orbital cellulitis is one of them and the oculoplastic practitioner will need to be aware of how it presents and how to manage it subsequently, as time is of the essence with this potentially life-threatening condition.

Essentially, orbital cellulitis refers to inflammation of the tissues *behind* the orbital septum, as opposed to pre-septal cellulitis, which is inflammation of tissue anterior to the septum. Pre-septal cellulitis is much less serious, but should still be treated appropriately. Orbital cellulitis is caused by a bacterial infection which typically spreads from the adjacent paranasal sinuses, but it can also be associated with trauma and via bloodstream spreading from other sources.

There are three main bacterial species which are commonly associated with orbital cellulitis:

- Staphylococcus aureus – most commonly spread from the skin
- Streptococcus pneumoniae – usually infects the sinuses and spreads
- Beta-haemolytic streptococci.

Common causes for orbital cellulitis include the spread of bacteria from the sinuses, or (more rarely) from infections of the skin, foreign bodies, dacryocystitis, infected orbital implants and dental abscesses.

It is worth reiterating that orbital cellulitis is a potentially life-threatening condition. If misdiagnosed or not treated appropriately, there could be serious consequences, especially in children in whom it most commonly presents and can degenerate very quickly – within hours. If there is any suspicion of orbital cellulitis, oral antibiotics must be administered as a matter of urgency. Therefore the patient should be admitted to hospital and kept nil by mouth initially (as they may need to go to theatre).

The patient will present with swollen, painful, erythematous eyelids, which may be so enlarged as to be completely closed. It may be difficult for the patient to open their eyelids making it hard to carry out visual acuity testing. However, where possible, it is still crucial to check the patient's vision. It may be helpful to use a surgical marking pen to mark the extent of the erythematous swelling so as to assess its progression.

It is important to gain an understanding of when the swelling started, and the nature of the progression of the symptoms, and record this in the notes. Predisposing previous history may include sinusitis or dacryocystitis.

Apart from swelling of the eyelids, ocular symptoms of orbital cellulitis may include proptosis, chemosis and limitation of eye movement (ophthalmoplegia). The patient may also present with other generalised symptoms including flu-like signs such as pyrexia (check their temperature), lethargy, nausea/vomiting and nasal drip.

A full ocular examination will be necessary and this should also include IOP, RAPD, pupil size and fundoscopy. The practitioner should be cautious about dilating the pupil, as this could mask a deterioration of visual symptoms (especially in children).

Other potential differential diagnoses may need to be excluded as they present with similar symptoms. These include other conditions with inflammatory causes (such as dacryocystitis, thyroid eye disease and idiopathic orbital inflammation) and vascular malformation, neoplastic tumour or trauma.

The patient should be CT scanned as a matter of urgency, particularly if there is any suspicion of orbital involvement. The resulting scan may show a distinct collection of pus and this needs to be surgically drained. It is important to check when the patient last ate and drank, as they may have to go to theatre as soon as possible to have pus drained. In this case, they will need to be nil by mouth.

It is also appropriate to undertake a full range of blood tests, especially a full blood count, as this is likely to show a raised white cell count (WCC). Other blood tests may rule out other aetiologies, such as thyroid eye disease.

A clinical photograph is useful for tracking the progression of the inflammation, and also in case medico-legal evidence is required in the future.

The main treatment will be intravenous antibiotics at the earliest practical opportunity. The specific choice of antibiotic may differ between protocols in different settings, but the consensus is that both penicillins and cephalosporins are the antibiotics of choice, given the bacterial species involved. The key point is that the antibiotics need to be administered intravenously as soon as possible – any delay could be extremely detrimental. Patients need to be closely monitored (especially children) and therefore need to be admitted to hospital. In the first 24–48 hours there needs to be some encouraging improvement in their symptoms. If there is no improvement (or a deterioration) in this period, further scanning and treatment adjustment may be required. Once the symptoms start to improve, the patient can be switched to oral antibiotics.

If the patient has to go to theatre to have drainage of any abscess, there will be some post-operative care considerations. They will probably have a drain placed in order to allow any further drainage of pus or blood. It is essential to reassure the patient with regard to such a drain, which will be protruding out of the wound and stitched in place. Usually the drain will stay in place for a couple of days after the drainage procedure and will need to be removed once the symptoms have subsided. A corrugated drain is the most common type used. Once the stitch has been cut, it will easily pull out. There will be a small wound where the surgery was undertaken and where the drain was positioned. Steristrips can be used to cover and pull this wound together.

Also, and very importantly, the patient's visual acuity, exophthalmometry, colour vision, IOP, fundal appearance, ocular motility and pupil/reaction should be monitored at least every hour for the first 24–48 hours post-operatively.

Exposed oedematous and potentially drying conjunctiva should be protected and lubricated.

Generally, most patients have a dramatic improvement in symptoms once the IV antibiotics have been commenced and any potential collection of infection has been drained. But, again, treatment must be instigated promptly and closely monitored. The oculoplastic practitioner may well have a part to play in observing the patient subsequently and will need to be responsive to changes to symptoms, whilst caring for the patient. Adequate pain control, anti-emetics and vigilant coordination of antibiotic treatment will be crucial. Equally, psychological support will be required for the patient and relatives, such as the parents of a child who has been affected.

Orbital floor fracture

The eye is protected from trauma to a certain degree by the bony surroundings of the orbital rim. However, if the globe/orbit is hit directly with an object, the force may cause damage to the bones of the orbit. This is mercifully rare, but eyes are occasionally subjected to squash balls, bottle corks, and (not too uncommonly) fists, causing injury. In this instance the energy of the blow is enough for the orbital floor to give way (instead of the eye) and this is just as well, or the outcome could be much worse.

The patient will often present with classic symptoms – firstly pain and discomfort, possibly associated with nausea and vomiting, swelling, bruising and haematoma. It may not be initially obvious that there is a floor fracture, but having gained a history and aroused some suspicion, you may decide to investigate a little further. It may be helpful to start by ascertaining the time and mechanism of the fracture.

Once the orbital floor gives way, some of the contents of the orbit may fall into the maxillary sinus, including the inferior rectus muscle. Consequently (apart from the discomfort and nausea this may initiate), the patient may find they are unable to look up on the affected side. This restriction in up-gaze is a classic sign of an orbital floor fracture. The patient will need to have a CT scan to confirm this and also to ascertain the extent of the fracture. Clinical photographs are useful to record the degree of the problem at the time of presentation.

It is also important to carry out a full ophthalmic assessment of the patient, checking that the eye has not been compromised in any way. Check for any numbness and loss of sensation (paraesthesia). A full orthoptic assessment will provide legitimate evidence of the extent of the entrapment and subsequent effect on eye movement. In adults it may be possible to undertake a forced-duction test. In this test the practitioner uses forceps (and under topical anaesthesia) the inferior rectus muscle is gently pulled in order to physically ascertain entrapment. However, this test can be painful and distressing for the patient, and they may not be able to tolerate it.

The key care aspects are to ensure that the patient is comfortable and as pain-free as possible, but also to deal with the nausea/vomiting if present. Intravenous analgesia and anti-emetics are fast-acting and will allow access for antibiotics and any other hydrating fluids that might be necessary.

The patient may find the whole experience unsettling and distressing, particularly in the case of children, so providing support and reassurance will be important. Orbital floor fractures may manifest slightly differently in children. After the immediate trauma, the orbital floor gives way in a similar way to an adult. However, in a child the bone is likely to spring back (like a trapdoor) and physically entrap the inferior rectus muscle, potentially leading to atrophy of the muscle. This can occur because of the springy nature of the orbital floor bone in children. It can cause a 'white eye' and incarceration of the muscle, which can lead to permanent damage to the muscle. Certainly, the need to surgically correct this is more urgent in children, for this reason.

Most orbital floor fractures require surgical intervention to repair. So, when it is appropriate to do so, the patient will need to be prepared for theatre and kept nil by mouth in readiness for a general anaesthetic.

Surgical repair is usually not required immediately, and this allows time for the eyelid swelling to reduce. The indications for surgery include persistent symptomatic diplopia and/or cosmetically significant enophthalmos (posterior displacement of the globe) or hypoglobus (downward displacement of the globe). The surgical correction often involves a lower eyelid approach with a subciliary conjunctival incision. The surgeon dissects down to the orbital rim and frees the periosteum of the bone, making their way to the orbital floor. Once there, the fracture will become obvious and then time will be spent releasing the trapped orbital contents from the fracture.

If the break is substantial enough, it may be necessary to bridge the fracture to prevent the contents falling back into the crack. A sheet of Medpor® (Stryker Medical) may be used to cover the break (or something similar); this is a biocompatible porous polyethylene implant that can be cut to shape and be anchored into place across the fracture. Alternatively, a titanium plate may be placed and screwed into the surrounding bone in order to span the extent of the fracture. There is also a combined product that incorporates both Medpor and a titanium plate (Medpor Titan®). This can be manipulated/bent and cut to shape to conform to the orbit and the fracture, and it can also be screwed into place if necessary. Small 5 x 1.2mm screws may be used to fix the plate. These may be self-tapping, which means there is no need for pre-placed drill holes to accommodate them.

As a practitioner, it is important to understand which type of implant (if any) has been placed in order to inform the patient. Immediately after the surgery, the patient's visiual acuity and eye movements need to be checked hourly for the first 24 hours. Post-operatively, the patient may experience some pain, swelling and cheek numbness, but this should subside over time.

Advise the patient not to blow their nose for at least four weeks so as to not cause orbital emphysema and a potential orbital compartment syndrome. There may be swelling within the eyelids and this may take a few weeks to reduce. Most patients recover well from the surgery and regain full eye movements.

Eyelid lacerations

The eyelid skin is the thinnest in the body and it is therefore no surprise that it is susceptible to damage. In addition, one of the main functions of the eyelids is to protect the eye and they are therefore in the frontline to a potential insult and injury. Conversely, the brow skin is notably thicker, but is equally prone to damage, given its exposed and prominent position.

Laceration(s) may come in various positions, sizes, numbers and depths. Given the many potential causes for eyelid lacerations, including hazardous occupations, active hobbies and sometimes just being in the wrong place at the wrong time, it is little wonder that any single accident can result in anything from the tiniest scratch to complex avulsion injuries. However, a high level of suspicion should be maintained as to the cause of the injury, particularly if it was not witnessed and/or involves a child. Until proven otherwise, a similarly high index of suspicion for a penetrating injury to the eye, orbit or even the brain should be afforded with an eyelid laceration.

Sharp injuries usually produce clean wounds which can be deep and involve other structures, whereas blunt wounds often create irregular lesions and potentially avulsion injuries (in which a physical structure is torn off by trauma or injury).

The required repair of injuries can vary from next to no treatment to major plastic reconstruction surgery. But, either way, a good understanding of the anatomy of the eyelid will be crucial in order to get the best outcome. The practitioner needs to undertake a thorough history and clinical examination, especially of the eye, in order to ascertain the extent of injury to the globe. Remember to check visual acuity. Until otherwise proven, the practitioner should always suspect other potential injuries. A full clinical examination should be undertaken, both in the EED and (if necessary) in the theatre at the time of the repair.

You will also need to look for any foreign bodies within the wound, particularly organic material such as wood which can harbour infection and isn't easy to detect (even on scans). If there is an obvious foreign body within the wound, it shouldn't be removed unless it is safe to do so. Remember, it might not be easy to estimate the degree or how much of the offending article may be in the laceration or exactly where it ends (i.e. whether it has penetrated the orbit).

From a nursing perspective, the injury may be painful and distressing, especially if it is a particularly complex laceration and/or there are other wounds or fractures in addition to the eye injury. Analgesia may be required to control the pain, but bear in mind that oral analgesics may be contraindicated if the patient is likely to need a general anaesthetic. In this case, the patient is required to be nil by mouth, so it may be better to administer analgesia intravenously. This also applies to the administration of antibiotics which are likely to be needed in order to prevent infection.

Given the nature of the injury, the eye may have been left exposed and therefore protection (in the form of lubricants) may be required. A viscous lubricant, such as Lacrilube, may offer sufficient protection and, in some cases, the patient may find a bandage contact lens easier to tolerate.

If the laceration is dirty or soiled, it may be necessary to clean the wounds using normal saline and gauze. It may also be a good idea to swathe the wound with antibiotic ointment until such time as it gets repaired. Covering the wound with a dressing either temporarily or for any length of time should be undertaken with a degree of caution. Ensure that the dressing is non-stick, as it will undoubtedly become attached to the wound, causing great discomfort on removal. Simple dressings, such as Mepitel (Molnlycke) or Melolin (Smith & Nephew), provide a protective layer and prevent attachment. Remember, if the wound is soiled, the patient is likely to require a tetanus toxoid (TT) injection.

Similarly (either at presentation or after cleaning/manipulating the wound), the wound may start bleeding and it may be necessary to control this immediately, before carrying out any further intervention. Simple pressure may be enough to control the bleeding or you may need to use a haemostat or cautery to stop it. It is also worth ascertaining whether the patient takes blood-thinning medication or is on anti-coagulants.

Shortly after the insult, the eyelids are likely to swell, making examination and repair more difficult. It may be necessary to take measures to reduce the swelling, such as applying a cool pack or even a bag of frozen peas. But remember to ensure that there is something (e.g. some gauze) between the cooling treatment and the wound.

As soon as it is viable to do so, the patient may need to go to theatre to undergo repair of the laceration(s) and potentially other injuries as well. They will need a pre-operative work-up and this may include bloods, ECG and basic observations. The patient may undergo the restorative surgery under a local (with or without sedation) or general anaesthetic and will need to be nil by mouth for at least 6 hours prior to surgery. Unfortunately, there may not always be adequate time to manage anti-coagulation therapy in order to reduce intra-operative bleeding. However, it may be useful to stop this a few days before surgery if possible, though the practitioner may need to liaise with the anti-coagulant team.

Repair of the wound may involve a variety of approaches, but there is usually some degree of suturing involved. Dissolving Vicryl stitches may be used for deeper layers and sometimes the skin, and nylon sutures for some other areas. Nylon/Prolene sutures are less likely to cause inflammation (and therefore scarring) but they will need to be removed.

Post-operatively, the wound needs to be kept clean. Simple saline 0.9% solution can be used for this, or, if the patient is at home, cooled boiled water decanted into a clean container. The cleaning should be as aseptic as possible, following the steps listed below:

- Make sure patient is comfortable and, if possible, semi-reclined
- Ensure adequate lighting and possibly use a magnifier
- Wash hands
- Open sterile cleaning pack (by the corners, with minimal contamination of the contents)
- Open and pour cleaning solution into Gallipot (whilst not touching the contents of the packet)
- Wash hands again and don sterile gloves
- Clean wound in one sweeping action, using cotton wool balls or gauze
- Then throw away cotton wool ball/gauze
- Repeat where necessary
- A cotton bud or Q-tip applicator may be useful to reach into awkward areas
- Be gentle, as it may still be sore to touch, and some wounds may still be fragile
- Don't excessively rub the wound, as this might cause bleeding
- Sutures can be removed when it is appropriate to do so. Certainly, nylon sutures can be taken out at about 7–10 days; others maybe at 10 days post-operatively. If you have any doubts about the wound, or if it is unstable, consider removing alternate sutures.

If a patient or relative is undertaking the cleaning, you should discuss this regime with them, and maybe even observe them doing the cleaning to check that they are doing it correctly. Over time, the wounds will settle, but adjunctive therapies, such as massage or application of silicone anti-scarring treatments, may be required to help improve the cosmetic appearance of the wound. It is important to reassure yourself and observe the patient's application of massage, as this will ensure that it is carried out effectively.

Some lacerations involve the medial canthal area and especially the lacrimal apparatus, which may require specific attention when repairing them. The lacrimal drainage system should be salvaged if possible and this is usually done in theatre at the time of the repair of the lacerations. A stent (as described in Chapter 8, p. 132) may also be used to help re-anastomose and align either end of the severed canaliculus and the eyelid. Therefore the patient may have a mono- or bi-canalicular stent in place after the surgery. It will be necessary to instruct the patient about this and the reasoning behind it.

Again, some stents can subsequently prolapse and the patient should be educated about what to do in such circumstances (see Chapter 8, p. 132).

Lacerations can affect other structures, including the levator muscle of the upper eyelid, and thus the patient can have a subsequent ptosis. This may be repaired at the time of the reconstruction or may need to be corrected at a later stage, once the inflammation has subsided. Similarly, the medial or lateral canthi may be detached as a consequence of the laceration. Again, it will be necessary to reattach them at the time of the reconstruction.

Other post-operative points include encouraging elevation of the patient's head so as to reduce swelling. A pressure dressing of a Jelonet, double eye-pad and bandage may be required in some instances. Care needs to be taken when applying the bandage. If it is too slack, it will be ineffectual and drop down over the patient's face; if it is too tight, it may cause pain and discomfort.

Application of a (double) eye-pad:

- Wash hands.
- Apply a liberal amount of antibiotic ointment or lubricant into the eye.
- Ensure the affected eye is closed.
- Apply Jelonet (cotton weave impregnated with yellow soft paraffin) (Smith & Nephew Healthcare) 5 x 5cm over closed eyelids (see Figure 12.2)
- Two sterile eye-pads will be required. The first is folded in half and is placed straight edge under the brow (see Figure 12.3).
- The second eye-pad is applied over the top and taped into place (using Medipore tape) (see Figure 12.4).

Emergency oculoplastic care

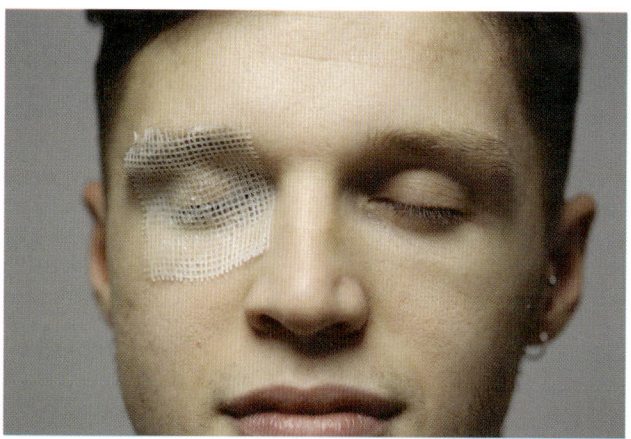
Figure 12.2: Eye-pad application: initially apply Jelonet

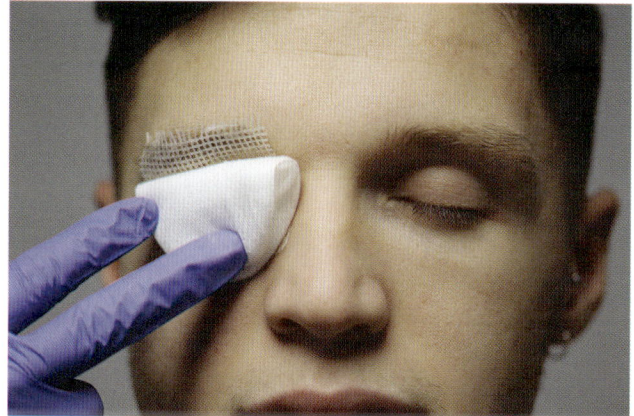
Figure 12.3: Apply folded eye-pad over Jelonet

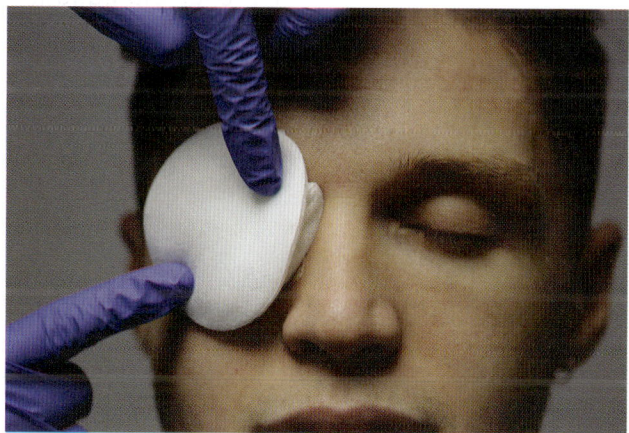
Figure 12.4: Apply eye-pad over folded eye-pad and then apply tape

Application of a head bandage:
- Identify whether there is a need to either replace or apply a bandage.
- Ascertain appropriate size and type of bandage needed.
- Ensure environment and timing are correct to apply bandage.
- Communicate the process to the patient.
- Wash hands, as per aseptic non-touch technique (ANTT), and apply non-sterile gloves.
- Remove existing bandage if necessary, being mindful that any soiling may cause it to stick to the underlying pad, and dispose of it appropriately.
- Identify whether it is necessary to remove or replace the eye-pad before continuing to apply bandage.
- It may be necessary to clean the area or the patient may benefit from having their hair cleaned or brushed.
- Observe the area for sores, especially if there has been a previous bandage or a possible allergic reaction.
- Check integrity of new bandage.
- Apply the bandage by unrolling (in a clockwise direction for the right eye and anti-clockwise for the left initially) around the head for two circuits. Then roll the bandage over the pad, then around the pinna of the ear around the nape of the neck and back round again.
- If the patient has long hair, it should be held out of the way.
- Carefully check the applied pressure of the bandage and especially check that it is not riding up around the ear.
- Once the bandage is completely applied, use tape to secure it.
- Check with the patient that the bandage is comfortable: it should be easy to slide a finger under the bandage.
- Dispose of any waste appropriately.
- Document the procedure and communicate to colleagues.
- Consider reviewing the patient after a short period to check the comfort and integrity of the bandage.

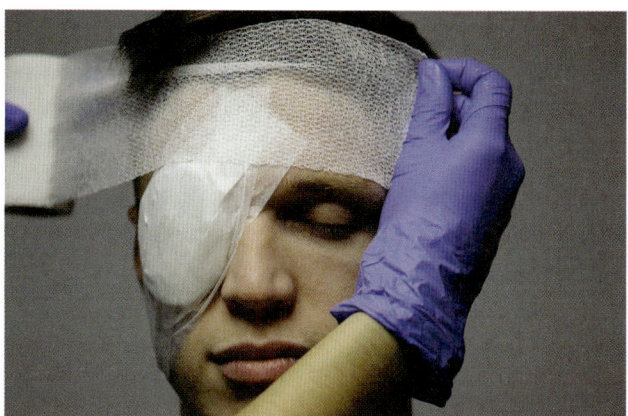
Figure 12.5: Initially unroll the bandage around the head

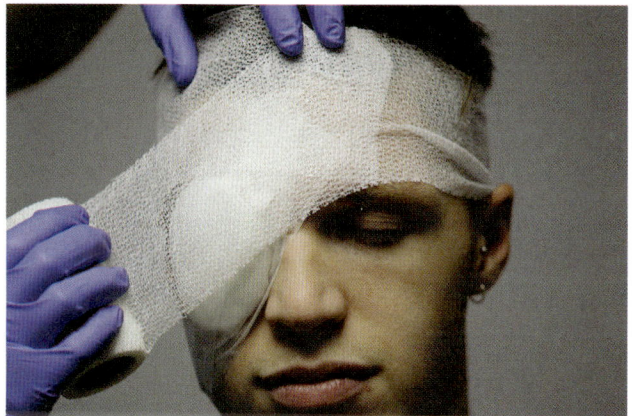
Figure 12.6: Bring the bandage down over the eye-pad

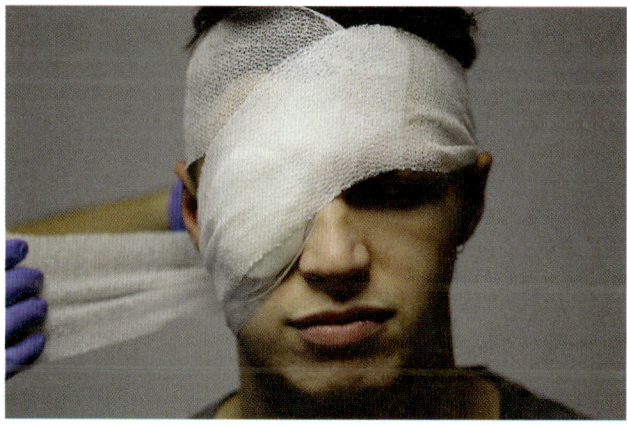
Figure 12.7: Roll bandage around head and over eye-pad several times

Animal bite wounds

Unfortunately, animal bites are becoming more common and may present as very serious injuries involving a combination of lacerations and puncture wounds. As always, the severity of the wounds will vary considerably, but the impact can be quite significant, both physically and psychologically. Bite injuries can largely be attributed to dogs, but may also involve cats and even humans. The occurrence of bites increases in the summer months, as the potential exposure to such animals and outdoor activities increases. Situations in which children are left unsupervised, while playing with animals, can lead to attacks.

At presentation, it is important to assess the patient and ascertain the nature and age of the injuries, taking particular note of the type of animal involved and the circumstances leading to the injury. Detailed notes should be recorded carefully and clearly. Clinical photographs should also be taken.

An extensive examination of the wounds and injuries should be commenced, and all details noted in the patient's records. Initially, the key concern is infection, so all wounds should be cleaned as far as possible. The practitioner also needs to remove any foreign bodies from the wounds. If there is any pus or discharge, a swab should be taken for culture and sensitivity.

It may be necessary to administer analgesia, but remember that the patient may need to be nil by mouth in order to go to theatre, so IV analgesia may be the best option. Similarly analgesia and anti-emetics may need to be administered in the same way.

The patient may be more susceptible to infection if they have other underlying medical conditions (such as diabetes) or are immunosuppressed. Antibiotic cover is certainly warranted in these individuals and the patient's tetanus status must be checked.

The antibiotics recommended for animal bites are quite specific but may vary slightly between different Trusts:

- In mild to medium infection, Co-Amoxiclav 625mg tds for 7 days (or Doxycycline 100mg bd and Metronidazole 400mg tds for those who are allergic to penicillin) for 7 days
- In severe infection, Co-Amoxiclav IV 1.2g tds and Clindamycin IV 600mg (or Clindamycin 600mg IV and Ciproflaxacin 500–750mg bd) for 14 days.

With dog bites in particular, it is important to note where the dog bite happened. Outside the UK, there is a slight risk of rabies. In the UK, rabies is extremely rare, but even in mainland Europe dogs can carry the disease. If there is any suspicion of infection, a rabies immunoglobulin/vaccine should be administered.

In some cases, x-ray or CT scanning may be required to investigate any underlying wounds or injuries.

In certain circumstances, it may also be necessary to investigate any potential vulnerable adult or child neglect issues pertaining to dog bites, and get clarity on the events leading to injury. If the practitioner has any suspicions regarding neglect, the case should be referred to the hospital safeguarding team and the social care team so that a child and family assessment can be undertaken.

The Dangerous Dogs Act (1991) lists the types and breeds of dogs that are deemed dangerous or are in fact banned in the UK. It also specifies the responsibilities of the dog owner and how dogs should be controlled. It may therefore be necessary to ascertain the type of dog involved in the attack and full details of the attack. If there is any concern that the dog is a dangerous breed or there appears to be evidence of poor management of the animal, this should be reported to the police.

Facial palsy

There are a number of possible causes of a facial palsy, and the onset of a palsy can be both devastating and sudden. A number of patients will therefore present initially at the EED with a facial palsy, obviously concerned and in urgent need of support and help. The goal for the practitioner is to establish the underlying cause of the palsy, establish the potential for recovery and ensure that the eye is adequately protected.

I go into more depth on facial palsy in Chapter 13, but (as always) a detailed history should be elicited from the patient, including onset and duration, symptoms of hearing loss or ear pain, any ENT history, trauma and past medical history.

The examination should evaluate the degree of lagophthalmos (inability to close the eye), corneal sensation, blink reflex and Bell's phenomenon. The corneal surface, lid position and cranial nerves should also be assessed.

The facial palsy can be graded using the House-Brackmann scale (House & Brackman 1985) and the impact upon the eye can be assessed. Consider taking clinical photographs.

Initial treatment will essentially protect the eye with frequent application of topical lubricants, taping of the eyes at night and possibly an eyelid weight to help with closure.

Retrobulbar haematoma

A rare but serious occurrence following orbital surgery, retrobulbar injection or blunt trauma (i.e. being hit in the face/orbit) is a subsequent compressive bleed within the orbit, behind the septum, that causes a compartment syndrome. The same issues

can be caused by a significant increase of pressure due to inflammation or an abscess or any of the following conditions:
- Atherosclerosis
- An intra-orbital aneurysm of the ophthalmic artery
- Haemophilia
- Leukaemia
- Thrombocytopenia
- Von Willebrand disease
- Hypertension
- Anti-coagulation.

No matter what the cause, the effect on vision can be devastating if a retrobulbar haematoma is left untreated. The presenting symptoms may be immediate and can include:
- Severe proptosis
- Tension within the orbit
- Resistance to retropulsion
- Reduction of ocular mobility (even complete stasis of the eye)
- Bulbar chemosis
- Increased and significant intra-ocular pressure
- Pain and discomfort
- Relative afferent pupil defect (RAPD) – see p. 188.

A retro-orbital bleed can cause a subsequent increase of significant pressure within the orbit, which can in turn cause a mechanical tamponade upon the orbital circulation and then the potential for a central retinal artery occlusion or optic atrophy causing blindness.

The pressure can be treated immediately with digital ocular massage, combined with IV Mannitol (osmotic diuretic) and Acetazolamide (Diamox).

However, if the vision is at risk and/or there hasn't been a significant improvement in symptoms using conservative means, surgical intervention may be required. A procedure known as lateral cantholysis and canthotomy may be undertaken to immediately relieve the pressure. Whilst this is unlikely to be undertaken by the oculoplastic practitioner, knowledge of the procedure and the equipment required will be useful.

In order to relieve the tension, the lateral canthal ligament (LCL) is detached from the orbit. If we consider the associated anatomy, the LCL is made up of dense fibrous tissue which attaches the upper and lower eyelid tarsal plates to the Whitnall's tubercle inside the orbital rim, deep to the septum. The LCL is inserted into the periosteum at Whitnall's tubercle, approximately 1.5mm behind the orbital rim. The mean horizontal length of the lateral canthus, from lateral commissure (the angle where the upper and lower eyelid meet) to lateral orbit, is about 7.5mm.

Once any intervention has been undertaken it will be necessary to continue to assess the patient's visual acuity, colour vision, eye movements, exophthalmometry, IOP and fundoscopy, at least every hour for 24–48 hours

Lateral canthotomy and cantholysis

The lateral canthotomy and inferior cantholysis procedure is used to release the eyelid and the underlying tension. It includes the following steps:

1. Injection of local anaesthetic – Marcaine 0.5% with Adrenaline.
2. Initially use an artery clip to 'crimp' (if available).
3. Firstly, the lateral canthotomy is a horizontal cut 1–2cm at the lateral canthal angle, extending laterally outwards, using scissors (Westcott/Stevens).
4. Using toothed forceps, retract the lower eyelid downwards to visualise or feel the lateral canthal tendon. (Use the scissors to 'feel' and strum the deep tissue – the crus.)
5. With the scissors directed along the lateral orbital rim (pointing away from the globe), dissect the inferior crus of the lateral canthal tendon and cut it.
6. The lower eyelid should be completely free laterally.
7. If necessary, perform a superior lateral canthal release.
8. Cauterise the wounds and do not close them.
9. There should be an immediate improvement in the tension.
10. In very rare cases, it may be necessary to perform an inferolateral anterior orbitotomy which is essentially an opening into the orbit behind the septum and the globe to release collected blood and/or pus.

The key point here is that this procedure, if required, needs to be done promptly and, if necessary, in the EED department. There will be no time to organise scans or theatre slots, as any potential delay could cause blindness and there will be minutes, not hours, to spare. Therefore, the practitioner needs to know what is required and have the instruments to hand immediately. In my experience, having surgical instruments ready and available can be problematic outside the operating theatre. It may therefore be helpful to have a pack or tray organised in advance for easy access.

At Manchester Royal Eye Hospital (MREH) we created a pack of instruments – the Manchester Emergency Cantholysis Kit (MECK) – for this very situation. We recommend that this pack contains:

- A pair of disposable Westcott scissors
- A pair of St Martin toothed forceps
- 5 x swabs (2 x 2)
- A disposable hand cautery
- A 5m syringe
- A 25g long needle
- (Separately) a tray/trolley to place pack on, as well as alco-wipes and sterile gloves.

With efficient diagnosis and prompt intervention, the potentially damaging effects of a retrobulbar haematoma can be avoided. Again, the patient will need to be closely assessed after the procedure, including visual acuity, colour vision, eye movements, exophthalmometry, IOP and fundoscopy, at least every hour for 24–48 hours.

The practitioner will need to support the patient and will also need to provide analgesia and topical antibiotics after the procedure. Once the orbit has settled a few weeks after the event, the eyelid can be repaired if necessary.

Burns

Facial burns are uncommon but can affect the eye, eyelids and surrounding structures. A considerable proportion of burns are associated with chemical injury. However, there can be various types of burns, including thermal, chemical, electrical and radiational.

Burns are classified, according to their extent, as:

- First degree – superficial, involving the epidermis
- Second degree – deeper partial-thickness burn, involving both the epidermis and dermis
- Third degree – a full-thickness burn, involving the deeper tissue.

If the burn includes the eyelids and surrounding adnexa, it may cause long-term scarring. Conjunctival cicatricial shortening and contracture of tissue, due to irreversible damage caused by a serious burn, can be extremely difficult to manage. Ocular motility, corneal scarring and poor cosmesis can all be associated with burns. Burns can also have a considerable psychological effect and the potential facial disfigurement can be life-changing.

Burns seen in the EED are generally only likely to affect the eyelids or the eye itself, simply because if the burn were any more serious or widespread the patient would be in the main A&E department, under the care of a plastic surgeon or maxillofacial surgeon.

However, the oculoplastic practitioner may also be called to the burns unit or the critical care unit to review or offer advice to a seriously ill patient with widespread burns.

In the first instance, the priority is to assess and protect the eye. The corneal scarring or ulceration may be secondary to significant eyelid injury. To some extent, the eye may be protected at the time of the injury, due to the blink reflex and Bell's phenomenon. The individual may also instinctively bring their arms up to their face, thus partly protecting the eyes.

Types of burns

Thermal burns are caused by hot liquids or exposure to flames. Liquid thermal burns can vary considerably, depending on the substance involved. Some liquids may cool very rapidly before making contact with the skin and the burns are therefore more superficial. This of course depends on the pressure, the distance away and the temperature at the point of release. Flame burns can often be deeper and the period of exposure may be longer.

Chemical burns are usually attributed to acid or alkali exposure, both of which can be devastating. Alkalis are more lipophilic, and penetrate more upon contact, than acids. Tissue death and necrosis is a significant issue associated with these types of injuries.

Electrical burns are contact burns, caused by exposure to an electrical current passing through tissue and relating to the eye, and can damage the cornea, conjunctiva and uveal tract.

Certainly, on presentation, there may be considerable swelling of the eyelids, depending on the type of burn and the nature of the injury. First-degree burns are not likely to cause any long-term damage, but there may be a lot of swelling and discomfort to start with. However, with second- and third-degree burns, the damage is likely to lead to contracture and lagophthalmos.

Treating burns

The practitioner needs to elicit a good history of events, whilst conducting a thorough examination. However, they also need to start vigorous irrigation of the affected area, particularly in the case of thermal and chemical burns. Copious flooding of the area (with Ringer lactate irrigation) is preferable, but saline and plain water may also be used. The history-taking may have to wait until the irrigation starts. It may also be necessary to keep irrigating until there is some indication that the pH has neutralised.

Copious amounts of lubricant, both for the eye and the surrounding tissues, is indicated in order to provide some comfort. Pain management, both topical and systemic, should be provided at the earliest opportunity. Antibiotic cover should also be considered due to the exposed nature of the tissue.

In the short term, caring for the patient with their head in the upright position is preferable where possible. Daily aseptic cleaning of the tissue should be a priority. In first-degree burns, a simple cleaning regime at home can be advocated, along with artificial tears and cool compresses.

It may also be necessary to undertake a temporary suture tarsorrhaphy to close the lids in order to protect the eye (see p. 167). In severe cases, surgical relaxing incisions may be an option to release contracted tissue.

Tissue necrosis may need to be managed, and any dead tissue may have to be removed with a blade, to stop it hindering wound healing. This is usually the role of the oculoplastic surgeon, but small areas of necrosis can be managed and treated by the practitioner under the supervision of the surgeon.

Unfortunately, there are very few dressings available that are specific to the eye and eyelids that can help with healing. Essentially, the dressing must always be non-stick, as removing dressings that have become attached to granulating tissue can be extremely painful. Some recognised dressings include Bactigras, Melolin and Mepilex Ag. However, some of the alternatives and recommended dressings are not very adaptable on the eyelids or face, such as hydrocolloid, hydrogel and alginate dressings. Nevertheless, some of these may help to create a moist atmosphere for healing whilst others also remove over-exudation and unwanted fluid from the wound especially in the early stages of healing. I have found foam dressings to be particularly useful as these remove exudate, but use them with a non-stick barrier (such as Mepitel) in between.

Infected wounds may be controlled with an application of silver-impregnated dressing, such as Aquacell Ag (ConvaTec).

In the long term, once the skin has epithelialised and granulated, surgical involvement may be required to correct defects, including full or split thickness skin grafting.

References

British Emergency Eye Care Society (BEECS) (2019). www.beecs.co.uk (last accessed 20.11.2019).

Fields, D., Tillotson, J. & Whittingham, E. (2015). *Eye Emergencies: a practitioner's guide.* Keswick: M&K Publishing.

House, J. & Brackman, D. (1985) Facial nerve grading system. *Otolaryngol Head Neck Surg.* **93**: 146-147

Long, B. & Koyfman, A. (2018). *Handbook of Emergency Ophthalmology.* Springer International Publishing.

13

Facial palsy and related care

Introduction

A facial palsy is a paralysis or weakening of the face, which is usually unilateral (though in rare cases it can be bilateral) and can cause extreme distress to the individual involved. The most common (single nerve) manifestation of a sudden weakening of the face is Bell's palsy (sometimes referred to as idiopathic facial nerve paralysis) which accounts for approximately 70% of all facial palsies. Its occurrence is approximately 25:100,000 in the UK (Bell's Palsy Association 2019).

The presenting symptoms include muscle twitching and weakening of the facial muscles on one side of the face, ptosis, pain, numbness, mouth droop, change of taste, dry eyes, pain, increased sensitivity to particular sounds (hyperacusis) and epiphora.

Bell's palsy

Bell's palsy is associated with the facial nerve (CN VII). The facial nerve travels from the pons of the midbrain to just under the pinna of the ear and spreads in several branches across the side of the face. The facial nerve supplies the muscles of the face and is associated with motor function and facial expression. It is also related to the sensation of taste from a proportion of the tongue (the anterior two-thirds), which explains why some palsy patients experience an associated loss of taste. It also supplies parasympathetic fibres to various ganglia within the head and neck.

Bell's palsy can have a sudden onset (within 48–72 hours) and has various potential causes (not yet truly known) associated with the facial nerve. The most likely cause is viral infection of the nerve associated with varicella-zoster and/or Epstein-Barr virus. The intracranial aspect of the facial nerve exits into the face via the stylomastoid canal, which is a narrow foramen through which the nerve passes. Inflammation caused by the virus can cause compression of the nerve within the foramen. This affects neurotransmission along the nerve, instigating a facial palsy/weakness. It may also be due to demyelination and on-going degeneration of the nerve.

If the patient has Bell's palsy, it is important for them to appreciate that the acute facial palsy is often self-limiting and most patients make a full recovery over a period of several months.

Other causes of facial palsy

There are several other possible causes for a facial palsy (including a stroke, meningitis, myasthenia gravis, Lyme disease, leprosy, diabetes, trauma, and surgical excision of acoustic neuroma and tumour) and it is essential that these are also considered. Most of these manifestations of facial palsy are associated with various other issues and symptoms. For example, in a stroke (which is the most common differential diagnosis) there is also likely to be weakness in the arms and legs and dysphagia (swallowing difficulties). A patient who has facial palsy as a consequence of a stroke will also have forehead wrinkling (unlike a Bell's palsy where the forehead will be smooth on the affected side).

Lyme disease

Lyme disease is a rare cause of facial paralysis and is triggered as a consequence of having been bitten by a tick (small arachnid), which is associated with woodland and heathland areas. The potential ensuing infection (not in all bites) with the bacterium *Borreliosis* can, amongst other symptoms (flu, pain, swelling, numbness), cause a facial palsy. Therefore, as part of the history-taking process it may be prudent to ascertain whether the patient works, or undertakes outdoor activities, in such areas and/or is aware of having been bitten.

Acoustic neuroma (vestibular schwannoma) surgery

A significant proportion of patients will have a facial palsy as the unfortunate consequence of surgery to remove an acoustic neuroma (Zanoletti, Faccioli & Martini 2016). The numbers vary from 7 to 50%, depending on the size of the tumour (the larger the lesion, the greater the incidence of post-operative facial palsy). This is a permanent palsy due to the facial nerve being irreparably damaged during the surgical excision of the tumour. There can also be hearing loss associated with the surgery.

These patients are likely to require life-long support and input. Various surgeries may be required to improve facial function and appearance. Furthermore, a considerable effort will be required to lubricate and protect the eye on the affected side.

Further support and information for this group of patients can be found at the British Acoustic Neuroma Association (2015).

History and clinical examination

When the patient presents with a unilateral facial weakness it is necessary to understand the causative mechanism and this will require a thorough history, including eliciting the following:

- Onset and duration of the palsy
- Symptoms of pain, discharge and hearing loss

- Past medical history
- History of trauma
- Any history specifically related to ENT issues
- Any history of dizziness, dysphagia or diplopia.

Clinical examination should be extensive and should include not just a facial and ophthalmic inspection but also a full body and cranial nerve assessment.

To assess CN VII (facial), the practitioner can ask the patient to undertake various expressions of the face and observe for any weakness – for example, puffing out the cheeks, pursing the lips, smiling, frowning, closing eyes tightly, showing teeth and lifting the brow. It is prudent to test the corneal reflex, as this may be indirectly affected by the palsy.

From an ophthalmic perspective, the examination should also specifically include several important assessment aspects:

- Lagophthalmos – this is how much opening there is between the upper and lower eyelids (palpebral aperture) both passively and actively (forcibly). In facial palsy, inability to close the eyelids can have a very significant effect, resulting in the cornea drying and becoming irritated. The extent of the dry eye and the condition of the cornea is ideally assessed using a slit lamp.
- Corneal sensation – this can be tested with the tip of a rolled corner of tissue. The sensation is usually reduced in facial palsy.
- Bell's phenomenon – this is a natural safety mechanism whereby the eye rolls upwards and outwards as a defensive mechanism when the eyes close. Again, this is reduced in facial palsy and may also compromise the eye. Whilst holding the eyelids open, ask the patient to close their eye. If they have a poor Bell's phenomenon, the eye will barely move.
- The eyelids – retraction, ectropion, ptosis.
- Blink reflex – this can again be reduced in facial palsy.

The patient may also present with more general issues which may include:

- Facial synkinesis (see below)
- Memory problems
- Facial tingling
- Headache
- Balance issues
- Neck ache.

Facial synkinesis

Facial synkinesis is another common clinical feature associated with prolonged facial palsy and is the development of associated or linked (but often unwanted) facial movements. This may be due to the nerve misfiring as it attempts to recover. For example, when smiling, the individual's eye might close (on the affected side) or the cheek may lift when they close their eyes. They may also experience hyperlacrimation (known as 'crocodile tears'). This can be due to the muscles affected being tight or having a higher tone (even though they may feel relaxed to the patient).

Synkinesis will require ongoing input and support for the patient and, from the practitioner's perspective, this will be necessary right from the outset. Encouraging general exercise can be beneficial – for example, walking, jogging and swimming. Yoga and meditation can also help reduce pain and facial tension, whilst decreasing anxiety and stress. A facial massager can be useful in encouraging increased blood supply to the face.

Investigations

Once a full history has been taken and the assessment has been completed and recorded in the patient's medical notes, it is appropriate to get clinical facial photographs taken.

A CT or MRI scan should be carried out if there is any indication of a cause other than Bell's palsy (such as trauma). If the cause is definitely Bell's palsy, scanning may not be necessary at the time of presentation, as the results won't affect the initial treatment. However, if there is no distinct improvement in symptoms after the initial course of treatment, scanning may be necessary. Any imaging undertaken should include the internal auditory canal (IAC) and the whole course of the facial nerve.

Electromagnetic testing of the affected muscles can be undertaken to assess the level of assault, but this is not a common investigation and again will not change the likely treatment.

A Schirmer's test can be undertaken to measure the degree of lacrimation. However, again, it is likely that the patient will be using lubricants, so this may not change the treatment regime (see Chapter 8, pp. 123, 124).

If there is any suspicion of any other cause for the facial palsy, it may be necessary to consider undertaking further blood investigations such as:

- Lyme titer – to test for lyme disease
- Varicella zoster titer
- FTA-ABS – fluorescent treponemal antibody absorption to test for syphilis (a very rare cause of facial palsy)

- Herpes simplex virus (HSV)
- EBV titer.

Tests for inflammatory markers for potential conditions such as sarcoidosis include:
- C-reactive protein (CRP) and erythrocyte sedimentation rate (ESR)
- Antineutrophil cytoplasmic antibody (ANCA)
- Angiotensin-converting enzyme (ACE)
- Anti-nuclear antibodies (ANA).

Once a diagnosis of Bell's palsy has been made, and the other potential causes have been ruled out, the degree of palsy can be classified. Various tools can be used to do this, but the most commonly referred to is the House-Brackmann (1985) grading system. This is actually a scoring system that assesses movement of the brow and angle of the mouth and assigns a score between 0 and 8 (normal being 8 and severe palsy being 0). It also uses subjective visual observations to arrive at an overall score:

Grade I – normal (8 out of 8)

Grade II – mild dysfunction, slight weakness/asymmetry at close observation, able to close the eye, normal symmetry of the forehead, no synkinesis, able to move mouth (7 out of 8)

Grade III – moderate dysfunction, obvious weakness but not disfiguring (5–6 out of 8)

Grade IV – moderately severe dysfunction, no movement of the forehead, inability to close the eye, synkinesis, hemifacial spasm (3–4 out of 8)

Grade V – severe dysfunction, only barely perceptible motion in the face, asymmetry with a droop of the mouth, decreased naso-labial fold, contracture, synkinesis, hemifacial spasm (2–3 out of 8).

Grade VI – total paralysis, no movement (0).

This scale is well regarded and has good levels of inter-rater reliability (Reitzen, Babb & Lalwani 2009).

Treatment for Bell's palsy

Initial strong recommendation and guidance (Baugh, Basura, *et al.* 2013) to treat Bell's palsy suggests systemic corticosteroids and antivirals as the first-line treatment. A reducing course of Prednisolone (50–60mg over 10 days) has been recommended (Baugh, Basura, *et al.* 2013) if initiated within 72 hours of the onset of symptoms.

The concurrent use of an antiviral agent with adjunctive steroid treatment, as outlined above, may have some limited additional benefit (Acyclovir being the most common drug of choice). Conversely, the use of an antiviral as a monotherapy (i.e. on its own) is not recommended.

Ophthalmic nursing considerations

The eye on the affected side may be open and exposed, and may also have reduced lubrication. Essentially, the eye will require protection until such time as the symptoms of Bell's palsy have reduced. For patients with long-term paralysis, it is even more important to protect the eye with life-long lubricants.

Prophylactic eye care, due to incomplete eye closure and lagophthalmos, is vital. The practitioner needs to emphasise its importance and spend time with the patient outlining the treatment regime and instillation technique. The patient may complain of symptoms relating to the eye, including itching, burning, foreign body sensation, blurring of vision and pain.

Lubrication and ocular surface hydration (with drops or ointment) should be prescribed and implemented. During the day, and in order not to blur the vision too much, drops may be sufficient. At night-time copious use of ointment will be crucial to protect the eye whilst the patient is asleep. Eye covers or goggles may be useful, especially during the night, but can be cumbersome, which may put some people off using them.

The practitioner should also assess the patient's drop instillation technique in order to evaluate the degree of effectiveness. This is especially important if the patient lives alone or you suspect they have any difficulties in getting the drop successfully and effectively instilled.

Taping the eye (especially overnight) can be useful, but again the technique needs to be supervised and assessed initially. If undertaken poorly, the eye can still remain open under the tape, and this may cause further issues such as corneal abrasion. I find that microporous type is the best option, as it is less sticky and more comfortable for the patient. I also place the tape lengthways horizontally across the lids, using 2 or 3 pieces, being careful to ensure that the eye is completely closed under the tape and the eyelashes are out of the way. A little blob of lubricating ointment before placing the tape will ensure that the eye has extra protection.

In some patients a botulinum toxin injection into the levator muscle complex can induce a complete ptosis. This will last for several months and will ensure more protection for the eye (along with lubricants). This can be undertaken in the clinic with minimal disruption. However, it will of course affect the patient's vision – especially if the visual acuity on the unaffected side is poor.

If the exposure is quite marked and is associated with significant keratopathy, surgery may be required. Initially a suture tarsorrhaphy to temporarily close the lids will offer some protection; this can be opened to assess the eye, and then closed again (see Chapter 2, p. 17). The patient will need to be prepared for the procedure which can be tolerated under a local anaesthetic.

In the middle to long term, patients with on-going facial paralysis and poor eyelid closure can be considered for an upper eyelid weight. These can either be stick-on weights or a more permanent gold or platinum weight surgically inserted into the upper eyelid. They have a concave shape, to follow the contour of the eyelid.

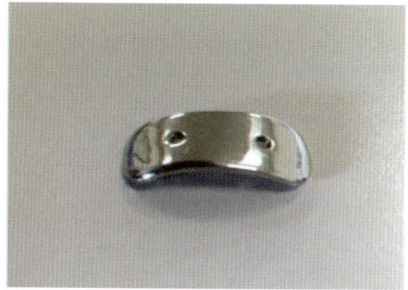

Figure 13.1: Platinum eyelid weight

The degree of weight required first needs to be assessed. The weights range from 0.6gm to 1.8gm; anything heavier becomes too bulky in/on the lid. We often trial an external stick-on weight for a few months to evaluate whether it is useful in protecting the eye. Once the patient is satisfied with this, a permanent weight can be surgically placed into the upper eyelid. The weight is inserted into a small pocket created within an upper eyelid skin crease incision, and the wound sutured closed.

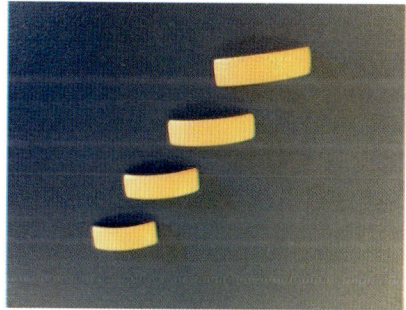

Figure 13.2: Range of stick-on eyelid weights

This operation has a good success rate and provides excellent protection, giving the patient an upper eyelid that is more able to close. However, very occasionally, the weight can cause problems (including migration and exposure) and may unfortunately have to be removed.

In extreme circumstances, a permanent lateral tarsorrhaphy can be performed. This involves the physical attachment of the upper and lower eyelids in the lateral corner to close the aperture of the eye, thus affording less exposure. The advantage is that if there is sufficient improvement in symptoms the procedure is reversible. The patient will require guidance and instruction regarding the potential reduction in visual field. For example, the patient will need to learn to turn their head, especially when crossing the road.

They may also require surgical correction of the lower lid ectropion (see Chapter 2, pp. 18ff) and any potential brow ptosis – usually a direct brow lift. This involves removing a section of skin and underlying muscle just above the brow and then suturing back together. The deficit created from removing the skin/muscle draws the brow superiorly and provides lift. This is a relatively straightforward corrective procedure but it has disadvantage of often leaving an obvious scar above the brow. This may, or may not, be acceptable to the patient so the issue of scarring needs to be mentioned and emphasised at the time of consent.

Non-surgical therapy for facial palsy

For long-term facial palsy (for example, patients who have had surgical excision of acoustic neuroma or stroke), the rehabilitation regime may also involve facial exercise therapy and clinics. Facial rehabilitation therapy may well involve a speech therapist and a physiotherapist. They will determine what exercises are appropriate by assessing the degree of facial palsy and providing an individual care plan. In the UK, patients can be referred to a facial rehabilitation clinic in the appropriate region.

At the clinic, the patient will receive further advice on dry mouth care, eating and drinking and speech therapy. Muscle rehabilitation will include massage techniques and stretching exercises for the facial muscles, and advice on how to control involuntary unwanted movements. The Facial Therapy Specialists UK website (2019) provides further information on where to find a therapist and other related information and courses.

Psychosocial effects of facial palsy

Facial paralysis places a tremendous psychological burden on the patient and can have a profound effect on their well-being. Our faces and facial expressions are fundamental factors in communication and social integration so it is not surprising that patients with facial palsy (especially long-term facial palsy) can suffer from depression, isolation, impaired relationships and reduced confidence. There may be particular embarrassment and anxiety associated with certain aspects of behaviour such as eating and drinking.

Oculoplastic practitioners may be able to offer support and links to bodies that may offer help. Organisations such as Changing Faces (2019) can offer advice and training on social coping mechanisms. The Bell's Palsy Information Website (2019),

Bell's Palsy Association (2019) and Facial Palsy UK (2019) also offer fantastic resources for patients and clinical staff.

A clinical psychologist may be required for individuals who find it difficult to cope. There are also regional facial palsy support groups that patients can be encouraged to attend. The Facial Palsy UK (2019) website is especially useful, providing a wealth of support, information and help for patients and those living with the condition.

References

British Acoustic Neuroma Association (2015). bana-uk.com (last accessed 24.11.2019).

Bell's Palsy Association (2019). https://www.bellspalsy.org.uk (last accessed 24.11.2019).

Bell's Palsy Information Website (2019). http://bellspalsy.ws/ (last accessed 25.11.2019).

Baugh, R., Basura, G., *et al.* (2013). Clinical Practice Guideline: Bell's Palsy. *Otolaryngology Head Neck Surgery.* **149**(3S), S1–S27.

Changing Faces (2019). https://www.changingfaces.org.uk (last accessed 25.11.2019).

Facial Palsy UK (2019). https://www.facialpalsy.org.uk (last accessed 25.11.2019).

Facial Therapy Specialists UK (2019). fts-uk.org (last accessed 25.11.2019).

House, J. & Brackmann, D. (1985). Facial Nerve grading system. *Otolaryngology Head Neck Surgery.* **93**, 146–47

Reitzen, S., Babb, J. & Lalwani, K. (2009). Significance and reliability of the House-Brackmann grading system for regional nerve function. *Otolaryngology Head Neck Surgery.* **140**, 154–58.

Zanoletti, E., Faccioli, C. & Martini, A. (2016). Surgical treatment of acoustic neuroma: Outcomes and indications. *Reports of Practical Oncology and Radiotherapy.* **21**(4), 395–98.

14
The orbit and related disorders

Introduction

The bony orbit houses the eye and associated adnexa, and provides protection for its precious contents, including the eye, extra-ocular muscles, peri-orbital fat, cranial nerves, blood vessels, glands and the optic nerve. This list includes many areas from which disease or a specific disorders can potentially arise. Furthermore, given the relationship between the orbit, its contents and surrounding anatomy (such as the brain, sinuses and nasal cavity), certain conditions and their possible spread to these other areas can pose a very serious risk.

In this chapter we will discuss the bony orbit and its fissures, and consider some of the more common peri-orbital presentations with their associated treatment and management. As always, it is vital to carry out the initial assessment and history-taking process carefully in order to collect all the evidence required to aid diagnosis. And, from a nursing perspective, there are a number of key care factors associated with orbital disorders and surgery that are important to be aware of.

Osteology

As one of the hardest structures in the body, bone provides internal structure and form, allowing for the attachment of muscles, ligaments and tendons, whilst providing protection and support. Within its structure, bone provides the main reserve of calcium in the body. Calcium is essential for several important physiological functions, including nerve conduction, blood-clotting and muscle contraction. Within the bone matrix, there are deposits of large inorganic mineral salts constitutionally made of calcium and phosphate called hydroxyapatite (see Chapter 10, on enucleation and orbital implants). By a process of calcification, these salts within the bony matrix crystallise, leading to hardening of the collagen fibres and essentially providing bone with its extrinsic structure.

Bone generally has a smooth outer shell (known as compact tissue) and a latticework inner structure that affords both strength and lightness (cancellous). Microscopically, bone is largely made up of longitudinal canals (haversian canals) surrounded by concentric lamellae (thin plates of bone). Within the canals run blood vessels, nerve fibres and delicate connective tissue. These canals can be seen to open out onto the surface of the compact bone, with microscopic orifices into which run blood vessels from the overlying layer of tissue called the periosteum.

Long thin cells, known as osteocytes, are found in the cavities between the lamellae, and these osteocytes have tiny finger-like extensions which are able to absorb nutrients and dispose of waste. Perpendicularly, canals containing blood, lymphatic vessels and nerves penetrate across the haversian bodies (Volkmann's canals) from the periosteum.

The periosteum covers the bone and is made up of two distinct layers that adhere firmly together. There is an outer layer that is entirely made up of connective tissue and contains nerves and blood vessels that supply the underlying bone; and an inner layer of elastic fibres, which is osteogenic (bone forming).

The periosteum plays a significant role in relation to oculoplastic surgery. It needs to be separated from the bone during certain surgical approaches to the orbit and it can even be harvested and relocated in reconstructive surgery. The periosteum within the orbit is most adherent at the orbital rim and less so further posteriorly within the orbit.

The bones of the orbit

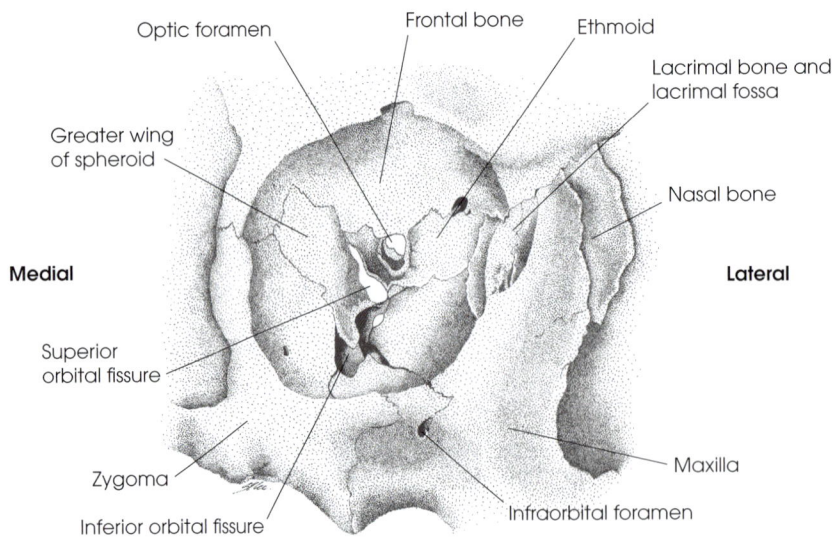

Figure 14.1: Bony orbit

In all, 22 bones make up the skull and 7 of them are associated with the bony orbit, within which the globe is situated. Put simply, the orbits can be visualised as two rectangles with opposing sides: medial (nasal) and lateral (temporal), superior (roof) and inferior (floor).

In reality the two orbits are cone-shaped (or pyramidal) and are separated by the ethmoid sinuses in the mid-line. The lateral orbital walls (in relation to both sides) are at right-angles (90°) from one another and travel backwards and inwards for a distance of 45–55mm (from the orbital rim to the optic strut). The lateral orbital walls and the medial orbital walls are perpendicular to each other, approximately 22mm apart. The orbital axis is approximately 22.5° (see Figure 14.1).

The orbit comprises the following bones:

- Frontal
- Sphenoid
- Ethmoid
- Lacrimal
- Maxillary
- Zygomatic
- Palatine.

Frontal bone

The frontal bone is made up of three component parts: orbital (roof), nasal and squamous (forehead). Considered in isolation, the frontal bone resembles a shell-like structure, with the convex squamous element making up the most significant part of the bone constituting the forehead. At its superior edge the frontal bone is adjacent to, and articulates with, the parietal bones of the cranium, divided by the coronal suture.

On its inferior border, just above the orbital rims on either side, are two curved elevations, the superciliary arches or brow ridges. Below the brow ridges is the prominent rounded edge of the supra-orbital margin. One-third of the way along the supra-orbital margin's medial edge (approximately 22mm from the nasal midline) is a small indentation (or, less commonly, a foramen) that transmits the supra-orbital nerve and blood supply known as the supra-orbital notch (Ashwini, Rao, Sharmila & Somayaji 2012). If you run your finger along the superior orbital rim, you might feel the notch medially. Posterior to the frontal bone and adjacent to the superciliary arches are the frontal sinuses. Between the two supra-orbital arches is an area known as the glabella.

The lateral aspects of the frontal bone anteriorly terminate at the zygomatic process. Inferior to this is a concavity called the temporal fossa and its articulation with both the sphenoid and zygomatic bones. Medially the frontal bone has a nasal element and is joined to the maxilla and nasal bones (frontonasal suture).

The frontal bone makes up a significant portion of the orbital roof. Running horizontally posteriorly, the concave portion of the frontal bone is generally triangular in shape. The upper surface of the orbital roof also represents part of the convex anterior fossa of the cerebral surface of the skull base. This is significant, as the thickness of the orbital roof bone is only 3mm (at its thickest). Whilst this is notably thicker than that of the floor of the orbit, it still represents a very small margin between the orbit and the brain – and this needs to be considered in relation to surgery, trauma and spread of infection. Conversely, with regard to trauma, the orbital roof rarely fractures (René 2006).

Also, notably, there are two small shallow fossas in the orbital roof anteriorly just behind the orbital rim, one laterally which houses the lacrimal gland and the other medially which is associated with the trochlear.

Sphenoid bone

The sphenoid bone articulates with most of the bones of the cranium and anchors them together (and is sometimes known as the 'keystone' bone for this very reason). It is butterfly-shaped, with 'wings' extending from a central portion. Two larger wings make up most of the surface of the bone and are known as the 'greater' wings. Inferiorly, two smaller appendages make up the 'lesser' wings.

The anterior surface of the greater wing of sphenoid is smooth and forms part of the posterior wall of the orbit. The inferior surface of the lesser wing of sphenoid makes up a section of the posterior part of the roof of the orbit, articulated to the orbital component of the frontal bone. It also makes up the upper boundary of the sphenoidal fissure, a narrow opening at the back of the orbit (the lower edge being the greater wing of sphenoid). The sphenoidal fissure leads from the orbit to the cranium and transmits several important vessels, including the 3rd, 4th, 5th and 6th cranial nerves, as well as the orbital branch of the meningeal artery, lacrimal artery and the ophthalmic vein.

The lateral aspect of the orbital part of the lesser wing of sphenoid also accommodates the optic nerve (and ophthalmic artery) through a small opening called the optic foramen. From a superior (cranial) view of the lesser wing of sphenoid, the optic nerve passes through the optic foramen across the chiasmatic groove and towards the brain.

The main body of the sphenoid bone contains two air spaces, separated by a septum, called the sphenoidal sinuses. These are approximately 2cm in diameter but do vary in size and are rarely symmetrical. These sinuses are relevant, especially in relation to sphenoidal sinusitis which, although rare, can be life threatening. Just superior to the sphenoidal sinus is a small bony indentation which houses the pituitary gland on the base of the brain, called the sella tunica.

Also of significance anatomically (but not bone related) is the fact that the cavernous sinuses are located on either side of the sella tunica and extend from the sphenoidal fissure. These are venous sinuses rather than bony air spaces and represent venous channels that receive the ophthalmic vein and some cerebral veins, amongst others, and also carry several cranial nerves. The venous sinuses are unlike ordinary veins, as their outer layer is formed by the dura of the brain and they don't possess a muscular wall. Interestingly, the cavernous sinus is the only part of the body where an artery (internal carotid artery) runs through a venous chamber. This is of clinical significance because:

- A rupture of the internal carotid artery within the sinus would likely create a cavernous sinus fistula, causing back-flow and engorgement of the eye vessels
- Pituitary enlargement (i.e. adenoma) could compress the cavernous sinus, causing ophthalmoplegia (weakness or paralysis of the extra-ocular muscles)
- A blood clot due to infection could cause a cavernous sinus thrombosis.

Ethmoid bone

Within the orbit, and medial to the sphenoid bone, is the ethmoid bone. This small bone lies between the nasal bone (posterior) and the sphenoid bone (anterior) and it consists of several parts: a horizontal (or cribriform) plate, a perpendicular plate, a small triangular process projecting superiorly (the crista galli), two labyrinths containing air cells and two lateral plates that form the orbital walls.

The ethmoid bone makes up part of the nasal cavity between the orbits. Its superior horizontal plate also forms part of the anterior fossa of the skull base and is perforated (olfactory foramina) to allow branches of the olfactory nerve (contributing to our sense of smell) to pass through. Descending centrally from the horizontal plate is the perpendicular plate that forms the nasal septum.

Two projections adjacent to the perpendicular plate form the superior and medial turbinates (or concha) in the nose. Between the concha and the orbital plate are the ethmoidal labyrinths, which contain several air spaces (cells) that vary in number and are typically classed into anterior, middle and posterior groups according to their position.

Two further smooth bony extensions extend obliquely from the horizontal plate; and adjacent to the ethmoidal sinuses is an oblong plate that forms the inner wall of the orbit. This plate is known as the lamina papyracea, as it is literally paper-thin.

Given its delicate nature, the ethmoid bone can break relatively easily. Its association with the skull base (the cribriform plate) can lead to a leak of cerebrospinal fluid and it may entrap the medial rectus muscle. It is also noteworthy that the orbital ethmoid bone is partially removed in an orbital decompression procedure (ethmoidectomy) in patients with thyroid eye disease (see Chapter 9).

Lacrimal bone

This is a small bone which houses the sac and nasolacrimal duct in its anterior inferior portion. Described as being fingernail-shaped, it is approximately 11–14mm in height. The lacrimal bone is part of the medial wall of the orbit and is quite fragile. Attached to its four borders are the frontal bone (superiorly), the ethmoid bone (posteriorly) and the frontal process of the maxilla (anteriorly). Inferiorly, it is divided into two, articulating with the orbital portion of the maxilla and the inferior nasal concha.

A ridge divides the orbital surface of the lacrimal bone vertically. This ridge, known as the lacrimal crest, has an anterior and posterior portion. The lower aspect of the bone unites to form part of the nasolacrimal duct.

On its inner nasal surface, the lacrimal bone forms, in part, the middle meatus of the nose. In dacryocystorhinostomy surgery, part of the lacrimal bone is removed to create a new drainage passage.

Maxillary bone

This is a large facial bone that incorporates several aspects, including holding all the upper teeth at its inferior edge, the roof of the mouth, the floor and lateral wall of the nasal cavity. It articulates with nine other bones – frontal, ethmoid, zygomatic, inferior nasal concha, palatine, lacrimal and vomer. The maxillary bone incorporates both sides of the face, and (bilaterally) the medial aspects of the orbital floor.

The orbital portion of the maxillary bone creates the medial part of the floor of the orbit, within which a groove runs along the floor. This groove houses the infra-orbital nerve and attaches posteriorly to the lacrimal bone. The infra-orbital nerve travels along the groove and out onto the surface of the cheek, through the infra-orbital foramen, along with the infra-orbital artery and vein. This exit corresponds approximately with the margin of the orbit (approximately 6–10mm from the margin), roughly in the midline of the cheek. This is significant, as this nerve can be easily damaged when involved with orbital surgical procedures, such as floor fracture repair, decompression surgery and exenteration (where the orbital contents and occasionally bone is removed). Damage to this nerve will cause numbness of the face/cheek.

Medially, the frontal surface of the maxillary bone extends superiorly to create the nasal projection of the bone and part of medial orbital rim. Posteriorly, the maxillary bone extends to the inferior orbital fissure which transmits the zygomatic branch of the maxillary nerve, pterygopalatine ganglion and the infra-orbital artery.

Posteriorly, behind the maxillary bone is the largest air sinus in the body, the maxillary sinus (on both sides of the face). The sinus can be associated with sinusitis and inflammation and can be a common route for infection, given its close relationship with other sinuses and the maxillary teeth. It can also be associated with cancer.

This is rare, but squamous cell carcinoma is the most prevalent form, followed by adenocarcinoma. These cancers can sometimes spread into the orbit, causing proptosis and other types of eye malpositioning.

The maxillary sinus can enlarge with age, and can also vary in size – even between the two sides of the face. It is common to see orbital contents fall into the maxillary sinus superiorly after an orbital floor fracture.

Zygomatic (malar) bone
There are two zygomatic bones on either side of the face that create the prominence of the face and cheek. The zygomatic bone is said to be shaped like a quadrangle and it makes up the lateral aspect and floor of the orbit. It has a concave surface that extends back to attach to the zygomatic process of the temporal bone posteriorly. Its superior portion creates the smooth rounded part of the inferior-lateral orbital rim. Its superior margin articulates with the frontal bone at the frontozygomatic suture.

Posteriorly, behind the zygomatic arch temporally, the bone articulates with the orbital surface of the maxilla and the greater wing of the sphenoid bone. Similarly, within the orbit, the zygomatic bone articulates with the frontal superiorly, the greater wing of sphenoid dorsally, and the maxillary bones inferiorly.

Palatine bone
This pair of small bones is situated at the back of the nasal cavity and the palatine bone makes up a proportion of the hard palate posteriorly. It is described as an L-shaped bone and its most superior aspect extends into the posterior orbit near the optic foramen.

The orbital periosteum (periorbita)
This is a layer of dense connective tissue that loosely lines the bones of the orbit and acts as an attachment for various muscles and tendons. At the orbital rims, sutures and edges of fissures/foramen, the periorbita is somewhat more adherent to the underlying bone. The periorbita stretches all the way back into the anterior orbital canal where some of it becomes continuous with the dura matter of the optic nerve.

To gain access to the orbital bone in surgery, the periorbita will need to be reflected off the bone, using an elevator. In some reconstructive procedures, where there is a shortage of tissue, a small flap of periorbita can be reflected off the bone and used to reattach tissue to recreate a medial or lateral canthus.

The orbital apex
The orbital apex reflects the posterior part of the orbit where the confluence of structures come together and either exit or enter the orbit through various fissures. It is seen as the communication between the orbit and the intracranial cavities, and

it has a high concentration of arteries, veins and nerves crammed into quite a small space. There is also a ring of dense tissue running around the apex of the orbits, the annulus of Zinn, from which various recti muscles arise. Not surprisingly, a lesion or inflammation in this area could compress these structures, causing reduction of sight, nerve palsy, reduction in eye movement and/or a relative afferent pupil defect.

Intraconal/extraconal space

The extra-ocular muscles and the orbit form a musculofascial cone, from the annulus of Zinn anteriorly to the globe. The area within this cone is referred as the intraconal space. The extraconal space is that outside the musculofascial cone and within the bony orbital space. Certain lesions that develop can be described as being either intraconal or extraconal, depending upon where they develop. This can be significant from a surgical perspective, as different symptoms may be displayed according to the position of the lesions.

Orbital assessment and examination

A recurring theme throughout this book has been that the importance of undertaking a thorough history and clinical assessment in order to ascertain the appropriate management of any case. However, it is arguably never more important than in cases that could involve the orbit.

When taking the history, it is important to ask the following questions:

- Duration of symptoms – how long has the problem been going on?
- Has the patient described any issues with their vision?
- Has there been any pain?
- Has there been any diplopia?
- Has there been any neurosensory loss?
- Are the symptoms aggravated by coughing or straining?
- What is the patient's past medical history?

Answers to these questions should help provide a picture of the presenting problem. It is essential to get an understanding of the patient's past medical history because a number of systemic diseases may be related to orbital issues that the patient may not readily associate with them. This could apply to sinusitis or thyroid disease, for example.

Krohel, Steward and Chavis (1981) explained the 'six Ps' when considering orbital assessment: Pain, Progression, Proptosis, Palpation, Pulsation and Periorbital changes. Nerad (2001) added a seventh 'P' to the list: Past medical history.

Along with history-taking, it is necessary to carry out a detailed clinical examination along with a full eye examination. Specifically orbit-related details will be required, along with a full eye examination.

This should include the following:

Exophthalmometry – in order to measure the degree of proptosis (eye protrusion). It is generally accepted that an asymmetrical proptosis of 2mm, compared to the other side, or a measurement greater than 21mm (23mm in individuals of African origin) is considered significant. Remember that those with large eyes (high myopes) may present with pseudoproptosis, giving the impression they have bulging eyes. Assessing proptosis using an exophthalmometer provides a measurement from the lateral orbital rim to the front of the cornea.

The proptosis can either be axial, meaning it is the proptosis in the midline (primary gaze) between the two eyes, i.e. on the same axis, and associated with intraconal lesions, or it can be non-axial and suggestive of an extraconal lesion. The proptosis can also either be unilateral (one side) or bilateral (both sides). Unilateral proptosis has many potential differential diagnoses, but bilateral proptosis is better recognised and is most commonly associated with thyroid orbitopathy, non-specific orbital inflammation and, more rarely, lymphoma, myeloma, leukaemia and arteriovenous shunts. Enophthalmos (and eye retracting back into the socket) may also be picked-up on exophthalmometry and can suggest, amongst several potential diagnoses, a blow-out fracture.

Be aware that there are several models of exophthalmometer that can be used to undertake exophthalmometry and they may provide different readings. Considering the inherent subjective inter-user variation, the practitioner should take note of the model used and the width setting, as well as the reading (see Chapter 12, p. 191).

Ocular pulsation – observe and palpate for an orbital pulsation, using the bell-end of a stethoscope to listen for bruits over a closed eye. If present, this may suggest an arteriovenous shunt.

Palpation of the orbital margins – on occasion an anterior orbital mass may be palpable as either a soft or hard, mobile or fixed, painful or non-painful lesion.

Retropulsion – digital pressure applied to a closed eye may elicit firm resistance if an orbital mass is present.

Valsalva manoeuvre – in arteriovenous-related orbital malformation, if the patient is asked to forcefully exhale against closed airways (i.e. pinching the nose and closing the mouth, as if blowing a balloon), they may elicit a proptosis which retracts back once they stop. This usually occurs as blood forcibly engorges vessels as a consequence of miswired arteries/veins (orbital varices) and fills the orbit, pushing the eye anteriorly. It may also happen when the patient strains or coughs, which is why this question needs to be asked when taking the history.

Full cranial nerve (CN) examination:

Cranial nerve	Name	Assessment
I	Olfactory	Sense of smell
II	Optic	Visual acuity, Ishihara, field test, fundoscopy
III	Oculomotor	Eye movements, pupil dilation, accommodation
IV	Trochlear	Eye movements
V	Trigeminal	Facial sensation and light touch V1 forehead, V2 cheek, V3 jaw, muscles of mastication
VI	Abducens	Eye movements, pupil dilation, accommodation
VII	Facial	Smiling, blowing cheeks, raise eyebrows, show teeth, taste
VIII	Vestibulocochlear	Hearing, whispering, Rinne and Weber test
IX	Glossopharyngeal	Taste, uvula deviation, gag response
X	Vagus	Taste, pharyngeal movement
XI	Accessory	Shrug shoulders, turn head from side to side
XII	Hypoglossal	Tongue

Lymph node assessment – a lymphadenopathy may be suggestive of a systemic disorder, such as lymphoproliferative disease.

Check intra-ocular pressure (IOP) both in the primary position and in upgaze.

Always evert the upper eyelid – lesions or an enlarged lacrimal gland may be identified.

Check the rest of the body for lesions and carry out breast examination to check for potential metastasis.

Other tests may include laboratory investigations (TFT, ANCA, ACE, FBC), chest x-ray, CT scan or MRI scan.

Selected orbital disorders

There are many potential differential diagnoses relating to orbital symptoms and I have briefly outlined a few of the more common diseases and lesions below.

Thyroid eye disease

Chapter 9 is dedicated to thyroid eye disease (Graves) and the presentation of thyroid-related orbitopathy.

Orbital cellulitis

This condition is discussed in Chapter 12 (Emergency oculoplastic care), pp. 193–195. This is an acute presentation, with associated malaise, pyrexia, eyelid swelling and oedema, axial proptosis, restriction of eye movements, decreased VA, reduced colour vision and increased IOP. Remember, this is an ophthalmic emergency and the patient requires antibiotics, immediately along with CT scanning.

If there is a defined abscess within the orbit, this may require draining surgically and the ENT team may need to wash out the associated sinuses at the same time.

Pre-septal cellulitis has arguably milder symptoms, and usually no proptosis. However, this can progress to orbital cellulitis and therefore needs antibiotics and close monitoring.

Lymphoma

This can present as a benign proliferation of lymphoid tissue within the orbit (commonly superolaterally), often involving the lacrimal gland. The most commonly identified presentation is a 'salmon-patch' lesion under the upper eyelid, but not necessarily in all cases. Alternatively, there may be a malignant lesion associated with the transformation of leucocyte B-cells. A proptosis that is firm upon retropulsion may provide a further clue. The proptosis can be slow and painless in progression. There may be an associated systemic disease, so check for other lesions and for lymphadenopathy. A biopsy will be required to confirm the diagnosis and treatment will probably involve radiotherapy and/or corticosteroids.

Non-specific orbital inflammatory disease (idiopathic)

Essentially this is a chronic inflammatory process within the orbit, with no obvious specific cause. There may be unilateral or bilateral orbital pain, lid swelling and diplopia. An orbital biopsy will be required for diagnosis and, occasionally, surgical debulking of the mass may be required. Treatment is usually immunosuppression with systemic steroids.

Dacryoadenitis

This condition involves inflammation of the lacrimal gland due to non-specific orbital inflammation. The gland is swollen causing an S-shaped deformity in the upper eyelid and can also be painful. Other possible causes of a swollen lacrimal gland (including a tumour) must be ruled out first. Treatment for isolated dacryoadenitis is oral non-steroidal anti-inflammatory drug or steroids

Dermoid cyst

This type of lesion occurs as congenital embryonic entrapment of surface ectoderm within suture lines around the orbit. Dermoid cysts are most commonly associated with the frontozygomatic suture, but can occur elsewhere. They present as a firm well-defined mass that may cause proptosis or ptosis and reduced eye mobility and can be painful. CT scanning will be required to ascertain the extent of the lesion. The lesion usually requires complete surgical excision and it may contain evidence of hair or teeth within it.

Cavernous haemangioma

This is the most common type of benign intraconal tumour of the orbit in adults and it is associated with a slow progressive axial proptosis. Cavernous haemangiomas are often very well-defined oval/round lesions within a capsule. These lesions need to be surgically removed.

Lacrimal gland tumour

There are various lacrimal gland tumours, the most common being pleomorphic adenoma. This presents as a reasonably well-defined nodular lesion that requires surgical removal and there is a good prognosis subsequently.

Conversely, the more rarely occurring adenoid cystic carcinoma and pleomorphic adenocarcinoma are less well-defined lesions associated with bony destruction. After diagnosis, they are best treated with radiotherapy, but unfortunately the prognosis is poor.

Rhabdomyosarcoma

This is the most common type of primary orbital tumour in children. The presentation is usually in children (slightly more common in boys) under the age of 10 years and is a rapidly growing progressive unilateral proptosis. There can be associated inferolateral displacement of the eye, as the lesion most commonly occurs in the superior orbit.

An orbital biopsy will confirm diagnosis, and treatment may involve excision in well-defined cases and combined radiotherapy and chemotherapy.

Metastases

This is a rare occurrence in the orbit, but can be associated with breast, lung, prostate and gastrointestinal primary tumours. It usually presents as a progressively rapid proptosis. CT scanning can show bony destruction of the associated area close to the lesion. An orbital biopsy will be required for diagnosis.

Neurofibroma

This type of tumour is discussed in Chapter 5, p. 85.

Optic nerve sheath meningioma

This is a rare benign tumour associated with the optic nerve meningeal sheath. It typically causes optic nerve compression and patients therefore often present with reduced VA and optic disc swelling, prior to any proptosis. If the VA remains stable, observation would be recommended in the first instance. But if the eye becomes blind or there is a threat to the optic chiasm, the tumour may require surgical excision.

Sphenoid wing meningioma
This is a tumour affecting the sphenoid bone, which can spread to affect the orbit, causing progressive painless proptosis and inferior displacement of the eye. Eventually optic nerve compression from the tumour can affect VA and therefore require surgical debulking. Access to the tumour is often only through a frontal craniotomy and via the skull base. Neurosurgeon support is therefore required.

Vascular lesions
An orbital varix is a congenital enlargement of venous blood vessels which can be increased with the Valsalva manoeuvre (see above, p. 229). This can present as an intermittent proptosis. Surgery is only indicated in severe or sight-threatening cases, as the procedure is often difficult.

Arteriovenous fistula
This presents as an abnormal anastomosis of arterial and venous circulation. A carotid-cavernous fistula is a 'high-flow' system that causes a reduction in VA, diplopia and often an audible pulsatile proptosis (bruit), orbital oedema, retinal vessel engorgement, raised IOP and chemotic conjunctiva. Catheter embolisation under x-ray control may be required.

Orbital biopsy and surgical approach to orbital lesions
In many cases the only way to confirm diagnosis of the presenting lesion is to undertake an orbital biopsy. Alternatively, the lesion may need to be removed or debulked (removed as much as is safely possible, but inevitably leaving some lesion behind).

I will outline the key nursing considerations below, but in order to understand the nursing care I need to briefly outline the most common surgical approaches to the lesion and whether to completely excise or biopsy.

Upper eyelid skin crease (Anterior orbitotomy)
This is commonly used as an approach for orbital biopsy and access to superior orbital lesions. The upper skin crease is identified and marked. Then, using either a blade or monopolar cutting cautery device, an incision is made along the crease. This trans-septal approach can provide access to anterior lesions and, once the surgery is completed, the wound is hidden in the crease line.

Transconjunctival
This is usually a lower eyelid approach to inferior lesions (or the orbital floor) which involves making an incision horizontally across the palpebral conjunctiva, either at the lower border of the tarsal plate or via the inferior fornix. A surgical plane is created between the orbicularis muscle and the orbital septum towards the floor. Once at the orbital floor, the periorbita can be lifted to gain access to the floor of the orbit.

Lateral orbitotomy
This approach facilitates access to the lateral and intraconal space posterior to the globe. In order to do so, a section of the zygomatic bone is removed, providing greater access. The procedure involves making an S-shaped incision (Stallard-Wright incision) that follows the length of the zygomatic bone from the superolateral orbital rim, under the brow, down to the upper cheek just posterior and superior to the zygomatic process. The bone is sawed horizontally, approximately 5mm above the frontozygomatic suture, and then just above the zygomatic arch inferiorly. The orbital wall is then removed and stored safely. Once the lesion has been removed, the bone is replaced. Pre-placed drill holes are used to suture the bone back in place.

Post-operative care involves ensuring that the patient doesn't knock this area and displace the bone. Also, immediately after surgery, a suction drain may be placed (for 2–3 days) into the orbital cavity in order to draw away any potential post-operative haemorrhage.

Medial orbitotomy
Sometimes referred to as the Lynch excision, this offers access to the medial orbit via a transconjunctival approach or, alternatively, a transcaruncular approach medially. In rare cases, it may be necessary to disinsert the medial rectus muscle.

Frontal craniotomy
For access to lesions at the superior apex of the orbit, and with the assistance of the neurosurgery team, a transfrontal approach may be used. This involves a frontal craniotomy (with bicoronal flap) and retraction of the frontal lobe of the brain, which then provides access to the orbital roof via the skull base. This is obviously major surgery that may take many hours to undertake, with serious risks and potential complications that will need to be discussed with the patient. A frontal craniotomy is most commonly used to debulk a sphenoid wing meningioma.

Key nursing considerations in relation to orbital surgery
Pre-operative care
Individuals who present with proptosis at the Outpatients department or Emergency

Eye department are probably aware that diagnosis and treatment of the pending issue will be paramount. Their symptoms have arisen quite rapidly or they may have been aware of a progressive problem. Often the associated procedures to access and remove orbital lesions can be quite long (several hours) and consequently require extended exposure to general anaesthetic with all the potential risks linked to surgery.

In the majority of patients, there will be a degree of urgency about investigating and taking measures to diagnose the lesion. This is likely to involve blood tests, routine observations and a pre-assessment. It will also involve some form of scanning, usually CT or MRI.

In the first instance, an orbital biopsy will be highly likely. Purely from a surgical perspective, the key concerns will be access to the lesion and likely peri-/post-operative complications, particularly bleeding. The practitioner therefore needs to ascertain whether the patient takes anticoagulation medication and take precautions to manage this as effectively as possible within the time available. Don't forget that, after the biopsy and confirmation of the diagnosis, for some patients there may be further surgery to remove or debulk the lesion.

Most orbital biopsies can be undertaken under a local anaesthetic, with or without sedation. Occasionally a general anaesthetic will be necessary if undertaking a more extensive procedure or if it is the patient's preferred option. If so, greater efforts will be required to ascertain the patient's medical health. Further investigation of the cardiac and respiratory history may be required to elicit whether there are any factors that could affect or compromise the patient's safety during the procedure, e.g. myocardial infarction, angina or COPD.

Other important aspects to explore include hiatus hernia, diabetes, kidney disease and liver disease. Social/environmental issues (including smoking, drug use and alcohol intake) are also relevant. A full review of the patient's medications will help gain an understanding of any underlying issues. It is also important to ascertain whether the patient has any allergies.

Once the patient has been identified as requiring a biopsy and/or other surgeries or treatment, there is unlikely to be much time to prepare them for the surgery. Many patients will be apprehensive and anxious, and arranging appropriate support will be difficult with so little notice. However, communication is key, and it will benefit the patient if they are given an understanding of the process, post-operative care and longer-term care and treatment.

Undertaking a review of the patient's 'activities of daily living' will enable the practitioner to understand where some potential issues may require further input and support.

The consent process will enable the patient to understand the nature of the procedure and what is involved. It should also include an outline of the potential risks associated with the surgery, including:

- Damage to the eye/vision (blindness)
- Bleeding
- Bruising
- Infection
- Numbness
- Scarring
- Eyelid malposition
- Pain and discomfort
- Insertion of a drain
- Need for further treatment/surgery
- Nausea/vomiting
- Risks associated with an anaesthetic.

The risks associated with surgery sound quite frightening so a degree of context and pragmatism needs to be applied when conveying these potential issues. Suggesting there is a risk that the patient could lose their vision will of course be very alarming, but balancing this explanation with associated statistics may help to ease the patient's concern.

The patient may have to be 'nil by mouth' prior to the procedure. Certainly, for a general anaesthetic, this can be 6 hours prior to the surgery.

Immediate post-operative care

After orbital surgery there are several key issues relating to care and recovery.

Pain

The majority of patients usually only experience mild to moderate pain following orbital surgery and this can be controlled with simple analgesics. Many patients leave theatre having had a regional peribulbar block put in at the end of surgery, which will provide relief immediately after the procedure. It is important to regularly assess the pain using a verbal rating scale, i.e. '0 is no pain, 10 is the worst pain imaginable – what is your pain score?' If at all possible, keeping the analgesic level maintained is more effective than allowing the pain to get out of control, which is much harder to manage. Eventually the local anaesthetic will wear off and only then will the practitioner get a true understanding of the degree of pain.

In moderate to severe pain management, the big issue is whether or not the pain could suggest an underlying problem. A relatively sudden onset of post-operative pain could be indicative of an intra-orbital bleed. This is a problem, and it is sometimes necessary to avoid using opiates to control severe pain in case they are masking a potentially serious issue. Certainly, moderate to severe pain warrants further investigation. The key point is not to ignore a sudden onset (or continuation) of post-operative pain. The practitioner should always consider the possible reasons for this pain, before providing strong analgesics.

Nausea and vomiting

Again, post-operative nausea and vomiting is unusual, but if present it is likely to be associated with the anaesthetic. Most anaesthetists prescribe anti-emetics at the end of surgery. If not, this should be explored and guaranteed before returning the patient to the ward or day-case department. Remember, different anti-emetics have different modes of action. Whilst one type may not work, an alternative may do.

If the nausea and vomiting is prolonged, it may be necessary to provide IV fluid replacement. Continuous retching and vomiting could cause the patient strain and stress and, more importantly, could risk triggering an orbital bleed. Therefore, it is important to make a consistent effort to control any vomiting and this should be regularly assessed in the early stages after surgery.

Visual acuity/pupil reaction

In the initial 24-48 hours after surgery it might be necessary to test visual acuity and pupil reaction every hour. This may be difficult, due to swelling and lubricant. It may also be somewhat painful for the patient, and therefore has to be done carefully and sensitively. It will be necessary to use an aseptic technique as much as possible when removing any dressings. A bedside Snellen chart might be required if the patient finds it difficult to get to the testing room.

Record the findings in the medical notes, and report any significant changes. A sudden reduction in VA or a change in pupil reaction could be suggestive of an orbital bleed. Remember, in the early stages, it is extremely important to check the VA/pupil, even if this means waking the patient from their sleep.

Keep nil by mouth

In some particularly difficult surgical cases, or where the procedure has been problematic, it may be necessary to keep the patient starved in case they have to return to theatre due to the risk of bleeding. If so, it is important to ensure adequate hydration and guarantee that a suitable intravenous regime has been prescribed. It is important to remind the patient why they need to remain nil by mouth so they understand the reasoning and don't feel tempted to eat or drink.

Reduce intra-ocular pressure

Some patients may require post-operative systemic diuretics to reduce the intra-ocular pressure. Acetazolomide (Diamox) is commonly used for this purpose and can be prescribed for oral or intravenous use. Of course, this will mean that the patient needs to go to the toilet more often, and this may be an issue in certain individuals who, for example, may have mobility issues. Acetazolamide can also have a hypokalaemic effect so the patient's potassium levels will need to be monitored if there is a long-term need for them to take the drug.

Reduced vision

Immediately after the surgery, one eye may be covered or patched for a period and this may have a debilitating effect on the patient, especially if the vision in the remaining eye is poor. This may mean offering them support and guidance in the short term until the pad is removed. It is important to undertake a falls assessment in patients who might be more at risk of falling. Whilst they are in hospital, helping the patient to orientate themselves to their surroundings and helping them to the toilet may provide reassurance.

Loss of sensation

The area where the surgery has taken place may be numb or might have reduced sensation. In many cases this is self-limiting and the nerves may well recover, but this may take several months. During the recovery period, and as the nerves regenerate, the patient may experience tingling and 'pins and needles' sensation.

However, for some patients the sensation in a particular area may never recover, and it is therefore important to emphasise this possibility at the consent stage.

Systemic corticosteroids

In order to reduce post-operative swelling, the patient may be required to take oral steroids. This is likely to be a short reducing course but may still have some undesirable side-effects. For example, diabetics may find that their blood glucose levels become more erratic, and they should be carefully monitored whilst taking the steroids.

Systemic antibiotics

Antibiotics may be prescribed prophylactically to prevent infection, and may be initially given IV, then converted to oral upon discharge.

Eye care

The operated eye will require care, lubrication and hygiene. In the days and weeks following the procedure, the eyes will need lubrication. In some instances, the eye may not close as well following surgery and there may be lagophthalmos. Lubricants to protect the eye (especially through the night) will be necessary.

The eyes will benefit from cleaning, and either normal saline or cooled boiled water with a clean swab will be useful for this. Remember to encourage the patient (or whoever else will be doing the cleaning) to wash their hands both before and after cleaning. During the process, encourage the patient to use the swab or cotton ball, sweep it across the lids in one direction and then discard.

It is important to ensure that any other eye medications, such as glaucoma drops, are instilled. Remember that the operated eye might be the best sighted eye, and so the patient may need assistance with mobility in the days following the surgery.

Wound care

The surgical wound also needs to be kept clean and regular attention with normal saline/cooled boiled water will be most useful to maintain this.

Vicryl sutures are often used to close wounds and they will dissolve in approximately 10–20 days. Vicryl rapide is a similar suture but this dissolves much more quickly, within 10 days. Alternatively, nylon sutures may be used, but of course these will need to be removed after 7–10 days. The Vicryl sutures may be removed at the first visit to the OPD after surgery, as they can cause a degree of inflammation and irritation.

Drain

In some circumstances after orbital surgery, a surgical drain is inserted into the potential residual space left by excision of the lesion (or abscess). Two main types of drain are used: either a corrugated undulating drain (like a corrugated roof on a greenhouse), cut to the desired width and length and inserted (and stitched) into the wound; or a closed suction drain which has a bulb on the end to collect fluids.

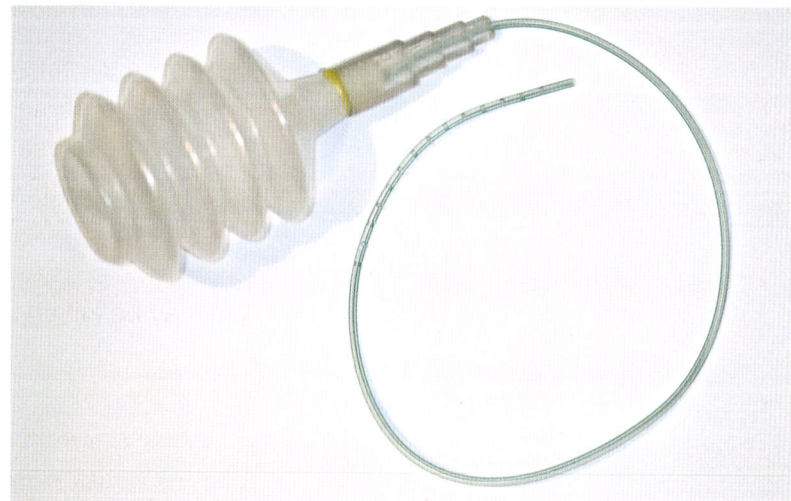

Figure 14.2: Surgical drain

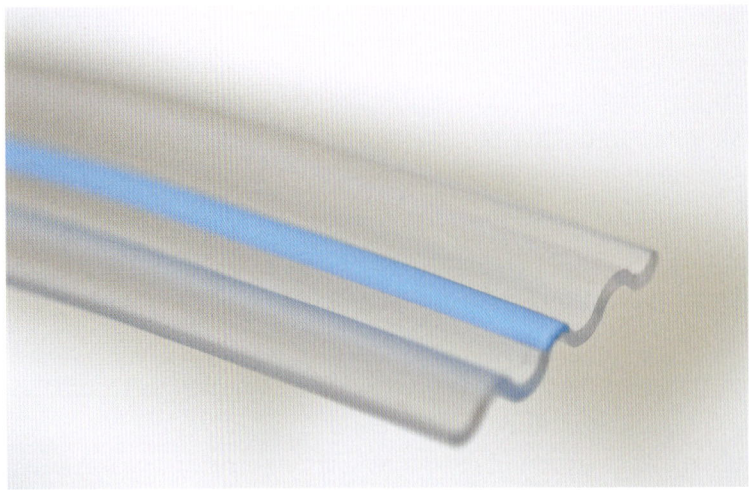

Figure 14.3: Corrugated drain

Drainage needs to be monitored and recorded whilst in place. Occasionally the drain can become dislodged and may have to be either reinserted or removed altogether.

Both types of drains used in the orbit are easy to maintain and usually easy to remove. Using an aseptic technique, they are held in place with a stitch. Once this has been cut, the drain should, with gentle traction, slip out. Monitor the patient in the hours following drain removal to ensure that the removal hasn't triggered a latent bleed.

Compression bandage

A bandage may be applied in the first hours or days after the procedure. In some cases, it may only be needed until the patient is wake and lucid after a general anaesthetic so that the vision can be checked post-operatively. When being extubated after a general anaesthetic, the patient may cough and strain which could initiate an orbital bleed, and the bandage can help prevent this.

Instructions on applying a head bandage appear in Chapter 12, p. 202. It is important that the bandage is not too tight, as this will cause discomfort and irritation. Also, if the bandage is to be kept on for several days it will very likely slip and require repositioning. It may therefore be helpful to show a relative or friend how to reapply the bandage for the patient.

It is important to monitor and record any soiling on the bandage, particularly any signs of bleeding or infection. Remember to tell the patient and/or relative this as well so if they see anything worrying they know it needs to be reported.

Head elevation

Sleeping with the head at a 45° angle can help reduce swelling, so sleeping with three pillows will be beneficial.

Swelling

In order to reduce swelling, ice packs can be made using crushed ice and a face cloth or tea-towel. Remember to be careful not to freeze the skin – limit the contact time of the ice packs. Also, remember some patients may be numb in the area as a consequence of the surgery and so may not feel how cold their skin has become.

Reassure the patient that swelling can be quite marked, especially within the eyelids, and this can take several months to subside. It is also important for the patient not to confuse oedema with infective swelling and they should be educated about the difference – an infection is often hot, painful and angry, with a discharge.

Nose blowing/Sneezing

Do not allow the patient to blow their nose for the first 10 days following surgery as this can force air into the orbit which could lead to vision loss. Similarly, if the patient thinks they need to sneeze, they should be encouraged to do so with an open mouth in order to reduce the pressure, which again could push air into the orbit.

Psychological context

It might be a difficult period for the patient having to undergo surgery and having uncertain outcomes and treatment. Keeping the patient informed, with honest and factual information, will provide some context and reassurance.

Simply providing a contact hospital email or telephone number will be reassuring and they should also be told what do in an urgent situation, especially out of normal working hours.

Considerations on discharge

On discharge after orbital surgery, some patients will need to be given the following instructions:

- Dressings – keep any dressing in place unless told to remove it.
- Wound hygiene – cleanliness is the order of the day; ensure appropriate hand hygiene if undertaking wound care or applying ointments or drops. Try to follow an aseptic technique where possible.
- Personal hygiene – showering the day after the surgery. Hot water and vigorous cleansing may encourage a bleeding risk. Hair washing might be best undertaken back-washed with assistance. Don't get soap into the wound.
- Avoid stress on going to the toilet and heavy lifting, such as gardening or carrying children.
- Avoid rubbing the eyelids.
- There will be sutures that may require removal. Sometimes the patient may get a small inflammation around a stitch (granuloma). In this case, the stitch may need to be removed and further antibiotic ointment will be required.

- No nose-blowing for the first 10 days following surgery, as this can force air into the orbit and be an infection risk.
- Cold ice compresses can help to reduce inflammation, but be careful not to induce frost-bite.
- Check for bleeding, sudden onset of pain or inflammation, discharge or other signs of infection.
- Medications can mostly be restarted within hours of the surgery, apart from anti-coagulants, which should wait until the next day after surgery.
- Arrange a follow-up date, time and place.
- Avoid driving for 48 hours after surgery, particularly after a general anaesthetic. If one eye is covered, consider whether the remaining vision is suitable for driving standard of Snellen 12/60?
- Avoid swimming for a couple of weeks following surgery, due to infection risk.
- Avoid hot drinks and food for 48 hours (heat and caffeine may cause bleeding).
- Following dressing removal, wound cleaning will be important and the application of antibiotic ointment onto the wound. Check the instructions and technique with the patient before they are discharged.
- Scars – consider using silicone anti-scarring treatment such as Kelo-Cote, Scar Away or Dermatix. These are not available on the NHS in the UK so the patient will need to buy them themselves and they may be too expensive for some patients.
- Provide details of who to contact with any questions or worries.

References

Ashwini, L., Rao, M., Sharmila, S. & Somayaji, S. (2012). Morphological and morphometric analysis of the supraorbital foramen and supraorbital notch: A study on dry human skulls. *Oman Medical Journal.* **27**(2), 129–133.

Krohel, G., Steward, W. & Chavis, R. (1981). *Orbital disease, a practical approach.* New York: Grune & Stratton.

Leatherbarrow, B. (2019). *Oculoplastic surgery.* 3rd edn. USA: Thieme.

Nerad, J. (2001). The diagnostic approach to the patient with proptosis. In *Oculoplastic Surgery,* pp. 348–85. New York: Mosby.

René, C. (2006). Update on orbital anatomy. *Eye.* **20**, 1119–29.

Sherman, D., Burkat, C. & Lemke, B. (2006). Chapter 21: Orbital anatomy and its clinical applications. *Duane's Ophthalmology* e-edition (version 2). Lippincott Williams & Wilkins http://www.oculist.net/downaton502/prof/ebook/duanes/pages/v2/v2c021.html (last accessed 27.11.2019).

15
Oculoplastic surgical competencies

Introduction

There are many facets that make up the advanced oculoplastic practitioner role, but from my perspective (and I believe, for many others who undertake a similar role elsewhere) the theatre and surgical aspects are perhaps the most important. Many oculoplastic practitioners will undertake minor surgical procedures themselves, others will assist the oculoplastic surgeon and a select few will perform more advanced surgery such as harvesting grafts.

In order to provide structure, consistency and safe practice, I have created my own surgical competencies. Over the years, many practitioners have asked me what these competencies look like and what information they contain. As surgery is such an integral part of the oculoplastic role, I felt it is appropriate to include them in this book.

These are my competencies, but you can use them as a basis or outline from which to create your own. They can be adapted, depending on the setting and who is undertaking the procedures. They are not exhaustive either. You may wish to add other roles to them and, over time, you may find that some aspects will no longer apply. I hope they will provide some guidance, and will also encourage you to develop your own oculoplastic practice.

1. Acting as Assistant Surgical Practitioner (ASP)

1.1. PROTOCOL FOR SKIN PREPARATION AND DRAPING OF THE OCULOPLASTIC PATIENT PRIOR TO SURGICAL INTERVENTION

EXPECTED OUTCOME:
The patient will have their surgical site prepared correctly and safely, using a recognised antiseptic solution and technique, and then have the area appropriately draped, using a sterile aseptic technique to provide an effective barrier between the sterile and non-sterile parts of the patient's body.

PERFORMANCE CRITERIA:
The assistant will be able to:
i. Discuss the considerations of skin assessment prior to surgical skin preparation
ii. Identify and discuss the procedural considerations
iii. Discuss factors relating to choice of skin preparation solution and outline the basic techniques required to carry out skin preparation
iv. Demonstrate an ability to prepare the skin and eye prior to ophthalmic surgery
v. Discuss the role of the assistant in draping and prepping the surgical patient using aseptic technique
vi. Demonstrate a safe practical ability to fully drape the surgical patient using recognised procedures and aseptic technique.

RATIONALE:
To prevent cross-infection and contamination of the surgical wound by removing soil and transient microorganisms and prevent bacterial re-growth (AORN 2016).

INDICATIONS:
Patients requiring surgical intervention.

CONTRAINDICATIONS:
Patients who do not require surgical intervention. Patients who may be allergic to specific skin preparations.

EQUIPMENT:
- Antiseptic skin solution (i.e. aqueous iodine 5% (Betadine) or if allergic Chlorhexidine) 10–20ml
- Prep-wells or Rampleys sponge-holding forceps and 5 x-ray detectable swabs (green) or sponges

- A tray and gallipot to hold equipment
- A range of the appropriate sterile disposable drapes for the oculoplastic procedure.

EQUIPMENT CONSIDERATIONS:

The x-ray detectable swabs used for the skin preparation will *not* be part of the overall individual count and will be 'handed-off' once used and prior to any surgical intervention.

ACTIONS AND ASSOCIATED RATIONALE:

1.1.1 The scrub practitioner should be appropriately prepared and sterile, using a recognised scrub technique, and should be wearing gloves and surgical gown.

- *To prevent and reduce the incidence of cross-infection and provide a barrier between the patient and the scrub practitioner.*

1.1.2 Correctly identify the patient prior to any intervention, using appropriate WHO (Haynes *et al.* 2009, NPSA 2009) checking criteria/protocol. Use the surgical 'timeout' to allow all the stakeholders in the theatre to assess the safety and identity of the patient.

- *To ascertain the patient's identity correctly prior to any surgical intervention. To correctly identify which antiseptic should be used on any individual patient. Skin is a major source of pathogens that cause surgical site infections (SSIs).*

1.1.3 Check that the patient has no history of being allergic or hypersensitive to the skin antiseptics proposed for use. For preparation a mixture of 50% aqueous iodine and 50% sterile water will be used on the face and around the eyes; for other areas of the body neat Povidone Iodine may be used, i.e. for skin graft sites. WHO (2016) suggest the use of alcohol-based preparations in preference to aqueous iodine but this is contraindicated in sensitive areas such as the eyes.

- *To correctly clean the surgical site: mechanically remove, chemically kill and inhibit contamination and colonising flora. Varying evidence as to the most appropriate antiseptic – Povidone Iodine effective against Strep gram-negative micro-organisms. Recent research suggests that Chlorhexidine may be more universally effective against a wider range of micro-organisms but it is not recommended for use on mucous membranes, i.e. conjunctiva (WHO 2016).*

1.1.4 Once the checking procedure is complete (surgical stop), the scrub nurse will pass the cleaning equipment. Using the Rampleys forceps, take one swab/sponge and place appropriately in/over the forceps so that it covers the distal end of the forceps. Using the forceps, soak some of the chosen antiseptic solution into the swab/sponge.

- *Rampley forceps are a suitable instrument to perform skin cleansing, providing a safe operating distance from the patient's skin to the operator's hand and preventing contamination. An appropriate amount of cleansing solution should be applied to the swab, not so little as not to provide sterility and not so much as to pool under the patient's head.*

1.1.5 The antiseptic should be applied with a degree of friction (but not so as to damage skin/tissue) in concentric circles and should extend from the planned incision site to the periphery of the area to be exposed in one continuous movement, not going over the same area twice (Lipp 2005, AORN 2016). Take care not to cause any undue damage to surrounding structures or equipment. Sensitive areas may have to be covered prior to application of antiseptic (Whalan 2006).

- *To prevent damage to the patient's skin from the forceps. If too little pressure is applied, the skin will not be appropriately cleaned. Cleansing using this method provides assurance that all the areas are cleansed and there is less chance of missing any sections.*

1.1.6 The area cleaned should be large enough to include all the potential incision sites and/or at other peripheral potential surgical sites the regime should be repeated (i.e. donor sites).

1.1.7 Once the act of cleansing an area is complete, the swab should be discarded and if necessary replaced with a new swab/sponge, until the whole area has been cleaned.

- *It may be necessary to use several swabs to clean the required area and maximise sterility.*

1.1.8 Time should be allowed for the antiseptic to dry (up to 2 minutes) and not be removed. When it is dry, the skin preparation is complete and the draping of the surgical area can begin (AORN 2016).

- *Allowing the solution to dry maximises its clinical effectiveness.*

1.1.9 Drapes commonly used for surgery are disposable, waterproof and breathable. The drapes are available in various shapes and sizes and provide a protective barrier between the patient and surrounding areas.

Usually the initial drape (head/neck) is placed under the head, while the patient's head is held up by an assistant. As with all draping, time should be taken to position the drape correctly and the drapes should be handled as little as possible. Scrub practitioners should be aware of their proximity to the surgical surroundings and provide themselves with sufficient space to perform the technique safely and not contaminate the drapes or the surgical site. The scrub practitioner may need to provide assistance with manipulating the drapes, i.e. two individuals working to position the drape. Do not allow the drapes to touch the floor (Whalan 2006).

- *Sterile draping provides a safe barrier between the sterile and non-sterile parts of the patient's body and maintains an adequate sterile field during surgery.*

1.1.10 Once the initial drape is under the head (and the head repositioned in the Rubens pillow), the inner part of the doubled drape will be placed over the head to cover the hairline and secured in place with an adhesive tape – taking care not to damage sensitive skin. Then a full-body disposable drape will be positioned over the patient and brought up to cover the neck and around the face to meet the head/neck drape. This will then be secured in place with adhesive tape. The only area of the patient left exposed is the face.

- *Only the appropriate area required is left open to reduce the risk of contamination by bacteria.*

1.1.11 If it is necessary to expose a donor site (e.g. the upper inner arm or abdomen), additional preparation and draping may be required. Additional smaller drapes may be used to compensate for any deficiencies in the sterile field.

- *Any exposed areas may potentially be contaminated and provide a risk of SSI.*

KNOWLEDGE REQUIRED:
- Anatomy and physiology of the skin
- An awareness of the implications of the type of anaesthetic and how it relates to the way the surgical site is prepared
- A competent ability and understanding of the aseptic technique in the surgical arena
- A working understanding of the type and nature of the surgery to be performed so as to be able to prepare the surgical field appropriately.

COMPLICATIONS:
Recognise the risk of an allergic reaction from the antiseptic solution, and potential pain and irritation. Modern adhesives used on disposable drapes may damage underlying skin when being removed – careful manipulation of the drapes will be required to reduce the risk of damage to the skin. Be aware of the potential actions that need to be taken if there is a significant reaction to the solution.

BOUNDARIES OF PRACTICE:
Any non-ophthalmic or oculoplastic patient.

LIMITATIONS:
Any non-ophthalmic or oculoplastic patient

References

Association of Peri-Operative Registered Nurses (AORN) (2016). Back to basics: Surgical skin asepsis. *AORN.* **103**(1), 96–100.

Atkinson, L.J. (1992). *Berry and Khon's operating room technique.* 7th edn. Missouri: Mosby.

Haynes, M. *et al.* (2009). A surgical safety checklist to reduce morbidity and mortality in a global population. *The New England Journal of Medicine.* **360**, 491–99.

Kumar, B. (1998). *Working in the operating department.* 2nd edn. New York: Churchill Livingstone.

Lipp, A. (2005). An evaluation of pre-operative skin antiseptics. *The British Journal of Perioperative Nursing.* **15**(1), 12–19.

National Association of Theatre Nurses (NATN) (1998). *Principles of safe practice in the perioperative environment.* Harrogate: NATN

National Patient Safety Association (NPSA) (2009). *WHO surgical safety checklist* (adapted for England and Wales). London: NPSA.

Whalan, C. (2006). *Assisting at surgical operations.* London: Cambridge University Press.

World Health Organisation (WHO) (2016). *Global guidelines for the prevention of SSIs.* Geneva: WHO.

1.2 TISSUE RETRACTION (OPHTHALMIC) USING HAND-HELD RETRACTORS

EXPECTED OUTCOME:

The operative field will be made more accessible to the surgeon by the safe and competent use of a surgical retractor.

PERFORMANCE CRITERIA:

The assistant will be able to:
i. Describe the types of retractors used in ophthalmic surgery
ii. Identify the appropriate retractor for the appropriate use/case
iii. Describe with due awareness the correct mechanical compression to the tissue so as not to cause undue damage
iv. Demonstrate an ability to retract for ophthalmic surgery, considering all appropriate factors, including: nature of the case, positioning and handling of the instrument, inappropriate use of the instrument
v. Identify the appropriate risk factors associated with tissue retraction.

RATIONALE:

Better surgical access, visualisation and ongoing observation of tissue through retraction and counter-retraction.

INDICATIONS:

Any oculoplastic surgical procedure where the tissues require retraction or counter-retraction to enable the surgeon to visualise the surgical field.

CONTRAINDICATIONS:

Only when *not* acting as scrub practitioner, i.e. not performing a dual role.

EQUIPMENT:

Appropriate instrument tray and retractors:
- Sewell
- Wright
- Malleable
- Langenbeck
- Desmarres
- Squint hook/Fison
- Eye protection for the practitioner.

EQUIPMENT CONSIDERATIONS:

Always check the integrity of the retractors; many can be damaged (through extensive use) and can damage tissue or break/bend during use.

Skin hooks have no place in oculoplastic surgery.

It is important to use the appropriate retractor with the right tissue and careful ongoing consideration should be given to the tissue. As the circumstances change during the procedure, it may be necessary to change the retraction instrument or the forces of retraction.

ACTIONS AND ASSOCIATED RATIONALE:

1.2.1 It is important that the practitioner assisting the surgeon is not the scrub nurse and that their responsibility is solely to assist, i.e. they are not performing a dual role.

- *Differentiation and understanding of the practitioner's role are essential to ensure safe and competent practice. It is not possible to safely undertake a scrub role while also retracting tissue.*

1.2.2 Identify the appropriate size and type of retractor for the type and nature of the tissue to be retracted. The three heavy retractors (Wright, Sewell and Langenbeck) will support a considerable amount of tissue within the orbit. The Sewell retractors, being curved, can allow access into small areas, but need to be handled with care, as the tip may not necessarily be within sight of the practitioner handling the instrument (Kirk 1994, Whalan 2006).

- *To allow the surgeon access to the deeper tissues. If an inappropriate retractor is used, in the wrong circumstances, it may damage tissue or bend/break.*
- *To understand the importance of treating tissues with care when retracting, particularly deeper tissues that may be damaged or torn by over-zealous retraction or by the tips of the instrument.*

1.2.3 Apply the retractor to the skin and tissue edges, maintaining an awareness of the mechanical compression of the tissues. Careful handling of retractors includes knowing how to support the hand for long periods of retraction. It is important to inform the surgeon if you require a rest or need to alter your hand position. Similarly, it is important to occasionally release the retractor to maintain blood flow (Nerad 2010).

- *To understand the effect of compression on the deeper tissues and the eye/globe.*
- *It is important to understand personal limitations and recognise fatigue in order to briefly rest or change position – failure to do so may lead to unexpected movement, and risk of damage to the patient or to the surgeon/practitioner.*

It may not always be possible to see the tip of the retractor and any amount of movement may mean a loss of tissue plane. It may require guidance from the surgeon and this will involve careful concentration.

1.2.4 The practitioner must learn to concentrate at all times when the retractor is in place. It is important to ensure that the lip of the retractor is in the correct plane (Whalan 2006). It is also very important to concentrate on the surgery and to watch the surgeon and the surgery at all times. If there is a need to change position (or remove the retractor), it may be necessary to use two hands to support the instrument while moving from one hand to the other.

- *Observing the surgery closely will enable you to predict ongoing requirements as the assistant, which will facilitate safer and more efficient surgery.*

1.2.5 On some occasions the retractors may be used not only to retract tissue but also to protect tissue from drills or saws. In this application the practitioner retracting tissue has to be aware that if a drill catches the retractor it may deflect either the drill or the retractor.

- *To appreciate the difficulties of tissue retraction when carried out near drills or saws, as they may have a tendency to deflect off the retractor, causing damage to surrounding tissue.*

1.2.6 Forceps and may be used to delicately move tissue and provide counter-retraction; this may require sensitive handling so as not to damage tissue (Atkinson 1992).

- *To understand the delicate nature of using fine forceps to hold tissue. Use pencil grip and only apply enough pressure to hold but not damage tissue.*

1.2.7 When passing any instruments to the surgeon, avoid passing them across the patient's face.

- *To avoid accidentally dropping the instrument on the patient's face.*

KNOWLEDGE REQUIRED:

- Anatomy and physiology of the orbit and surrounding structures
- The need to retract tissues to allow access to the deeper tissues
- Familiarity with the retractors available
- Being used to handling the retractors
- Understanding the importance of treating the tissues with care. The larger the retractor used, the less pressure will need to be exerted on the blade of the retractor.

COMPLICATIONS:

Carefully remove and insert the retractor and be aware of tissues being caught in the instrument.

It may sometimes be necessary for the surgical assistant to provide tissue retraction and apply suction simultaneously. In this situation the assistant needs to be mindful of the application of suction protocol and have been proven competent by their clinical supervisor in both these practices prior to the intervention. This should only be done under direct supervision by a member of the surgical team.

BOUNDARIES OF PRACTICE:

The surgeon will always be present to provide direct supervision. If the surgeon is not present, the retractor will be removed and the surgeon informed.

LIMITATIONS:

Any situation where the assistant does not feel competent or comfortable, or where there is a risk to patient (or staff) safety. Or any situation where the assistant is expected to perform beyond the parameters outlined in this protocol, which could in turn put the patient (or staff) at risk.

References

Atkinson, L.J. (1992). *Berry and Kohn's operating room technique*. 7th edn. Missouri: Mosby.
Kirk, R. (1994). *Basic surgical skills*. Edinburgh: Churchill Livingstone.
Nerad, J. (2010). *Techniques in ophthalmic plastic surgery: A personal tutorial*. Saunders/Elsevier
Whalan, C. (2006). *Assisting at surgical operations*. London: Cambridge University Press.

1.3 APPLYING MECHANICAL SUCTION TO THE OPERATING FIELD

EXPECTED OUTCOME:

The assistant will safely and competently apply suction to the wound/operating field and the surgical area will be kept free from the build-up of fluid/debris.

PERFORMANCE CRITERIA:

The assistant will be able to:

i. Demonstrate a working knowledge of the types of suction equipment available and how they work
ii. Identify the various types of suction tips available to the surgeon/assistant
iii. Demonstrate a safe, competent ability to apply suction to an area to remove fluid, show how to safely handle the suction tip and preserve the integrity of the surrounding tissue.

RATIONALE:

Better access, visualisation and ongoing observation of tissue through mechanical suction.

INDICATIONS:

Where fluids are obstructing the surgical view/access and therefore the surgeon's view.

CONTRAINDICATIONS:

Suction being applied in areas where delicate structures/tissue or potential specimens may be damaged. When the user feels that the apparatus may not be functioning appropriately.

EQUIPMENT:

- A suction machine or wall- or pendant-mounted suction (Schraeder wall outlet) (disposable collection jar, filter, float) suction tubing and a suction cannula or tip.
- Fraiser
- Yanker
- Baron.

The suction unit is connected to the vacuum pipeline inlet. Suction units provide a maximum flow 40L/min at a vacuum 53kPa (Kumar 1998).

EQUIPMENT CONSIDERATIONS:

Suction cannulas (tips) can often get blocked, particularly if they are reused. Disposable suction cannulas are extensively used. Suction is often used as a smoke evacuation device, which is not appropriate.

ACTIONS AND ASSOCIATED RATIONALE:

1.3.1 It is important that the practitioner assisting the surgeon is not the scrub nurse and that their responsibility is solely to assist, i.e. not carrying out a dual role.

- *Differentiation and understanding of the practitioner's role is essential to ensure safe and competent practice. It is not possible to safely undertake a scrub role while also applying suction.*

1.3.2 Identify areas requiring evacuation of fluid. These may be indicated by the operating surgeon and using the appropriate suction cannula gently applies suction in the appropriate area. Care must be taken not to damage surrounding/adjacent tissue.

- *To maintain a clear operative field that minimises pooling of fluid, which would make it harder for the surgeon to operate. The suction can damage very delicate tissue if used inappropriately.*

1.3.3 Many types of suction cannula have an occlusion hole where the device is held in the hand. This allows for control of suction to the area. When the hole is not occluded, the suction is lessened. Otherwise when occluded it provides suction at full power (Williams 2001). The assistant has to be aware of using the suction when drilling.

- *If necessary, the occlusion hole may be uncovered to release tissue that may be engaged in the suction tip.*
- *If the suction tip comes into contact with the drill this can damage the drill bit or the suction tip, or the drill may be deflected and this may cause indirect damage to adjacent tissue.*

KNOWLEDGE REQUIRED:

- Understanding of the principles of suction aspiration
- Understanding of the difference between sump suction and direct suction
- Understanding of the equipment required to provide efficient suction, and ability to troubleshoot when a problem arises
- Understanding of the anatomy and physiology of the orbit and surrounding tissues.

COMPLICATIONS:

It may be necessary for the surgical assistant to provide tissue retraction and suction simultaneously. In this situation the assistant would have to be mindful of the application of suction protocol and have been proven competent by their clinical supervisor in both these practices prior to the intervention. This should only be done under direct supervision by a member of the surgical team.

BOUNDARIES OF PRACTICE:

The surgeon will always be present to provide direct supervision. If the surgeon is not present, the suction device would be removed and the surgeon informed.

LIMITATIONS:

Any situation where the assistant does not feel competent or comfortable, or where there is a risk to patient (or staff) safety. Or any situation where the assistant is expected to perform beyond the parameters outlined in this protocol, which could in turn put the patient (or staff) at risk.

References

Kumar, B. (1998). *Working in the operating department.* 2nd edn. New York: Churchill Livingstone.

Nerad, J. (2010). *Techniques in ophthalmic plastic surgery: A personal tutorial.* Saunders/Elsevier

Williams, M. (2001). How do you keep your patient safe? Biological issues that impact on procedures. *British Journal of Peri-operative Nursing.* **11**(3), 124–30.

1.4 HOLDING TISSUE WITH FORCEPS

EXPECTED OUTCOME:
That the assistant will be able to competently and safely hold tissue and/or retract (or counter-retract) tissue during surgery with the appropriate forceps.

PERFORMANCE CRITERIA:
The assistant will be able to:
i. Describe the types of forceps used in ophthalmic surgery
ii. Identify the appropriate forceps for the appropriate type of tissue
iii. Describe with due awareness the correct mechanical compression of the tissues when using the forceps
iv. Demonstrate an ability to use forceps to hold and retract tissue for ophthalmic surgery, considering all appropriate factors, including: nature of the case, positioning and handling of the instrument, inappropriate use of the instrument
v. Identify the appropriate risk factors associated with using forceps to hold tissue.

RATIONALE:
To directly assist the surgeon or, if working autonomously, to enable the practitioner to hold tissue to perform surgery.

INDICATIONS:
An operative procedure during surgery to allow the surgeon better access, visibility and/or manipulation of tissue to enable actual surgical procedures to take place.

CONTRAINDICATIONS:
When the tissue is too delicate or friable to be handled with forceps, which could lead to further damage to the tissue. Beware of damaging histological specimens.

EQUIPMENT:
An appropriate instrument tray with forceps provided:
- Moorfields
- 0.12 forceps or Bishop Harmon
- 0.5 forceps
- 0.3 forceps
- Paufique
- Adson.

EQUIPMENT CONSIDERATIONS:
Smooth forceps generally cause more trauma to tissue, due to low friction and greater

forces required to hold tissue. Forceps with teeth offer a better grip with less crushing of tissue.

ACTIONS AND ASSOCIATED RATIONALE:

1.4.1 Identify the need for tissue to be manipulated with the forceps, and consider other types of retraction. This may be indicated by the surgeon. If using retractors, consider the protocol for the use of hand-held retractors.

- *There may be an alternative to physically holding tissues, which may be safer and less traumatic to the tissue. Using inappropriate forceps on delicate tissue may cause irreparable damage. Paufique or Adson forceps are the most commonly used for oculoplastic surgery.*

1.4.2 Otherwise, identify the appropriate forceps for the type of tissue, and the reason for the tissue to be held. Forceps with teeth should be used for most tissues commonly encountered in ophthalmic surgery (Nerad 2010). If there is any doubt, the assistant should ascertain the appropriate forceps for the task from the operating surgeon:

- Moorfields – conjunctiva
- 0.12 or Bishop Harmon forceps – delicate tissue
- 0.5 – delicate tissue including fat
- 0.3 – delicate tissue
- Paufique – general tissue holding
- Adson – heavy tissue holding.

1.4.3 Always hold the forceps like a pen, gripping with thumb and forefinger. Remember not to hold them too close to the tips (Whalan 2006).

- *To ensure a firm grip where the hand is less likely to slip and impede the use of the instrument or restrict access.*

1.4.4 Wherever possible, attempt to support the assisting hand, either with the other hand or something else (Leatherbarrow 2019).

- *Supporting the forcep-holding hand will reduce shake and unsteadiness.*

1.4.5 As the assistant grasps the tissue with the forceps, they should use gentle pressure to close the tips. When grasping tissue, select the plane of tissue that is least susceptible to damage. In other words, it is better to grasp the dermis or subcutaneous fat rather than the skin edge directly.

- *So as not to damage delicate tissue, the teeth of the instrument should not leave marks on the tissue.*

KNOWLEDGE REQUIRED:
- Anatomy and physiology of the orbit, eye and surrounding adnexa, and also the skin
- Familiarity with the types of forceps available to use and the appropriate tissue they should be used on
- Understanding of the importance of handling tissue with care and appreciating the limitations of particular instruments
- Understanding and appreciation of the forces required to hold particular tissue.

COMPLICATIONS:
It may not always be easy to recognise the nature or condition of particular tissue and it will be important to observe carefully the effect of holding particular tissues.

BOUNDARIES OF PRACTICE:
The surgeon will always be present to provide direct supervision. If the surgeon is not present, the forceps and/or traction device would be removed and the surgeon informed.

LIMITATIONS:
Any situation where the assistant does not feel competent or comfortable, or where patient (or staff) safety is at risk. Or any situation where the assistant is expected to perform beyond the parameters outlined in this protocol, which in turn could put the patient (or staff) at risk.

References

Leatherbarrow, B. (2019). *Oculoplastic surgery* 3rd edn. Thieme USA.
Nerad, J. (2010). *Techniques in ophthalmic plastic surgery: A personal tutorial.* Saunders/Elsevier
Whalan, C. (2006). *Assisting at surgical operations.* London: Cambridge University Press.

1.5 USE OF THE THEATRE-OPERATING MICROSCOPE (CEILING-MOUNTED OR FREE-STANDING) TO ASSIST THE SURGEON OR TO PERFORM MINOR OCULOPLASTIC AND/OR OPHTHALMIC PROCEDURES

EXPECTED OUTCOME:

That the specialist practitioner will be able to use the ceiling-mounted (or free-standing) theatre microscope either to assist the surgeon during ophthalmic/oculoplastic cases or to perform minor operations.

PERFORMANCE CRITERIA:

The assistant will be able to:

i. Demonstrate a working knowledge of the ceiling-mounted or free-standing microscope
ii. Have a basic knowledge of how to trouble-shoot if the need arises
iii. Understand how to care for and clean the microscope
iv. Demonstrate an ability to manipulate and use the microscope during a surgical procedure
v. Demonstrate an ability to use the assistant's eyepiece safely and competently during surgery.

RATIONALE:

To directly assist the surgeon or, if working autonomously, to undertake specific procedures that require the use of a microscope (see below).

INDICATIONS:

Operation requires the use of the operating microscope. Many general ophthalmic procedures are performed using a theatre microscope and/or require an assistant (who also uses the microscope).

In addition, the oculoplastic specialist nurse may use the operating theatre microscope when performing electrolysis for trichiasis and removing certain small lesions.

CONTRAINDICATIONS:

Other types of microscopes for use in other types of surgery, e.g. neuro or ENT. These microscopes have different functions and perform at different focal lengths.

EQUIPMENT:

An operating theatre microscope (either ceiling-mounted or free-standing) for use in ophthalmic surgery.

EQUIPMENT CONSIDERATIONS:

Theatre microscopes vary by individual design and may therefore operate very differently from one another.

ACTIONS AND ASSOCIATED RATIONALE:

1.5.1 The specialist practitioner will gain an understanding of the general design and function of the particular model of microscope used in the theatre. This will include being able to understand and competently:

- Turn the microscope on
- Understand the manual manipulation of the unit to gain an appropriate view
- Connect and correctly use the foot pedal
- Adjust the illumination
- Use the red reflex
- Use the assistant's eyepiece and adjust the inter-papillary distance (IPD).
- *Most operating microscopes incorporate the same essential components, including a binocular optical lens system which can be controlled either by hand or by foot, but individual models will vary considerably in layout and design. The practitioner needs to be aware of the differences between devices, but also appreciate the basic principles that are common to all microscopes.*

1.5.2 The user must also be able to troubleshoot any problems that arise and understand how to care for the microscope. The user must be able to use the foot-pedal that accompanies the microscope and be able to use the X-Y and focus functions. The specialist practitioner must be able to competently perform surgical procedures using the microscope.

- To be able to troubleshoot during the procedure if it becomes necessary, as the practitioner will be occasion-scrubbed and will not be able to use their hands to manually move the microscope.

KNOWLEDGE REQUIRED:
The user will have to demonstrate an understanding of the theatre microscope and its place in ophthalmic surgery.

COMPLICATIONS:
A basic ability to troubleshoot will be necessary.

BOUNDARIES OF PRACTICE:
In certain situations, the surgeon will be present to provide direct supervision of the use of this equipment. However, the use of the microscope will also be needed in certain situations where the user will not be directly supervised. In this instance the user will always be mindful of the boundaries and limitations of practice outlined within this protocol.

LIMITATIONS:

Any situation where the assistant does not feel competent or comfortable, or where patient (or staff) safety is at risk. Or any situation where the assistant is expected to perform beyond the parameters outlined in this protocol, which could in turn put the patient (or staff) at risk.

References

Atkinson, L.J. (1992). *Berry and Kohn's operating room technique.* 7th edn. Missouri: Mosby.

1.6 SAFE CUTTING OF SUTURES IN OPHTHALMIC/OCULOPLASTIC SURGICAL PROCEDURES.

EXPECTED OUTCOME:
The assistant will demonstrate a safe ability to cut sutures using the appropriate suture-cutting scissors.

PERFORMANCE CRITERIA:
The assistant will be able to:
i. Demonstrate a working knowledge of the types of sutures used for ophthalmic/oculoplastic surgery and their characteristics and presentation
ii. Identify and understand the different methods of suture tying
iii. Demonstrate the appropriate, safe and correct way to use suture-cutting scissors
iv. Demonstrate an ability to safely cut sutures used in surgery, including with the use of the theatre-operating microscope (see 1.5).

RATIONALE:
Cutting sutures in ophthalmic procedures is a delicate and precise manual task, and poor technique may cause a risk to the patient or damage instruments.

INDICATIONS:
Any suture that is indicated by the surgeon (and confirmed by the assistant) as needing to be cut, or any sutures that require cutting during minor surgical procedures.

CONTRAINDICATIONS:
Caution must be exercised when sutures are difficult to see within the wound and in these instances it may be more appropriate for the surgeon to cut them.

EQUIPMENT:
The appropriate oculoplastic/orbital tray:
- Suture-cutting scissors
- Westcott scissors
- Vanna scissors.

EQUIPMENT CONSIDERATIONS:
Certain scissors are indicated for use in several applications, i.e. for dissecting tissue, and are not therefore the ideal choice for cutting sutures.

ACTIONS AND ASSOCIATED RATIONALE:
1.6.1 The assistant will recognise the suture being used (and the application) and ascertain whether the suture will require cutting, or the assistant will be instructed to cut a particular suture as guided by the surgeon.

- *To make sure that the appropriate suture is cut.*

1.6.2 The appropriate suture-cutting scissors will be chosen: for the very finest sutures (e.g. 10/0 vicryl), Westcott scissors; for most other heavier sutures, straight suture-cutting scissors. Westcott-type scissors (sometimes known as 'finger' or 'spring' scissors) should be used between the index finger and thumb. The curvature of the Westcott scissors should be directed away from the wound, i.e. curved upwards. The assistant should also use either their opposing index finger or some other point to steady the cutting hand prior to use. When cutting all other sutures, straight, sharp scissors should be used (Nerad 2010).

- To choose the appropriate suture-cutting scissors. Only scissors with a sharp tip and straight blade should be used for cutting most heavy sutures (Leatherbarrow 2019); and for finer sutures, use Westcott scissors.

1.6.3 The assistant using suture scissors should use the tripod technique (Whalan 2006). Place the middle finger in the left ring of the scissor and the thumb in the right ring of the scissor and use the index finger to support the scissor. Again, the assistant should use the other hand (index finger) to support the cutting hand.

- *To allow for safe and steady cutting of the suture by the assistant. Westcott scissors are not recommended for cutting sutures (Nerad 2010) but may be suitable for the very finest suture material – rather than heavier scissors, which it may be argued, could be too large for fine sutures.*
- *Many surgical reference books consider the tripod technique to be a safe way of cutting sutures*

1.6.4 It is recommended to use the scissors to gently slide down some of the length of the suture to the cutting position. The assistant may wish to ascertain the cut length of the suture prior to cutting. It is good practice for the assistant to pause momentarily to confirm they are cutting the appropriate suture, at the right length, prior to cutting.

- *To allow the assistant to gauge and orientate themselves to the suture, so as to cut it at the appropriate point.*
- *Cutting sutures erratically may damage the suture material or may lead to the assistant accidentally cutting some other structure – the cutting of the suture should be careful and calculated.*

1.6.5 When using a theatre microscope, the assistant should carefully orientate themselves prior to cutting the suture and be mindful of other sutures or material that may accidentally be cut. Close the scissors slowly, rather than snipping abruptly or erratically.

- *When working with the theatre microscope, it's easy to become disorientated, especially when working in such a small field of view. The assistant should therefore keep looking at the position of their hand in relation to the area the surgeon is working in.*

KNOWLEDGE REQUIRED:
- An understanding of the types of sutures used in ophthalmology and their characteristics
- An awareness and understanding of the surgery being performed
- An understanding of the types of scissors used to cut sutures.

COMPLICATIONS:
None.

BOUNDARIES OF PRACTICE:
With most suture cutting, the assistant will be directly supervised by the surgeon. However, in some minor procedures the practitioner will be working with no direct supervision.

LIMITATIONS:
Any situation where the assistant does not feel competent or comfortable, or where patient (or staff) safety is at risk. Or any situation where the assistant is expected to perform beyond the parameters outlined in this protocol, which could in turn put the patient (or staff) at risk.

References

Leatherbarrow, B. (2019). *Oculoplastic surgery.* 3rd edn. USA: Thieme.
Nerad, J. (2010). *Techniques in ophthalmic plastic surgery: A personal tutorial.* Saunders/Elsevier
Whalan, C. (2006). *Assisting at surgical operations.* London: Cambridge University Press.

2. Infiltration and administration of subcutaneous local anaesthetic into the eyelid and/or surrounding area (including donor sites)

EXPECTED OUTCOME:

The practitioner will safely and competently inject/infiltrate local anaesthetic into the subcutaneous plane. The eyelid and/or surrounding area will be anaesthetised subcutaneously using appropriate local anaesthetic.

PERFORMANCE CRITERIA:

The assistant will be able to:
i. Demonstrate the ability to outline the site for injection
ii. Discuss and demonstrate an ability to prepare the injection and the injection site using ANTT
iii. Discuss and demonstrate the method of delivery of the injection and infiltration
iv. Identify the risk factors and complications of administering local anaesthetic
v. Discuss the pharmacology and characteristics of the anaesthetic being used
vi. Demonstrate how to prepare the patient prior to the injection and make the appropriate safety checks
vii. Demonstrate the ability to physically administer the local anaesthetic competently and safely into the subcutaneous tissue of the eyelid (or donor sites) and the surrounding area
viii. Demonstrate an ability to provide an adequate assessment of the anaesthesia after administration.

RATIONALE:

To enable minor operative procedures to be performed with minimal discomfort to the patient.

INDICATIONS:

Patients requiring minor operative surgery:
- Electrolysis for trichiasis
- Incision and curettage of chalazia
- Incision and/or excision of lesions
- Excision of skin tags or skin appendages
- Application of TCA to xanthelasma
- 3 snip procedure/ Kelly's punctoplasty

- Punctal cautery
- Everting sutures (inc. transverse)
- Donor sites for full thickness skin grafts
- Donor sites for dermis fat grafts.

CONTRAINDICATIONS:

Any patient with a history of hypersensitivity to Lidocaine or any of its derivatives. Any patient under the age of 16 years old (without direct supervision). Any pregnant patient. Any patient with a history of heart block or porphyria.

NEED FOR CAUTION:

In cases of epilepsy, severe liver/renal disease, respiratory depression, congestive cardiac failure, cardiac arrhythmias and hypovolaemia.

EQUIPMENT:

- Blue tray or transferable trolley
- 5ml syringe, green needle/drawing up needle, long orange needle (25g)
- Dilute preparation may also be considered – 3ml syringe and sterile normal saline
- Local anaesthetic
- Sterile prep tray with swabs
- Cleaning swab for the skin, iodine
- Gloves.

EQUIPMENT CONSIDERATIONS:

Observe aseptic non-touch technique (ANTT) policy at all times.

ACTIONS AND ASSOCIATED RATIONALE (not necessarily in this order):

2.1 The practitioner will identify the patient against their wristband, consent form and the theatre list and will confirm the correct patient for the planned procedure – WHO checklist (2009). The practitioner will also identify and confirm the side/site for surgery. The site will have been marked prior to surgery. This is confirmed with the patient and against the consent form and the theatre list.

- *To identify the correct patient and confirm the appropriate surgery requiring local anaesthetic.*

2.2 The practitioner will check the patient has none of the contraindications as outlined above (this may have been ascertained preoperatively).

- *To reduce the potential risk of the patient reacting adversely to the administration of the local anaesthetic.*

2.3. The practitioner will wash their hands using ANTT technique. The practitioner will clean the plastic prep tray (or trolley) using an alcohol cleanser and will gather the appropriate equipment as outlined above. Then the prep pack will be opened using aseptic technique and the equipment will be emptied onto the sterile tray.

- *To ensure that the practitioner follows the Trust ANTT guidelines.*

2.4. The practitioner will check the local anaesthetic with themselves and with another qualified nursing or medical colleague and will then draw up the anaesthetic using the sterile 5ml syringe and drawing-up needle. The drawing-up needle will be exchanged for a long orange needle (25G).

- *To ascertain that the correct drug is being administered, which is appropriate to the patient.*
- *The long orange needle (25G) is appropriate for the safe and less painful administration of local anaesthetic.*

2.5 For certain procedures, a dilute solution of local anaesthetic with normal saline may be used to provide a more comfortable injection.

- *To reduce the pain of administration of the local anaesthetic.*

2.6 The practitioner will don protective gloves. The practitioner may prepare the area with an antiseptic before administering local anaesthesia.

- *To protect the practitioner and the patient from potential cross-infection by blood contaminants.*
- *To optimise the skin condition and protect against potentially harmful bacteria.*

2.7 The practitioner will indicate to the patient that they are going to administer the local anaesthetic.

- *To prepare the patient for the imminent administration of the local anaesthetic. The practitioner will need to predict any potential movement of the patient upon insertion of the needle.*

2.8 The practitioner will insert the needle through the skin and advance the needle parallel to the skin (at an angle of approximately 20°) into the subcutaneous tissue for approximately 5mm and then stop and draw back on the syringe. The practitioner will then slowly inject the local anaesthetic into the area requiring anaesthesia by raising a bleb and, if necessary, advancing the needle within the bleb to other areas requiring anaesthesia.

- *When injecting into the eyelid, staying more or less parallel to the eyelid/skin reduces the potential risk of perforating the globe.*
- *Drawing back on the syringe prior to injecting anaesthetic will indicate to the practitioner that they have not directly cannulated a blood vessel (blood would*

enter the syringe). This enables the practitioner to avoid injecting anaesthetic intravenously.

- *To allow the anaesthesia to infiltrate/diffuse the appropriate tissues and to avoid the formation of a haematoma.*

2.9 Having injected the patient, the practitioner will withdraw the needle and will immediately discard it in a sharps bin. They will also, using a swab, gently apply pressure on the anaesthetised area and may massage appropriately.

- *To ensure safe and appropriate sharps management.*

2.10 After approximately 5 minutes, and before any surgical intervention, the practitioner will assess the level of anaesthesia (this may be done using forceps and asking the patient whether or not they can feel any contact with the forceps against the skin). It may be identified that further local anaesthetic will be required and the practitioner may need to prepare for that.

- *To ensure the anaesthetic has worked effectively.*

KNOWLEDGE REQUIRED:
- Pharmacology of local anaesthetic
- Anatomy and physiology of the skin and the eyelid
- Awareness of the possible side effects and contraindications of the anaesthetic and how to react if the need arises
- Identification of risk factors
- ANTT guidelines
- Sharps management policy
- Medicines management policy.

COMPLICATIONS:
Anaphylactic reaction to the local anaesthetic – urgent intervention and call for help.
Haematoma – apply firm pressure to prevent further bleeding. Contact a member of the medical team. Consider postponing the surgery.
Pain during surgery – consider infiltrating more anaesthetic. If in doubt, consider abandoning the procedure and seek advice from the medical team.

BOUNDARIES OF PRACTICE:
Where the patient is known to have large amounts of scar tissue and is deemed difficult to anaesthetise.

LIMITATIONS:
Ensure that maximum dose is not exceeded. Any situation where the assistant does

not feel competent or comfortable, or where patient (or staff) safety is at risk. Or any situation where the assistant is expected to perform beyond the parameters outlined in this protocol, which could in turn put the patient (or staff) at risk.

References

Leatherbarrow, B. (2019). *Oculoplastic surgery.* 3rd edn. USA: Thieme.
British Medical Association and the Royal Pharmaceutical Society of Great Britain (2009). *British national formulary.* Oxfordshire: Pharmaceutical Press.

3. Closing of subcutaneous layers, stapling or suturing of the skin

EXPECTED OUTCOMES:

The practitioner will close surgical wound edges so that they are in apposition, allowing for primary epithelialisation.

PERFORMANCE CRITERIA:

The practitioner will be able to:

i. Identify the types and characteristics of suturing materials used
ii. Discuss and demonstrate the different suturing techniques that can be applied
iii. Demonstrate a competent and safe ability to suture the subcutaneous layers, using the appropriate suturing material, technique and instruments
iv. Demonstrate a competent and safe ability to suture the skin, using the appropriate suturing material, technique and instruments
v. Demonstrate a competent safe ability to use and deploy staples into the skin for wound closure, using a disposable stapling device.

INDICATIONS:

To close surgical incisions and wounds including the following:
- Full thickness skin graft donor sites
- Split thickness skin grafts
- Suturing of STSG in exenteration wounds
- Dermis fat graft donor sites
- Blepharoplasties
- Levator aponeurosis advancement
- Direct brow lift
- Fascia lata donor site on the lateral aspect of the thigh
- Closure following excision/incision of lesions in minor surgery.

CONTRAINDICATIONS:

Suturing of layers deep to the subcutaneous layer.

Stapling will not be appropriate for some types of wound closure and it only tends to be used in closure of temporalis fascia patch grafts.

EQUIPMENT:
- Appropriate instrument tray
- Sutures or staples.

EQUIPMENT CONSIDERATIONS:

For most ophthalmic suturing, Castroviejo needle holders are used. For heavier suturing, most practitioners use Webster suture holders.

ACTIONS AND ASSOCIATED RATIONALE:

3.1 Assess the wound and the type of closure required. If necessary, confirm chosen technique with the medical staff/surgeon. Confirm the suture material to be employed. Suture techniques that may be employed to suture skin include:

- **Simple interrupted** (percutaneous): small wounds under no tension
- **Vertical mattress** – provides both deep and superficial support for wounds, and everts the skin edges
- **Continuous:** (running percutaneous) – longer wound that is under no tension; or locking percutaneous, for longer wounds under moderate tension
- **Subcutaneous** – for the deeper layers.
- *The correct suture technique and material will be employed for the wound closure. Cutting and reverse cutting sutures are the most suitable for skin closure. Using the inappropriate material may lead to dehiscence of the wound, increased inflammation and more chance of scarring.*

3.2 The needle, when selected, should be carefully and appropriately loaded in the Castroviejo or Webster needle holders. Adopt a pencil grip for holding Castroviejo needle holders and a thumb/ring finger grip for Webster needle holders. Adopt the appropriate suturing technique outlined as per Leatherbarrow (2019) and Nerad (2001).

- *Avoid over-tightening the suture, 'approximate do not strangulate'.*
- *To avoid the needle moving within the holders.*
- *To promote healing and minimise scarring.*

3.3 When suturing skin, ensure that the wound edges are everted. Ensure proper anatomical realignment of issues. Avoid undue wound tension.

- *Do not leave dead space as this may lead to infection.*
- *To avoid tissue and/or wound breakdown and to allow for skin edge approximation, the practitioner may have to undermine the wound.*

3.4 Handle the tissue with care, using the appropriate forceps (see 1.4).

- *To avoid crushing and damaging the tissue.*

3.5 In subcutaneous suturing the needle should be buried – the needle is first passed from the deep to superficial in the wound and then from superficial to deep. Do not over-tighten the sutures. Knot the suture with three throws. Additional throws may be required with nylon sutures. Cut the suture 3–6mm distal to the knot.

- *To avoid the suture 'cheese-wiring' through the skin.*
- *Avoid over-tightening the suture – 'approximate do not strangulate'.*

3.6 Stapling: Similar rules and methods apply as above. The skin edges must already be approximated with underlying subcutaneous sutures. The wound should not be under any tension. Using Adson forceps, the wound 2–3mm anterior to the insertion of the staple will be lifted slightly. Use the disposable stapler to apply staples as per manufacturer's instructions.

- *Staples do not hold a wound under tension.*
- *Adson forceps are used to help the staple to grip and insert into the skin.*

3.7 When closing levator aponeurosis wounds, it will be necessary to pick up the underlying orbicularis when closing the wound.

- This is in order to reform a new skin crease.

KNOWLEDGE REQUIRED:
- Skin anatomy and physiology
- Suture material available
- Suture and stapling technique
- Basic surgical skills.

COMPLICATIONS:
Where 'dog-ears' are produced, use forceps to pull the side of the dog-eared wound edge vertically. Then trim the excess skin so that the wound will close symmetrically.

BOUNDARIES OF PRACTICE:
The surgeon may be present to provide direct supervision. The exception to this will be for the closure of minor surgical wounds. Only simple interrupted sutures will be used, and any difficulties will be reported immediately to the medical team.

LIMITATIONS:
Any situation where the practitioner does not feel competent or comfortable to provide the appropriate level of expertise, and finds the provision of this particular practice is beyond their level of competence.

References

Leatherbarrow, B. (2019). *Oculoplastic surgery*. 3rd edn. USA: Thieme.

Nerad, J.A. (2001). *Requisites in ophthalmology: Oculoplastic surgery*. Missouri: Mosby.

4. Applying diathermy for wound haemostasis

EXPECTED OUTCOMES:
The nurse practitioner will control any intra- or post-operative bleeding.

PERFORMANCE CRITERIA:
The practitioner will be able to:
i. Demonstrate knowledge and understanding of assisting with surgical haemostasis, and assist in locating the origin of bleeding
ii. Determine the safe and correct use of equipment required for surgical haemostasis
iii. Demonstrate an ability to employ the appropriate technique to assist in maintaining haemostasis
iv. Determine and demonstrate the safe and correct use of electrosurgery.

INDICATIONS:
Bleeding vessels and the diathermy of identified vessels in the vicinity of the surgery that may have a propensity to bleed if incorporated into the surgery.

CONTRAINDICATIONS:
Patients who take anti-coagulation therapies and/or aspirin may be at greater risk from bleeding.

EQUIPMENT:
- An electrosurgical diathermy unit, headpiece and lead
- Hand-held diathermy device.

EQUIPMENT CONSIDERATIONS:
There are many diathermy machines available.

ACTIONS AND ASSOCIATED RATIONALE:

4.1 The practitioner will familiarise themselves with the individual function and capability of the types of electrosurgical machine available for use. The practitioner will also be familiar with the methods of diathermy available: coagulation, figuration, blend, cut, etc.

- *To appreciate the boundaries and scope of the electrosurgical diathermy machine.*
- *To appreciate the mode required to achieve haemostasis.*

4.2 The practitioner will also have an appreciation of how the theory of electrosurgical diathermy works. Simple tamponade of bleeding areas may reduce, help to control or even stop bleeding using Q-tip cotton buds or a swab.

- *Sometimes it may be just as effective to allow the functional clotting to take place, rather than overdo the amount of mechanical bipolar, which can damage surrounding tissue.*

4.3 The bipolar forceps and lead will have been connected appropriately to the diathermy machine.

- *To allow for proper functioning of the bipolar forceps.*

4.4 The electrosurgical machine will have the appropriate settings for bipolar diathermy (as per the instruction manual) or through guidance by the surgeon.

- *To understand the physiological mechanisms of haemostasis and how these can be augmented by using diathermy in surgery.*
- *To appreciate the effectiveness, dangers and limitations of diathermy, the user must understand the instrument they are using and how it works.*

4.5 The bleeding vessel will be identified by the practitioner whilst performing surgery outlined in this risk assessment document or by the surgeon during oculoplastic/ophthalmic surgery.

- *Keeping a clear blood-free field of view enables good surgery and reduces the possibility of mistakes. Therefore maintaining haemostasis is vitally important at all times (Leatherbarrow 2019).*

4.6 The appropriate forceps will be used for the type of vessel being cauterised.

- *To avoid the risk of using heavy forceps for delicate tissue, which will damage surrounding healthy tissue.*

4.7 The diathermy forceps will be held with a pencil grip and placed over the bleeding vessel until all apparent bleeding stops. Charring of the tips of the hand-piece may interfere with the efficiency of the instrument. If this happens, they will need to be cleaned (Wicker 2000).

- *To understand the appropriate settings for the level of energy required to safely achieve diathermy of a bleeding vessel. To achieve and produce haemostasis.*

KNOWLEDGE REQUIRED:

- Awareness of other forms of coagulation
- Appreciation of the clotting cascade and the factors that influence this
- A good understanding of the capability of the electrosurgical machine being utilised in theatres
- Appreciation of the elements of health and safety associated with the use of electrosurgical devices.

COMPLICATIONS:

Surgical smoke or plume is created when using electrosurgery on tissue and it is reported that surgical smoke can be harmful to those who inhale it (Biggins 2002). Therefore, the practitioner and those assisting the surgery should be encouraged to wear masks and use available smoke plume removal devices – not just surgical suction machines (Wicker 2000).

BOUNDARIES OF PRACTICE:

The surgeon will nearly always be present to provide direct supervision, and if not, no diathermy will be performed. The only exception to this will be when the practitioner is performing minor surgery – this may be applied without direct supervision.

LIMITATIONS:

Any situation where the practitioner does not feel competent or comfortable to provide the appropriate level of expertise, and finds the provision of this particular practice is beyond their level of competence.

References

Atkinson, U. (1992). *Berry and Kohn's operating room technique.* 7th edn. Missouri: Mosby.

Biggins, J. (2002). Congress presentation: The hazards of surgical smoke: not to be sniffed at! *The Journal of Peri-operative Practice.* **12**(4), 136–43.

Leatherbarrow, B. (2019). *Oculoplastic surgery.* 3rd edn. USA: Thieme.

Nerad, J.A. (2001). *Requisites in ophthalmology: oculoplastic surgery.* Missouri: Mosby.

Wicker, P. (2000). Electrosurgery in peri-operative practice. *The Journal of Peri-operative Practice.* **10**(4), 221–26.

5. Minor surgical procedures

5.1. ELECTROLYSIS FOR TRICHIASIS

EXPECTED OUTCOMES:

The practitioner will demonstrate an understanding and competent ability to apply electrolysis treatment to eyelashes that are abrading the eye (trichiasis).

PERFORMANCE CRITERIA:

The practitioner will be able to:

i. Correctly identify those lashes that require treatment, prior to surgery, using a slit lamp and gaining a history from the patient
ii. Take informed written consent and mark the appropriate site/side for surgery
iii. Demonstrate the ability to administer local anaesthetic
iv. Discuss the condition of trichiasis and how it manifests in patients
v. Use the ceiling-mounted microscope
vi. Identify the appropriate equipment required and its safe usage
vii. Discuss related anatomy and the physiology of the eyelid
viii. Prepare the patient and discuss the procedure
ix. Correctly use the appropriate machine and correctly earth the patient
x. Demonstrate the ability to competently, safely and correctly carry out the procedure
xi. Discuss possible complications of the procedure
xii. Discuss the post-operative care of the patient
xiii. Discuss the limitations of practice.

INDICATIONS:

Trichiasis.

CONTRAINDICATIONS:

Any condition other than trichiasis.

EQUIPMENT:

- Diathermy machine (various models)
- Electrolysis needles and hand-piece
- Epilation forceps
- Prep tray
- Local anaesthetic.

EQUIPMENT CONSIDERATIONS:

Diathermy machines have various settings by which electrolysis can safely be undertaken, it is important that the practitioner is aware of the settings and does not exceed them.

ACTIONS AND ASSOCIATED RATIONALE:

5.1.1 Identify aberrant lashes prior to surgery, gain written consent and mark the appropriate sight/side for surgery, using the correct Trust consent form.

5.1.2 Instil Oxybuprocaine into the affected eye.

5.1.3 Administer local anaesthetic to the appropriate area requiring surgery (as per protocol 2). Check and prepare the equipment for use.

- *To ensure treatment is focused on the appropriate eyelashes and follows Trust guidelines and protocol.*

5.1.4 Check that the patient has a pad on, to return the current back to the machine.

- *To avoid patient receiving a burn.*

5.1.5 Wash hands and don sterile gloves.

- *To follow ANTT guidelines to protect both the patient and practitioner and reduce the incidence of infection.*

5.1.6 Using the theatre-operating microscope (as per protocol 1.5), identify the lashes requiring treatment. The practitioner will then check the level of anaesthesia with the patient.

- *To ensure that the area is appropriately anaesthetised.*

5.1.7 The practitioner will then pass the electrolysis needle down the side of the shaft of the eyelash requiring removal. The electrical current is applied for 2–10 seconds. The appearance of blanching or bubbles at the eyelid indicates that sufficient current has been supplied. The eyelash may well fall out when the electrolysis needle is removed, or it can be removed using epilation forceps – it should be easy to remove.

- *To destroy the cells that create eyelashes or fine hairs.*
- *It may be appropriate to use a lid guard or ocular shell whilst at the same time trying to apply delicate electrolysis treatment.*
- *The practitioner must, through experience, gain an understanding of the correct use of the electrolysis needle so as to reduce the potential risk of damaging the globe.*

5.1.8 This will be repeated as necessary.

5.1.9 Apply and prescribe topical antibiotics to the eyelids for one week post-operatively.

- *To reduce the risk of post-operative infection*

5.1.10 Care must be taken to protect the globe from accidental injury by not advancing the electrolysis needle too far into the follicle. Following surgery, the practitioner will record the surgical episode in the medical notes, including:

- Date of surgery
- Nature of the surgery and the reason for it
- The name of the practitioner
- The local anaesthetic used
- Treatment areas, shown on a detailed diagram
- An outline of the surgery performed
- Post-operative treatment and follow-up
- Signature.
- *To provide an accurate record of the surgery performed.*

KNOWLEDGE REQUIRED:

- Anatomy and physiology of the eyelids and globe
- The principles of electrolysis of the eyelashes
- Possible complications and contraindications of applying electrolysis to the eyelashes
- Post-operative care
- Action to take if any complications occur
- Effect of electrolysis on homeostasis.

COMPLICATIONS:
Reaction to the local anaesthetic (see protocol 2). Damage to the eye. Recurrence of the problem – may need further treatment. Electrolysis treatment may not be entirely effective when there is extensive trichiasis; other forms of treatment may be required i.e. removal of lash-bearing skin. There is often a need to repeat the treatment. Certain diathermy machines cannot be directly used with patients who have a cardiac pacemaker, and this should be identified prior to any treatment. Risks of swelling, pain, infection, bleeding and bruising.

BOUNDARIES OF PRACTICE:
This procedure will be carried out by a competently assessed practitioner. Any patient deemed unsuitable will be told and the procedure will be cancelled. All patients listed for this surgery should be appropriately reviewed, assessed for fitness for surgery, consented and marked prior for surgery by the practitioner carrying out the procedure. However, the practitioner may not be directly supervised during the procedure.

Competency will also need to have been achieved for, and used in conjunction with:

- Infiltration and administration of subcutaneous local anaesthetic into the eyelid and/or surrounding area to enable minor operative procedures to be performed (protocol 2)
- Use of the theatre-operating microscope (protocol 1.5).

LIMITATIONS:

Any situation where the practitioner does not feel competent or comfortable to provide the appropriate level of expertise, and finds the provision of this particular practice is beyond their level of competence.

References

Leatherbarrow, B. (2019). *Oculoplastic surgery.* 3rd edn. USA: Thieme.

Nerad, J.A. (2001). R*equisites in ophthalmology: Oculoplastic surgery.* Missouri: Mosby.

5.2 INCISION AND CURETTAGE OF CHALAZIA

EXPECTED OUTCOME:
The practitioner will demonstrate an understanding and competent ability to perform incision and curettage of chalazia.

PERFORMANCE CRITERIA:
The practitioner will be able to:

i. Use their acquired knowledge to diagnose/identify a chalazion, using appropriate eyelid anatomy and physiology
ii. Discuss the pre-operative checks required and gain informed written consent from the patient and mark the appropriate site/side
iii. Identify the appropriate equipment required
iv. Discuss the appropriate patient preparation prior to the procedure
v. Demonstrate the ability to administer local anaesthetic
vi. Demonstrate the ability to use a chalazion clamp and evert the eyelid
vii. Demonstrate the ability to use a scalpel and 15 blade to incise the chalazion from the posterior eyelid
viii. Demonstrate the ability to curettage the wound
iv. Discuss the post-operative care
v. Identify boundaries and limitations of practice.

INDICATIONS:
Upper or lower eyelid chalazia (or meibomian cysts).

CONTRAINDICATIONS:
Any lesions which are not chalazions – notably Hordeolum (an acute inflammation of the meibomian gland) or suspicious lesions that may be basal cell carcinoma. These would require biopsy.

EQUIPMENT:
- An incision and curettage set – including various chalazion clamps
- Prep pack
- 11 blade
- Double pad and Jelonet dressing
- Antibiotic ointment
- Local anaesthetic.

ACTIONS AND ASSOCIATED RATIONALE:
5.2.1 Identify the location of the chalazia prior to surgery, gain written consent and mark

the appropriate site/side for surgery using the correct Trust recognised paperwork and protocol. Immediately prior to surgery, it will be appropriate to use the WHO safety checklist to confirm the patient's details.

- *To confirm correct identity of the patient and the surgical site/side prior to surgery.*

5.2.2 Instil Oxybuprocaine into the affected eye.

- *To reduce the discomfort of the procedure.*

5.2.3 The practitioner may mark the specific area where the chalazion is, prior to the infiltration of any anaesthetic. The practitioner may clean the skin of the affected side with an antiseptic solution (check allergies). The majority of chalazia will point to the back of the tarsal plate and should be incised posteriorly. If the chalazia point towards the skin, it would beneficial to open the lesion from the skin side, but this should be introduced in the consent process (consider scarring).

- *Infiltration of local anaesthetic can often obscure the exact location of the lesion once injected.*
- *It's most appropriate, where possible, to approach the chalazia posteriorly in order to reduce scarring anteriorly.*

5.2.4 Administer local anaesthetic to the appropriate area requiring surgery (as per protocol 2.4). Check and prepare the equipment for use. The practitioner will require an overhead light to provide illumination. The practitioner will then check the level of anaesthesia with the patient, using a pair of forceps.

- *To anaesthetise the eyelid and allow surgery to be performed.*

5.2.5 Wash hands (ANTT) and don sterile gloves.

- *To reduce the incidence of infection.*

5.2.6 The practitioner will then position the appropriately sized chalazion clamp over the lesion and, if taking a posterior approach, will evert the eyelid once the clamp is secure. If taking an anterior approach, the clamp may still be used but there will be no need to evert the lid.

- *To ensure treatment is focused on the appropriate area of the eyelid and follows Trust guidelines and protocol.*
- *To enable optimal visualisation and control of bleeding during the procedure.*
- *To provide the optimal presentation of the chalazion prior to any intervention.*
- *To reduce movement of the clamp and therefore the lesion prior to incision.*

5.2.7 The practitioner will use their non-dominant hand to gently hold the chalazion clamp and will then use the 11 blade correctly loaded into a handle (or use a disposable blade) to incise the length of the chalazion vertically. Some references suggest making a cross incision.

- *This will optimise the excision in order to curette the maximal amount of exudate out of the wound.*
- *Using a cross incision may reduce the possibility of the wound closing and the chalazion reforming.*

5.2.8 The practitioner will then use a curette(s) of the appropriate size to remove the contents and inner wall of the chalazion. This will be repeated as necessary. Care must be taken to protect the globe from accidental injury throughout the procedure.

- *To remove the chronic matter from inside the meibomian gland.*

5.2.9 Once the curettage is complete, apply a stat dose of antibiotic ointment and remove the chalazion clamp.

- *To reduce further risk of post-operative infection.*

5.2.10 Place a double pad and Jelonet ® paraffin dressing (Smith & Nephew) on the closed eye for 2 hours post-operatively. Initially the patient, if they are able, may be encouraged to apply firm pressure over the pad with the heel of their hand for 10 minutes post-operatively. (The pad may be changed later in the daycase area if there is discomfort.)

- *To reduce any immediate post-operative bleeding and reduce bruising/ haematoma formation.*

5.2.11 Apply topical antibiotics to the eye/eyelids for one week post-operatively as prescribed.

- *To reduce further risk of post-operative infection.*

5.2.12 Following surgery, the practitioner will record the surgical episode in the medical notes, including:

- Date of surgery
- Nature of the surgery and the reason for it
- The name of the practitioner
- The local anaesthetic used
- Treatment areas, shown on a detailed diagram
- An outline of the surgery performed
- Post-operative treatment and follow-up
- Signature.
- *To provide an accurate record of the surgery performed.*

KNOWLEDGE REQUIRED:

- Anatomy and physiology of the eyelids and globe
- The principles of the formation of chalazia
- Possible complications and contraindications of the potential surgery
- Post-operative care

See minor operation table for a comparison of the minor operative procedures.

COMPLICATIONS:

Reaction to the local anaesthetic (see protocol 2). Damage to the eye. Recurrence of the problem – may need further treatment/intervention. Action to take if any complications occur. Risk of swelling, pain, infection, bleeding, bruising.

BOUNDARIES OF PRACTICE:

This procedure will be carried out by a competently assessed practitioner. Any patient deemed unsuitable will be told and the procedure will be cancelled. All patients listed for this surgery should be appropriately reviewed, assessed for fitness for surgery, consented and marked before surgery by the practitioner carrying out the procedure. However, the practitioner may not be directly supervised during the procedure.

LIMITATIONS:

Any situation where the practitioner does not feel competent or comfortable to provide the appropriate level of expertise, and finds the provision of this particular practice is beyond their level of competence.

References

Nerad, J.A. (2001). *Requisites in ophthalmology: Oculoplastic surgery.* Missouri: Mosby.

Table 5.1: Comparison of the minor operative procedures.

Manifestation	Indications	Surgical	Rationale	Comment
Chalazion (meibomian cyst, internal hordeolum)	• Non-tender, painless nodule • Sub-acute may be erythematous and painful initially • May become inflamed, involving the entire lid or cheek • Not usually at the lid margin and more commonly within the tarsal plate	• Approached posteriorly by everting the eyelid • 15 blade and meibomian clamp • Make a vertical incision • Curette the contents	• Specific competency (p.280) • At present, only lesions over 6 months old may be supported/funded by commissioning bodies; otherwise an individual funding request may be required (IFR)	• Caused by the blockage of the meibomian gland • More chronic lesions may become fibrosed • Occasionally the anterior lesions need to be approached surgically from the front of the eyelid • Chronic lesions may require a steroid injection

Cont.

	• May become chronic, staying for several months • Usually 'points' posteriorly, but occasionally may be more anterior • May burst and discharge • Usually filled with sebaceous material			• Chronic lesions or lesions that recur in the same place should be biopsied • Some lesions may have an overlying palpebral conjunctival granuloma that requires excision
Stye (external hordeolum)	• Infection of the glands of Zeis or Moll associated with the hair follicle • Red, irritated and painful acute infection • *Staphylococcus* infection	• Incision and curettage of the lesion may be indicated but is rarely required	• As above	• Short period of infection and self-limiting (within 1–2 weeks) • Short course of topical antibiotics may suffice
Xanthelasma	• Common benign lesion • Arises from the invasion of the dermis by xanthoma cells • White/yellowish subcutaneous lesions • Commonly arise medially in the upper and lower eyelids • Xanthelasmata is associated with raised cholesterol and this should be checked by GP	• Application of trichloroacetic acid 90% with a cocktail stick • Surgical removal with an elliptical excision and wound closed with prolene sutures	• Specific clinical competency (p.298) • COSHH regulations for the handling and safe disposal of TCA • At present, the procedure may not be funded by commissioning bodies – it may be pertinent to check this and an individual funding request (IFR) may be required	• Surgical removal of xanthelasmata may be problematic due to position and size with the potential to cause webbing or eyelid malposition • Any lesion over 5mm in diameter may not be suitable for surgical excision and it may be necessary to assess whether there is enough surplus skin to ensure wound closure • Application may be the first-line treatment before considering surgical approaches • TCA is corrosive and is dangerous to handle; it is also harmful to the environment so should be disposed of carefully

Cont.

				• TCA only to be applied to the xanthelasmata and avoid healthy skin
• TCA destroys the proteins in cells
• The xanthelasmata may need several treatments of TCA
• Xanthelasmata may return after a period of time despite TCA treatment
Cyst of Moll (sudoriferous or apocrine hidrocystoma)	• Small (up to 10mm in diameter), circular, translucent, firm and painless lesion
• Often form near the puncta	• 'De-roof' the lesion
• Ensure the capsular bag is removed
• Aspiration may not be effective as the lesion may re-fill
• If possible, the lesion can be excised in its entirety but this may take time and often the fragile capsular bag may burst
• Ensure that you cauterise the base of the wound	• Part of protocol 5.3, Removal of skin lesions (p.289)	• Carry out careful consideration of the surrounding structures such as the puncta
• It may be necessary to probe the puncta to ensure the canaliculi are protected
• If in any doubt, it may be necessary to refer to the oculoplastic team
• Consider sending removed material for histopathology
• Any lesion that involves both the anterior and posterior lamella or the entire lid margin may require complete excision (i.e. wedge excision) and require referral to oculoplastic team
Epidermal inclusion cyst	• Round, elevated, off-white/yellowish painless lesion
• Cysts measure up to 8mm in diameter
• Arise from the hair follicle and contain keratin	• Incision and expression of the cyst
• It may be possible to excise the lesion intact (i.e. within its cystic bag)	• Part of protocol 5.3, Removal of skin lesions (p.289)	• Carry out careful consideration of the surrounding structures such as the puncta
• It may be necessary to probe the puncta to ensure canaliculi are protected
• If in any doubt it may be necessary to refer to oculoplastic team

Cont.

				• Consider sending removed material for histopathology • Any lesion that involves both the anterior and posterior lamella or the entire lid margin may require complete excision (i.e. wedge excision) and require referral to oculoplastic team
Milia	• Multiple tiny epidermal inclusion cysts • They often arise in crops	• The lesions may be removed with the point of a 21G hypodermic needle and forceps • Slightly larger lesions may require to be cut with a blade and/or Westcott scissors	• Part of protocol 5.3, Removal of skin lesions (p.289)	• Some lesions may require cautery • It may be necessary to remove the lesions over several visits • Histopathology to confirm diagnosis
Squamous papilloma (skin tag, acrochonrdon or fibroepithelioma)	• Common pedunculated skin lesions that may arise anywhere on the face • Occasionally sessile	• Simple excision from the base of the lesion using forceps and Westcott scissors, making sure to take a reasonable margin • For sessile lesions ensure that you take an elliptical and subcutaneous excision; a deep Vicryl suture may be required to bring skin edges together • Hand cautery to the base	• Part of protocol 5.3, Removal of skin lesions (p.289) • Diathermy protocol (p.273) • Suturing protocol (p.270)	• Some rare squamous papillomas originate from within the inner lining of the puncta and require oculo-plastic involvement • Any lesion that involves both the anterior and posterior lamella or the entire lid margin may require complete excision (i.e. wedge excision and referral to the oculoplastic team • Send for histo-pathology as (very rarely) there may be malignant cells in the base of some lesions
Seborrheic keratosis (basal cell papilloma)	• Benign proliferations of normal cells • Appear as greasy, shiny lesions that can look 'stuck on'	• Simple excision from the base of the lesion, using forceps and Westcott scissors, making sure to take a reasonable margin	• Part of protocol 5.3, Removal of skin lesions (p.289) • Diathermy protocol (p.273) • Suturing protocol (p.270)	• Any lesion that involves both the anterior and posterior lamella or the entire lid margin may require complete excision (i.e. wedge excision) and

Cont.

		• They may be light brown in colour • Several sub-types • Some may have 'church-spire' projections	• For sessile lesions, make sure to take an elliptical and subcutaneous excision; a deep Vicryl suture may be required to bring skin edges together • Hand cautery to the base		require referral to oculoplastic team • Send for histopathology
Naevi (singular naevus)		• Non-specific, circumscribed chronic lesion • Often pigmented • Several subtypes • They may appear on the lid margin	• Many of these lesions can be left in situ and do not require excision • Shave biopsy using a blade	• Part of protocol 5.3, Removal of skin lesions (p.289)	• Histopathological identification may be required to identify particular subtypes and to rule out any malignant element
Cutaneous horn		• Describes a lesion that has a horn-like projection of keratin arising from the skin • Can be associated with malignancy in approximately 20% of cases	• It's important to remove a sufficient base to ensure the subcutaneous component is also removed • Make an ellipse around the base, 2–3mm around the lesion, using a blade • 'Boat-out' the subcutaneous component (excising the lesion like the hull of a boat, deeper in the middle than the edges) • Diathermy may be required • Undermining of the wound may be required to bring the wound edges together	• Part of protocol 5.3, Removal of skin lesions (p.289) • Diathermy protocol (p.273) • Suturing protocol (p.270)	• Histopathological identification may be required to identify particular subtypes and to rule out any malignant element
Basal cell or squamous cell carcinoma		Malignant skin lesion: • Ulceration • Telangiectasia • Lid destruction	Assess the extent of the lesion and gain a full history from the patient:	• Part of protocol 5.3, Removal of skin lesions (p.289) • Diathermy protocol (p.273)	• Upon the result, consider excision with a margin • Mohs excision

Cont.

	• Nodular appearance • Madarosis (loss of eyelashes) • Crusting • Bleeding • Itchy • Induration (firm)	• Photographs • List for incisional biopsy • Take a small representative sample or punch biopsy		• Organise reconstruction • Oculoplastic referral • Provide support and advice for the patient

5.3. REMOVAL OF EYELID SKIN LESIONS (INCLUDING EXCISIONAL AND INCISIONAL BIOPSY)

EXPECTED OUTCOMES:
The practitioner will demonstrate an ability to safely and competently remove specified skin lesions.

PERFORMANCE CRITERIA:
The practitioner will be able to:
i. Use their acquired knowledge to diagnose/identify skin lesions that may be treated through surgical intervention using appropriate eyelid anatomy and physiology
ii. Discuss the pre-operative checks required and the consent procedure
iii. Identify the appropriate equipment required to remove the lesion
iv. Outline the surgical approaches to removing various lesions whilst considering cosmesis, potential risks and limitations in clinical ability
v. Discuss the appropriate patient preparation prior to the procedure
vi. Demonstrate the ability to administer local anaesthetic (see protocol 2)
vii. Demonstrate the ability to safely and competently remove an eyelid lesion
viii. Discuss and outline the post-operative care
vix. Identify boundaries and limitations of practice

INDICATIONS:
See minor operations table, Competency 5.2, p. 283.

Skin tags (achrocordons), epidermal inclusion cysts, sebaceous cysts, milia, papillomata, suspicious-appearing lesions that may benefit from incisional/excisional biopsy, follicular and seborrhoeic keratosis.

CONTRAINDICATIONS:
All other benign or malignant lesions that required more considered medical/surgical intervention and are beyond the clinical competency of the practitioner. Any lesion involving or in close proximity to either the upper or lower punctum and/or the medial canthal region.

EQUIPMENT *(Varying depending on requirements to remove specific lesions)*:
- Minor lid tray (including 11 or 15 blade)
- Prep tray, swabs and Q-tips
- Disposible vanna scissors
- Suture (if required)
- Double pad and gauze/paraffin dressing

- Antiseptic solution
- Benoxinate
- Local anaesthetic
- Bipolar cautery/diathermy
- Hand-held diathermy.

ACTIONS AND ASSOCIATED RATIONALE:

5.3.1 Identify the location and type of the lesion prior to surgery, gain written consent and mark the appropriate site/side for surgery using the correct Trust recognised paperwork and protocol.

- *To ensure the appropriate treatment is prescribed and the patient is aware of the risks and benefits of treatment.*
- *To check that the patient is fully aware of the treatment plan and the viable alternatives.*

5.3.2 Once in theatre, the patient will be identified, surgical procedure correlated against the patient surgical safety checklist and the consent verified with the patient and the theatre team.

- *The WHO safety check list provides a basis on which to verify the patient and the treatment plan.*

5.3.3 Instil Oxybuprocaine into the affected eye.

- *To reduce the discomfort of administering local anaesthetic and skin cleansing.*

5.3.4 The practitioner may mark the specific area where the lesion is, prior to the infiltration of any anaesthetic. The practitioner may clean the skin of the affected side with an antiseptic solution.

- *Infiltration of local anaesthetic can often obscure the exact location of the lesion once it is injected.*

5.3.5 The practitioner will administer local anaesthetic to the appropriate area requiring surgery (as per protocol 2).

- *To anaesthetise the eyelid and allow surgery to be performed in comfort.*

5.3.6 The practitioner will wash their hands and don sterile gloves.

- *To reduce the incidence of cross-infection and provide a barrier against blood-borne pathogens.*

5.3.7 The practitioner will then check the level of anaesthesia with the patient, using a pair of forceps. Clean sterile paper disposable drapes should be placed appropriately on the patient.

- *To confirm that the patient is comfortable and doesn't require any further anaesthesia.*
- *To provide a barrier between the patient and operating area.*

5.3.8 The practitioner will then use the 11 or 15 blade correctly loaded into a Bard Parker handle to incise/excise the lesion (or use a disposable blade):

- Skin tags (Achrocordon): An elliptical incision immediately around the base of the skin tag may be necessary, undermining the lesion minimally, or a simple shave excision may be an alternative. Further undermining of the skin edges may be required before suturing back together or the area may be left to granulate by secondary intention.

- Epidermal inclusion cyst and sebaceous cyst: Using forceps and Vannas/Westcott blunt-tipped scissors, the practitioner will gradually undermine the cyst and remove intact if possible or it may be more appropriate to 'de-roof' the lesion. Cautery may be required. Further undermining of the skin edges may be required before suturing back together or the area may be left to granulate by secondary intention.

- Milia (tiny epidermal inclusion cysts): Simple small shave excisions may be all that is required or the use of a green needle to remove the individual lesions. Some lesions may require a suture. Cautery may be required for each lesion. The wounds can be left to granulate by secondary intention.

- Follicular and seborrhoeic keratosis: An elliptical incision immediately around the base of the lesion, undermining the lesion minimally, or a simple shave excision may be an alternative. Cautery may be required. Further undermining of the skin edges may be required before suturing back together or the area may be left to granulate by secondary intention.

- Incisional biopsy: An identified area of the lesion will be removed to provide a representative section of the lesion for histopathology.

5.3.9 Cautery may be used following excision of the lesion (either using a hand-held or bipolar electro-cautery device).

- *To reduce/stop unnecessary bleeding and optimise visualisation*

5.3.10 This will be repeated as necessary. Care must be taken to protect the globe and other structures from accidental injury throughout the procedure.

- *There may be more than one lesion to remove.*
- *It is vitally important to prevent damage to the eye or loss of vision*

5.3.11 It may be necessary to suture the wound closed and this may also involve undermining of local skin to allow the skin edges to approximate. A suture that dissolves will be most likely to be used, e.g. Vicryl.

- *To allow for better wound healing and improve cosmesis,*
- *Dissolving sutures are likely to cause less post-operative inflammation and swelling, and in turn cause less scarring.*

5.3.12 Once the excision is complete, apply a stat dose of topical antibiotic. In some cases it may be appropriate to place a double pad and Jelonet ® paraffin dressing (Smith & Nephew) in place for 1–2 hours post-operatively. Initially the patient, if they are able, may be encouraged to apply firm pressure over the pad with the heel of their hand for 10 minutes post-operatively. (The pad may be changed later in the daycase area.) Apply topical antibiotics to the eye/eyelids for one week post-operatively as prescribed.

- *To provide better asepsis and overall reduce the risk of infection.*
- *To stop any immediate post-operative bleeding and reduce the formation of a haematoma.*

5.3.13 Following surgery, the practitioner will record the surgical episode in the medical notes, including:

- Date of surgery
- Nature of the surgery and the reason for it
- The name of the practitioner
- The local anaesthetic used
- Treatment areas, shown on a detailed diagram
- An outline of the surgery performed
- Post-operative treatment and follow-up
- Signature
- Completion of histopathology report if required.
- *To provide an accurate record of the surgery performed.*

KNOWLEDGE REQUIRED:

- Anatomy and physiology of the eyelids and globe
- The principles of the formation of the different lesions
- Possible complications and contraindications of the potential surgery
- Post-operative care
- Action to take if any complications occur.

COMPLICATIONS:
Reaction to the local anaesthetic (see protocol 2). Damage to the eye. Recurrence of the problem – may need further treatment/intervention. Risk of swelling, pain, infection, bleeding, bruising.

BOUNDARIES OF PRACTICE:
This procedure will be carried out by a competently assessed practitioner. Any patient deemed unsuitable will be told so and the procedure will be cancelled or appropriate advice sought from a medical practitioner. All patients listed for this surgery would be appropriately reviewed, assessed for fitness for surgery, consented and marked before surgery by the practitioner carrying out the procedure. However, the practitioner may not be directly supervised during the procedure.

LIMITATIONS:
Any situation where the practitioner does not feel competent or comfortable to provide the appropriate level of expertise, and finds the provision of this particular practice is beyond their level of competence.

References

Nerad, J.A. (2001). *Requisites in ophthalmology: Oculoplastic surgery.* Missouri: Mosby.

Competency will also need to have been achieved for the following protocols:

2.1 Infiltration and administration of subcutaneous local anaesthetic into the eyelid and/or surrounding area to enable minor operative procedures to be performed

4.0 Applying diathermy for haemostasis

3.0 Suturing of subcutaneous layers, stapling or suturing of the skin.

5.4. EVERTING SUTURES FOR THE CORRECTION OF INVOLUTIONAL ENTROPION (see Chapter 2, p. 27)

EXPECTED OUTCOME:

The practitioner will demonstrate an understanding and competent ability to place everting sutures for the correction of involutional entropion.

PERFORMANCE CRITERIA:

The practitioner will be able to:
i. Discuss the anatomy and physiology of the eyelid
ii. Discuss the effect and causes of involutional entropion and differentiate it from cicatricial entropion
iii. Outline the equipment required for the procedure
iv. Demonstrate an ability to administer local anaesthetic
v. Demonstrate the ability to competently and safely place everting sutures
vi. Describe the possible side effects of carrying out the procedure
vii. Describe the post-operative care
viii. Identify boundaries and limitations of practice.

INDICATIONS:

Involutional lower eyelid entropion.

CONTRAINDICATIONS:

Cicatricial entropion, congenital entropion and patients under the age of 18 years.

EQUIPMENT:

- Either a minor lid tray or a pair of needle-holders, toothed forceps and suture scissors
- Prep tray
- Local anaesthetic
- 3 x 4/0 Vicryl sutures (double ended) or 5/0 Vicryl (double ended).

EQUIPMENT CONSIDERATIONS:

5/0 Vicryl may be used, but the smaller needle may make the procedure more difficult.

ACTIONS AND ASSOCIATED RATIONALE:

5.4.1 Identify the location and type of entropion prior to surgery, gain written consent and mark the appropriate site/side for surgery using the correct Trust recognised paperwork and protocol.

- *To ensure the appropriate treatment is prescribed and the patient is aware of the risks and benefits of treatment*

- *That the patient is fully aware of the treatment plan and the viable alternatives.*

5.4.2 Once in theatre, the patient will be identified, surgical procedure correlated against the patient surgical safety checklist and the consent verified with the patient and the theatre team.

- *The WHO safety check list provides a basis to verify the patient and the treatment plan.*

5.4.3 Instil Oxybuprocaine into the affected eye(s).

- *To reduce the discomfort of administering the local anaesthetic and carrying out the skin cleansing.*

5.4.4 The practitioner may clean the skin of the affected side with an antiseptic solution. Administer local anaesthetic to the lower eyelid (as per protocol 2) and/or the subconjunctival inferior fornix injection. Prior to starting the surgery, the practitioner will check the level of anaesthesia with the patient, using a pair of forceps.

- *Infiltration of local anaesthetic can often obscure the exact location of the lesion once injected.*

5.4.5 Wash hands and don sterile gloves.

- *To reduce the incidence of cross-infection and provide a barrier against blood-borne pathogens.*

5.4.6 A clean sterile paper may be used to provide a sterile area to work within or disposable drapes may be required.

- *To provide a barrier against infection and a surgical field to work in.*

5.4.7 The practitioner will then take one of the 4/0 Vicryl sutures and load one of the needles (back-handed) into the Castroviejo needle holders. With the non-suturing hand, the practitioner will use forceps to hold the lower eyelid and pass the 4/0 needle away from the eye (i.e. back-handed) full-thickness through the lower eyelid. Initially through the lower deep conjunctival fornix, passing anteriorly (picking up lower lid retractors) and superiorly to emerge from the skin just below the eyelashes.

- *The action of the placed suture will cause the eyelid to evert.*

5.4.8 This will be repeated with the other end of the suture. Once placed 1–2 mm adjacent to the previous arm of the suture, it will be tied and the end of the suture cut.

- *The degree of tightening of the sutures will govern the amount of correction or eversion required. Equally, the deeper the suture is placed in the fornix, the more inversion will be noted.*

5.4.9 This is carried out laterally, medially and centrally on the lower eyelid. In some patients only 1 or 2 sutures may be required to get the desired effect.

- *This provides uniform stabilisation of the eyelid.*

5.4.10 Care must be taken to protect the globe and other structures from accidental injury throughout the procedure.
- *The eye and eyesight should be carefully monitored throughout.*

5.4.11 Once the surgery is complete, apply a stat dose of antibiotic and thereafter into the eye/eyelids for one week post-operatively (as prescribed).
- *To prevent post-operative infection.*

5.4.12 Following surgery, the practitioner will record the surgical episode in the medical notes, including:
- Date of surgery
- Nature of the surgery and the reason for it
- The name of the practitioner
- The local anaesthetic used
- Treatment areas, shown on a detailed diagram
- An outline of the surgery performed
- Post-operative treatment and follow-up
- Signature.

- *To provide an accurate record of the surgery performed.*

KNOWLEDGE REQUIRED:
- Anatomy and physiology of the eyelids and the globe
- The principles of everting sutures
- Possible side-effects and complications of everting sutures
- Post-operative care
- Action to be taken if complications occur.

COMPLICATIONS:
Overcorrection: sutures will have to be removed and replaced. Particular attention must be paid to overcorrecting the medial stitch so as not to evert the lower eyelid punctum.
Haematoma: Apply pressure; contact a member of the oculoplastics team if concerned. It will be necessary to cancel the procedure if the haematoma impedes the placement of sutures.

BOUNDARIES OF PRACTICE:
This procedure will be carried out by a competently assessed practitioner. Any patient deemed unsuitable will be told so and the procedure will be cancelled or appropriate advice sought from a medical practitioner. All patients listed for this surgery should be

appropriately reviewed, assessed for fitness for surgery, consented and marked before surgery by the practitioner carrying out the procedure. However, the practitioner may not be directly supervised during the procedure.

LIMITATIONS:

Any situation where the practitioner does not feel competent or comfortable to provide the appropriate level of expertise, and finds the provision of this particular practice is beyond their level of competence.

References

Nerad, J.A. (2001). *Requisites in ophthalmology: Oculoplastic surgery.* Missouri: Mosby.

Competency will also need to have been achieved for the following protocols:

2.1 Infiltration and administration of subcutaneous local anaesthetic into the eyelid and/or surrounding area to enable minor operative procedures to be performed.

3.0 Suturing of subcutaneous layers, stapling or suturing of the skin.

5.5 APPLICATION OF TRICHLOROACETIC ACID 90% (TCA) TO XANTHELASMATA

EXPECTED OUTCOME:

The assistant will be able to competently and safely apply trichloroacetic acid to a xanthelasma.

PERFORMANCE CRITERIA:

The practitioner will be able to:
- **i.** Discuss the anatomy and physiology of the skin and the eyelids
- **ii.** Demonstrate a knowledge of the development, identification and nature of xanthelasmata
- **iii.** Demonstrate an understanding of the pharmacodynamics and contra-indications of trichloroacetic acid, and its safe handling and disposal
- **iv.** Demonstrate an ability to administer local anaesthetic
- **v.** Demonstrate a competent ability to apply trichloroacetic acid to a xanthelasma
- **vi.** Describe the possible side effects and considerations of carrying out the procedure
- **vii.** Describe the post-operative care
- **viii.** Identify boundaries and limitations of practice.

INDICATIONS:

Xanthelasma palpebrarum.

EQUIPMENT:

- A prep tray
- 'Cocktail sticks'
- Trichloroacetic acid – the present concentration is 90% ($C_2HC_{13}O2$)
- Gloves
- Local anaesthetic.

ACTIONS AND ASSOCIATED RATIONALE:

5.5.1 Identify the location and extent of xanthelasmata prior to surgery, gain written consent and mark the appropriate site/side for surgery using the correct Trust recognised paperwork and protocol.
- *To ensure the appropriate treatment is prescribed and the patient is aware of the risks and benefits of treatment.*
- *That the patient is fully aware of the treatment plan and the viable alternatives.*

5.5.2 Once in theatre, the patient will be identified, surgical procedure correlated against the patient surgical safety checklist and the consent verified with the patient and the theatre team.
- *The WHO safety check list provides a basis to verify the patient and the treatment plan.*

5.5.3 Instil Oxybuprocaine into the affected eye(s).
- *To reduce the discomfort of administering the local anaesthetic and carrying out skin cleansing.*

5.5.4 The practitioner may clean the skin of the affected side with an antiseptic solution. Administer local anaesthetic to the lower eyelid (as per protocol 2). Prior to starting the surgery, the practitioner will check the level of anaesthesia with the patient, using a pair of forceps.
- *To provide local anaesthesia and allow the surgical procedure to take place.*

5.5.5 Wash hands and don non-sterile gloves.
- *To reduce the incidence of cross-infection and the risk of burns to the skin from the TCA.*

5.5.6 TCA is presented in a glass bottle. The details of the contents will be checked, along with the expiry date. Approximately 1ml TCA will be decanted into a small receptacle and the glass bottle will be re-sealed and will be returned to a safe area.
- *To utilise a small but safe amount of TCA, reducing risks if it is accidentally spilt.*
- *To establish that the practitioner is using the correct product and strength.*

5.5.7 Remove gloves, wash hands and don a new set of sterile gloves.
- *To reduce the incidence of cross-infection and the risk of burns to the skin from the TCA.*
- *After decanting, TCA residual acid can remain on the gloves and may cause burns – hence the need to replace the gloves.*

5.5.8 Using a clean 'cocktail stick', gently apply a minimal amount of TCA onto the very end of the stick and remove excess, then dab onto the xanthelasma. The treated areas of the pale yellowish pigmented xanthelasma will turn white within a few seconds after contact with the acid. The practitioner should continue, moving onto the next area to be treated, and so on, until the whole lesion is treated. Avoid all healthy tissue with the acid – only treat the xanthelasma.
- *To safely and efficiently apply the TCA to the xanthelasma.*
- *Depigmentation indicates that the acid is working and the practitioner continues to treat unreacted areas.*

5.5.9 Once complete, gently clean the area and/or apply antibiotic ointment.
- *To reduce the incidence of infection.*

5.5.10 The remaining TCA will be disposed of appropriately, following Trust Policy.

5.5.11 Following surgery, the practitioner will record the surgical episode in the medical notes, including:

- Date of surgery
- Nature of the surgery and the reason for it
- The name of the practitioner
- The local anaesthetic used
- Treatment areas, shown on a detailed diagram
- An outline of the surgery performed
- Post-operative treatment and follow-up
- Signature.

- *To provide an accurate record of the surgery performed.*

KNOWLEDGE REQUIRED:
- Anatomy and physiology of the eyelid
- The principle of applying TCA to xanthelasmata
- Possible side-effects and complications of applying TCA to xanthelasmata
- Local policy for using and disposing of TCA
- Post-operative care
- Action to be taken if complications occur.

COMPLICATIONS:
Accidental misuse of trichloroacetic acid: dilute copiously with saline if used or spilt in the wrong area.

Never hold or pour TCA anywhere near the patient.

Encourage the patient to keep their eyes closed throughout the procedure.

BOUNDARIES OF PRACTICE:
This procedure will be carried out by a competently assessed practitioner. Any patient deemed unsuitable will be told so and the procedure will be cancelled or appropriate advice sought from a medical practitioner. All patients listed for this surgery should be appropriately reviewed, assessed for fitness for surgery, consented and marked before surgery by the practitioner carrying out the procedure. However, the practitioner may not be directly supervised during the procedure.

LIMITATIONS:
Any situation where the practitioner does not feel competent or comfortable to provide the appropriate level of expertise, and finds the provision of this particular practice is beyond their level of competence.

References

Haygood, U., Bennet, J.D. & Brodell, R.T. (1998). Treatment of Xanthelasma Palbebrum with bichloroacetic acid. *Dermatological surgery.* **24**(9), 1027–31.

Leatherbarrow, B. (2019). *Oculoplastic surgery.* 3rd edn. USA: Thieme.

Nerad, J.A. (2001). *Requisites in ophthalmology: Oculoplastic surgery.* Missouri: Mosby.

Competency will also need to have been achieved for the following protocol:

2.1 Infiltration and administration of subcutaneous local anaesthetic into the eyelid and/or surrounding area to enable minor operative procedures to be performed.

5.6 PUNCTAL CAUTERY TO OCCLUDE PUNCTA

EXPECTED OUTCOME:
The practitioner will demonstrate an understanding and competent ability to undertake punctal cautery.

PERFORMANCE CRITERIA:
The practitioner will be able to:
i. Discuss the related anatomy and physiology of the eyelid and the lacrimal system
ii. Outline the requirements for punctal cautery especially in relation to severe dry eyes
iii. Outline the equipment required for the procedure
iv. Demonstrate an ability to administer local anaesthetic
v. Demonstrate the ability to competently and safely perform punctal cautery using a hand-held cautery device
vi. Describe the possible side effects and considerations of carrying out the procedure
vii. Describe the post-operative care required
viii. Identify boundaries and limitations of practice.

INDICATIONS:
Severe dry eyes and reduced tear production, not managed by other conventional methods.

CONTRAINDICATIONS:
This procedure is difficult to reverse so it is important that other conventional methods are explored first.

EQUIPMENT:
- A minor tray or individually a St Martins forcep.
- Hand-held cautery device
- Q-tips
- Prep tray
- Local anaesthetic.

EQUIPMENT CONSIDERATIONS:
Electro-cautery can be used, but with low settings – each machine will vary. It will also be necessary to remove any existing punctal plugs before commencing cautery.

ACTIONS AND ASSOCIATED RATIONALE:
5.6.1 Identify which puncta are to be treated prior to surgery, gain written consent and mark the appropriate site/side for surgery using the correct Trust recognised paperwork and protocol.

- *To ensure the appropriate treatment is prescribed and the patient is aware of the risks and benefits of treatment.*
- *To ensure that the patient is fully aware of the treatment plan and the viable alternatives.*

5.6.2 Once in theatre, the patient will be identified, surgical procedure correlated against the patient surgical safety checklist and the consent verified with the patient and the theatre team.

- *The WHO safety check list provides a basis to verify the patient and the treatment plan.*

5.6.3 Instil Oxybuprocaine into the affected eye(s).

- *To reduce the discomfort of administering the local anaesthetic and carrying out skin cleansing.*

5.6.4 The practitioner may clean the skin of the affected side with an antiseptic solution. Administer local anaesthetic to the lower eyelid (as per protocol 2). Prior to starting the surgery, the practitioner will check the level of anaesthesia with the patient, using a pair of forceps.

- *To provide local anaesthesia and allow the surgical procedure to take place.*

5.6.5 Wash hands and don sterile gloves.

- *To reduce the incidence of cross-infection and provide a barrier against blood-borne pathogens.*

5.6.6 A clean sterile paper may be used to provide a sterile area to work within or disposable drapes may be required.

- *To provide a barrier against infection and a surgical field to work within.*

5.6.7 The punctum is located. Using a pair of forceps to hold the eyelid, the hand-held cautery is inserted vertically into the punctum perpendicular to the eyelid (Leatherbarrow 2010).

- *To ensure that the tip of the cautery enters the punctum at the appropriate angle.*

5.6.8 Once in the punctum, the switch of the hand-held cautery is pressed and the tip will become hot. There will be a thermal reaction at the punctum, causing it to blanch. At this point, the hand-held cautery should be removed (approximately 3–4 seconds).

- *The local reaction provides evidence that the hot tip of the cautery has burned the punctum, causing it to be occluded.*

5.6.9 Once finished, it is necessary to check how effective the reaction has been by examining the punctum.

- *It may be necessary to repeat the procedure if there is a suspicion that the punctum has not completely closed.*

5.6.9 Once the excision is complete, apply a stat dose of topical antibiotic. Apply topical antibiotics to the eye/eyelids for one week post-operatively (as prescribed).

- *To reduce the risk of post-operative infection.*

5.6.10 Following surgery, the practitioner will record the surgical episode in the medical notes, including:

- Date of surgery
- Nature of the surgery and the reason for it
- The name of the practitioner
- The local anaesthetic used
- Treatment areas, shown on a detailed diagram
- An outline of the surgery performed
- Post-operative treatment and follow-up
- Signature.
- *To provide an accurate record of the surgery performed.*

KNOWLEDGE REQUIRED:
- Anatomy and physiology of the lacrimal system and eyelid
- The mechanism of dry eyes and how punctal cautery will benefit the patient
- Possible side-effects and complications of punctal surgery
- Post-operative care
- Action to be taken if complications occur.

COMPLICATIONS:
Burning/destruction of adnexal tissue.

BOUNDARIES OF PRACTICE:
This procedure will be carried out by a competently assessed practitioner. Any patient deemed unsuitable will be told so and the procedure will be cancelled or appropriate advice sought from a medical practitioner. All patients listed for this surgery would be appropriately reviewed, assessed for fitness for surgery, consented and marked before surgery by the practitioner carrying out the procedure. However, the practitioner may not be directly supervised during the procedure.

LIMITATIONS:
Any situation where the practitioner does not feel competent or comfortable to provide the appropriate level of expertise, and finds the provision of this particular practice is beyond their level of competence.

References

Leatherbarrow, B. (2019). *Oculoplastic surgery*. 3rd edn. USA: Thieme.

Nerad, J.A. (2001). *Requisites in ophthalmology: Oculoplastic surgery*. Missouri: Mosby.

Competency will also need to have been achieved for the following protocol:
2.1 Infiltration and administration of subcutaneous local anaesthetic into the eyelid and/or surrounding area to enable minor operative procedures to be performed.

6. Endoscopic procedures

6.1 NASAL ENDOSCOPY AND REMOVAL OF SILICONE STENTS

EXPECTED OUTCOME:
The practitioner will be able to competently and safely perform basic nasal endoscopy.

PERFORMANCE CRITERIA:
The practitioner will be able to:
i. Discuss the anatomy and physiology of the nose and the lacrimal system
ii. Demonstrate a knowledge and understanding of the endoscope (and illumination system)
iii. Demonstrate an ability to competently and safely handle the endoscope
iv. Demonstrate an ability to safely and correctly use nasal sprays
v. Describe and demonstrate a knowledge of how, where and under which circumstances a silicone stent would be used
vi. Demonstrate an ability to correctly identify a silicone stent intranasally
vii. Demonstrate an ability to competently and safely remove a silicone stent
viii. Identify boundaries and limitations of practice

INDICATIONS:
Nasal examination of patients who have either been listed for or have undergone nasolacrimal surgery.

EQUIPMENT:
- Endoscopic light source and light pipe
- Rigid zero or 30-degree rigid endoscope
- Prep tray with saline
- Xylometazoline (Otrivine) (non-prescription)
- Lidocaine and Phenylephrine or Plain Lidocaine Nasal Spray (has to be prescribed).

EQUIPMENT CONSIDERATIONS:
There are various types of endoscopic light sources available; the practitioner should be familiar with the equipment.

This is a diagnostic procedure. No surgery will be performed by the practitioner. It is most commonly performed in the outpatients treatment room, but may also be carried out in theatre.

ACTIONS AND ASSOCIATED RATIONALE:
6.1.1 Once in theatre or OPD, the patient will be identified, procedure correlated

against the patient surgical safety checklist and the consent verified with the patient and the team.
- *The WHO or LocSIP safety check list provides a basis to verify the patient and the treatment plan.*

6.1.2 Instil Oxybuprocaine into the affected eye(s).
- *To reduce the discomfort of administering the local anaesthetic and carrying out skin cleansing.*

6.1.3 In the OPD the patient will be correctly identified by the practitioner and asked to sit in the examination chair. It should be possible to completely recline the chair should the need arise. The patient will be prepared for the administration of the nasal sprays: given a tissue, and sat back with head in the head-rest.
- *To be able to put the patient in a slight reverse Trendelenburg if they feel faint.*
- *The patient needs to be comfortable during the procedure.*

6.1.4 The nasal cavities will be appropriately prepared with a nasal decongestant/local anaesthetic. Nasal spray bottle will be gently placed in the nare of the nose by either the practitioner or the patient. The patient will be informed that the practitioner will count to three and on three they will spray 2–3 squirts of the nasal fluid. At that point the patient will sniff up the spray. The patient will be warned prior to use that, whilst the procedure may not be uncomfortable, the sprays do taste unpleasant and inevitably some of the spray will go down the patient's throat (and may therefore numb the back of the throat, making swallowing difficult). The patient will be given 5–10 minutes for the spray/s to work. The Lidocaine/Phenylephrine spray will be administered in the same way.
- *To allow a safe, decongested view of the nasal cavity. Local anaesthetic spray will make the viewing more comfortable for the patient. The patient can insert the nasal spray themselves if they feel confident.*
- *The local anaesthetic spray will often numb the patient's throat – this can be disconcerting for the patient, and the practitioner must prepare and reassure the patient about its use.*

6.1.5 Whilst waiting for the sprays to work, the practitioner will connect the endoscope to the light pipe and this to the light source as per the manufacturer's instructions. The endoscope will be tested and checked to ascertain that the view is clear down the scope.
- *If the endoscope is broken or not properly cleaned, the view will be obstructed. In this case, use another scope and remove the original one from action until the problem is resolved.*

6.1.6 The practitioner will explain to the patient how the endoscope will be used. The patient will be encouraged to breathe through their mouth (normally). The practitioner will hold the nasal endoscope firmly in the right hand and at the same time look down the endoscope by bringing the eyepiece to their eye. Or, if preferred, the scope can be used with a TV monitor. The view should be clear and bright.

- *To avoid the patient's breath misting the end of the scope, obscuring the view.*

6.1.7 The practitioner will then advance toward the nare of the nostril that requires examination and, using the left hand, supported by the bridge of the patient's nose, guide the endoscope gently into the nasal cavity. The practitioner will then perform the nasal examination. It may be necessary to clean the endoscope with saline and a cotton wool ball.

- *Looking down the scope whilst advancing toward the nose allows for safer endoscopy.*
- *Using both hands to support the scope will enable a steady advancement of the endoscope and will provide a better view.*
- *During the examination, the endoscope will get contaminated. Cleaning with an appropriate wipe will enable the practitioner to continue.*

6.1.8 All findings should be correctly noted and written in the patient's medical notes.

- *To provide an accurate record of the procedure performed.*

RATIONALE FOR THE ACTIONS ABOVE:
To ascertain the basic nasal anatomy for the surgeon prior to any surgical intervention or post-surgical review. To correctly view the appropriate side.

KNOWLEDGE REQUIRED:

- Anatomy and physiology of the nose and lacrimal system
- Understanding of the endoscope and how it functions
- Understanding of the function, presentation, side-effects and contraindications of both Xylometazoline and Lidocaine/Phenylephrine sprays.

COMPLICATIONS:
Epistaxis: Stop the nasal endoscopy immediately and apply basic first aid to stop the bleeding. Ask the patient to sit forward and apply firm pressure to the bridge of the nose. Get assistance from a member of the medical team. You may need to insert a nasal pack (always have one available).

Pain: The procedure may cause pain if nasal mucosa are touched that have not been anaesthetised. More local anaesthetic spray may be used under the direction of the medical team.

Numb throat due to the local anaesthetic: Encourage the patient and tell them that the numbness will wear off, but they should avoid all hot food and drinks for 1 to 2 hours so as to not burn themselves in the meantime.

BOUNDARIES OF PRACTICE:

This procedure will be carried out by a competently assessed practitioner. Any patient deemed unsuitable will be told so and the procedure may be cancelled or appropriate advice sought from a medical practitioner during the clinic. All patients for this diagnostic procedure would be appropriately reviewed and have this recorded in the notes and again by the practitioner prior to any intervention. However, the practitioner may not be directly supervised during the procedure.

LIMITATIONS:

Any situation where the practitioner does not feel competent or comfortable to provide the appropriate level of expertise, and finds the provision of this particular practice is beyond their level of competence.

References

Leatherbarrow, B. (2002). *Oculoplastic surgery.* London: Dunitz.

Nerad, J.A. (2001). *Requisites in ophthalmology: Oculoplastic surgery.* Missouri: Mosby.

6.2 PROTOCOL FOR REMOVAL OF SILICONE STENTS USING A NASAL ENDOSCOPE

EXPECTED OUTCOMES:

To safely and competently remove silicone stents from the nasal cavity or via the puncta using a nasal endoscope.

INDICATIONS:

A patient with Crawford stents following dacryocystorhinostomy (DCR) surgery (see Chapter 8).

CONTRAINDICATIONS:

A practitioner who has not been shown to be successfully competent in protocol 6.1. Patients who have had a silicone stent placed either for canalicular stenosis or post-surgical repair of the canaliculus following trauma, as the silicone stent may well be difficult to locate (usually positioned below the inferior turbinate) and view down the endoscope.

EQUIPMENT:

An assistant is needed to help cut the stent between the puncta, and:

- Oxybuprocaine 0.5%
- An overhead light
- Crocodile forceps
- Squint hook – why?
- Conjunctival scissors
- Endoscopic light source and light pipe.
- Rigid zero or 30-degree rigid endoscope
- Prep tray with saline
- Xylometazoline (Otrivine) (non-prescription)
- Lidocaine and Phenylephrine or plain Lidocaine Nasal Spray (has to be prescribed).

ACTIONS AND ASSOCIATED RATIONALE:

6.2.1 Once in theatre or OPD, the patient will be identified, procedure correlated against the patient surgical safety checklist and the consent verified with the patient and the team.

- *The WHO or LocSIP safety check list provides a basis to verify the patient and the treatment plan.*

6.2.2 Instil Oxybuprocaine into the affected eye(s).

- *To reduce the discomfort of the removal and cutting of the bi-canalicular stent.*

6.2.3 In the OPD the patient will be correctly identified by the practitioner and asked to sit in the examination chair. It should be possible to completely recline the chair should the need arise. The patient will be prepared for the administration of the nasal sprays: given a tissue, sat back with head in the head-rest and asked to blow their nose on the affected side.

- *To be able to put the patient in a slight reverse Trendelenburg if they feel faint.*
- *The patient needs to be comfortable during the procedure.*

6.2.4 The nasal cavities will be appropriately prepared with a nasal decongestant/local anaesthetic. The nasal spray bottle will be gently placed in the nare of the nose by either the practitioner or the patient. The patient will be informed that the practitioner will count to three and on three they will spray 2–3 squirts of the nasal fluid. At that point the patient will sniff up the spray. The patient will be warned prior to use that, whilst the procedure may not be uncomfortable, the sprays do taste unpleasant and inevitably some of the spray will go down the patient's throat (and may therefore numb the back of the throat, making swallowing difficult). The patient will be given 5–10 minutes for the spray/s to work. The Lidocaine/Phenylephrine spray will be administered in the same way.

- *To allow a safe, decongested view of the nasal cavity. Local anaesthetic spray will make the viewing more comfortable for the patient. The patient can insert the nasal spray themselves if they feel confident about doing so.*
- *The local anaesthetic spray will often numb the patient's throat – this can be disconcerting for the patient, and the practitioner must prepare and reassure the patient about its use.*

6.2.5 Whilst waiting for the sprays to work, the practitioner will connect the endoscope to the light pipe and this to the light source as per the manufacturer's instructions. The endoscope will be tested and checked to ascertain that there is a clear view down the scope.

- *If the endoscope is broken or not appropriately cleaned, the view will be obstructed. In this case, use another scope and remove the original one from action until the problem is resolved.*

6.2.6 The practitioner will inform the patient as to how the endoscope will be used. The patient will be encouraged to breathe through their mouth (normally).
The practitioner will hold the nasal endoscope firmly in the right hand and at the same time look down the endoscope by bringing the eyepiece to their eye. Or, if preferred, the scope can be used with a TV monitor. The view should be clear and bright.

- *To avoid the patient's breath misting the end of the scope, obscuring the view.*

6.2.7 The practitioner will then advance towards the nare of the nostril that requires examination and, using the left hand supported by the bridge of the patient's nose, guide the endoscope gently into the nasal cavity. The practitioner will then perform the nasal examination. It may be necessary to clean the endoscope with saline and a cotton wool ball.

- *Looking down the scope whilst advancing toward the nose allows for safer endoscopy.*
- *Using both hands to support the scope will enable a steady advancement of the endoscope and will provide a better view.*
- *During the examination, the endoscope will get contaminated. Cleaning with an appropriate wipe will enable the practitioner to continue.*

6.2.8 The practitioner will then perform the nasal examination and attempt to view the untied ends of the silicone stent. Once located, the practitioner will use the crocodile forceps and the endoscope to take hold of the silicone stent.

- *To remove the silicone stent safely and avoid the patient accidentally aspirating the stent.*

6.2.9 Once secured by the practitioner, the assistant will use the squint hook to take hold of the exposed stent in the medial canthal area of the eye and cut it with the blunt-tipped scissors. When this has been successfully achieved, the practitioner will be able to safely remove the stent from within the nose.

- *The stent will need to be cut to allow it to be removed.*
- *An assistant will be necessary to help with this part of the procedure.*

6.2.10 It may be necessary to clean the endoscope with saline and a cotton wool ball if it gets contaminated during the examination.

- *Cleaning the endoscope with an appropriate saline-impregnated wipe will enable the practitioner to continue.*

6.2.11 All findings should be correctly noted and written in the patient's medical notes. On the odd occasion when the silicone stent cannot be viewed intra-nasally, it may be possible to rotate the stent out of the punctum with forceps and then cut and remove it.

- *To provide an accurate record of the procedure performed.*

KNOWLEDGE REQUIRED:

- Anatomy and physiology of the nose and lacrimal system
- Understanding of the endoscope and how it functions

- Understanding of the function, presentation, side-effects and contraindications of both Xylometazoline and Lidocaine /Phenylephrine sprays
- Understanding of DCR surgery and how Crawford stents are placed.

COMPLICATIONS:

Epistaxis: Stop the nasal endoscopy immediately and apply basic first aid to stop the bleeding. Ask the patient to sit forward and apply firm pressure to the bridge of the nose. Get assistance from a member of the medical team. You may need to insert a nasal pack (always have one available).

Pain: The procedure may cause pain if nasal mucosa are touched that have not been anaesthetised. More local anaesthetic spray may be used under the direction of the medical team.

Numb throat due to the local anaesthetic: Encourage the patient and tell them that the numbness will wear off, but they should avoid all hot food and drinks for 1 to 2 hours so as to not burn themselves in the meantime.

Unable to locate silicone stent: Inform the surgeon.

BOUNDARIES OF PRACTICE:

This procedure will be carried out by a competently assessed practitioner. Any patient deemed unsuitable will be told and the procedure may be cancelled or appropriate advice sought from a medical practitioner during the clinic. All patients for this procedure would be appropriately reviewed and have this recorded in the notes and again by the practitioner prior to any intervention. However, the practitioner may not be directly supervised during the procedure.

LIMITATIONS:

Any situation where the practitioner does not feel competent or comfortable to provide the appropriate level of expertise, and finds the provision of this particular practice is beyond their level of competence.

References

Leatherbarrow, B. (2019). *Oculoplastic surgery.* 3rd edn. USA: Thieme.

Nerad, J.A. (2001). *Requisites in ophthalmology: Oculoplastic surgery.* Missouri: Mosby.

7. Harvesting full-thickness skin graft (FTSG)

EXPECTED OUTCOME:
The assistant will be able to demonstrate the ability to harvest a full-thickness skin graft from the inner upper arm, pre-auricular or supra-clavicular area in a safe manner. This will include the ability to administer local anaesthetic into the area, mark the area required and harvest the graft. Following removal, the assistant should be able to maintain haemostasis and close the wound appropriately. This will be under direct supervision by a senior member of the medical team.

PERFORMANCE CRITERIA:
The practitioner will be able to:
i. Demonstrate a good knowledge of the anatomy and physiology of the skin.
ii. Demonstrate the ability to administer local anaesthetic into the area as per protocol 2.1
iii. Demonstrate the ability to adequately prepare the site and identify the appropriate area from which to harvest the skin graft
iv. Demonstrate the ability to drape the area as per protocol 1.1
v. Using a pre-prepared template, mark the area appropriately for harvesting
vi. Administer local anaesthetic as per protocol 2
vii. Demonstrate the ability to excise and dissect the full-thickness skin graft
viii. Demonstrate the ability to use diathermy to control haemostasis as per protocol 4
ix. Demonstrate the ability to (if necessary) carry out further dissection and undermining of the wound to allow closure
x. Demonstrate the ability to suture the wound, using mattress sutures (interrupted vertical) as per protocol 3
xi. Discuss appropriate dressings.

INDICATIONS:
Surgical defects requiring full-thickness skin grafts to cover the area.

CONTRAINDICATIONS:
Harvesting skin grafts from any other sites.

EQUIPMENT:
- Instrument tray
- Drapes
- Overhead or headlight
- Diathermy

- Post-operative dressing
- Sutures.

ACTIONS AND ASSOCIATED RATIONALE:

7.1 Identify what procedure is to be carried out prior to surgery, gain written consent and mark the appropriate site/side for surgery using the correct Trust recognised paperwork and protocol.

- *To ensure that the appropriate treatment is prescribed and the patient is aware of the risks and benefits of treatment.*
- *To ensure that the patient is fully aware of the treatment plan and the viable alternatives.*

7.2 Once in theatre, the patient will be identified, surgical procedure correlated against the patient surgical safety checklist and the consent verified with the patient and the theatre team.

- *The WHO safety check list provides a basis to verify the patient and the treatment plan.*

7.3 The appropriate area of the inner upper arm, supra-clavicular or pre-auricular areas from which the FTSG can be harvested will be identified and the area to be harvested will be marked.

- *There are several potential donor sites that can be used – preference may depend upon skin colour, skin condition and accessibility.*

7.4 Local anaesthetic will be administered into this area as per protocol 2.

- *To provide local anaesthesia and enable the surgical procedure to take place.*

7.5 The area is prepped and draped as per protocol 1.1.

- *To provide a barrier and to prevent risk of cross-infection.*

7.6 A template is received from the surgeon, and the actual area of the skin graft to be harvested is marked with a skin marker using the template.

- *A template is used to provide an outline of the skin required, so as to harvest the appropriate amount of skin.*

7.7 A surgical blade (No 15) is used to create a full-thickness incision around the edge of the marked area. Paufique forceps (or other toothed forceps) and a 15 blade are used to carefully dissect the full-thickness skin away from the subcutaneous tissue.

- *Using the scalpel blade provides an element of control (of the thickness) when harvesting the skin.*

7.8 The full-thickness skin graft is wrapped in a saline-soaked swab and passed to the scrub nurse or it may be thinned by the practitioner using Westcott scissors.

- *The harvested skin is debulked until the rete pegs are observed.*
- *Skin that isn't appropriately debulked may later cause increased risk of scarring and chronic thickening.*

7.9 Dissect the skin edges away from the underlying tissue. Using forceps and spring scissors, until the skin edges appose comfortably.

- *The wound edges will appose without tension, reducing the risk of dehiscence.*

7.10 Ensure haemostasis prior to suturing using bipolar diathermy.

- *Bleeding will be controlled and will prevent underlying haematoma.*

7.11 Suture the wound as per protocol 3.

7.12 Once sutured, clean the wound and apply an appropriately sized dressing.

- *To protect the wound from infection.*

KNOWLEDGE REQUIRED:

Competency must be demonstrated in the following areas:

- Full-thickness skin graft harvesting technique
- Marking the graft site
- Identification of risk factors
- Identification of contraindications
- Identification of complications
- Understanding of the action to be taken in all of the above
- Anatomy and physiology of skin.

COMPLICATIONS:

Buttonhole may occur in the graft. In this case, the practitioner must inform the surgeon.

BOUNDARIES OF PRACTICE:

The surgeon will always be present to provide direct supervision.

LIMITATIONS:

Any situation where the practitioner does not feel competent or comfortable to provide the appropriate level of expertise, and finds the provision of this particular practice is beyond their level of competence.

References

Leatherbarrow, B. (2019). *Oculoplastic surgery.* 3rd edn. USA: Thieme.

Nerad, J.A. (2001). *Requisites in ophthalmology: Oculoplastic surgery.* Missouri: Mosby.

Competency will also need to have been achieved for the following protocols:

1.1 Preparation and draping of the surgical patient
2 Infiltration and administration of subcutaneous local anaesthetic into the eyelid and/or surrounding area to enable minor operative procedures to be performed
3 Suturing of subcutaneous layers, stapling or suturing of the skin
4 Applying diathermy for haemostasis.

8. Harvesting of dermis fat graft from the abdomen or buttock

EXPECTED OUTCOME:
The practitioner will be able to demonstrate the ability to harvest a dermis fat graft (DFG) from the abdomen or buttock. This will include the need to be able to administer saline subcutaneously, mark the area and harvest the graft. Following removal of the fat graft, the assistant will demonstrate an ability to stabilise haemostasis and close the wound appropriately.

PERFORMANCE CRITERIA:
The practitioner will be able to:
i. Demonstrate a good knowledge of the anatomy and physiology of the skin
ii. Demonstrate an ability to mark the site
iii. Demonstrate an ability to prepare and drape the area
iv. Discuss the application and use of cutaneous dermis fat grafts
v. Demonstrate an ability to inject saline into the skin to create a peau d'orange (dimpled) effect
vi. Demonstrate an ability to mark an elliptical incision and dissect the tissue and fat
vii. Demonstrate an ability to gauge the appropriate size fat graft
viii. Demonstrate an ability to provide appropriate haemostasis
ix. Demonstrate an ability to close the wound, including deep closure
x. Discuss appropriate dressings and wound care post-operatively.

INDICATIONS:
Volume replacement in the orbit, lower eyelid spacer, lower eyelid adhesions.

EQUIPMENT:
- Oculoplastic instrument tray
- 10ml saline – 25g needle
- 4/0 Vicryl
- 4/0 Nylon
- Dressing
- Bipolar diathermy.

ACTIONS AND ASSOCIATED RATIONALE:
8.1 Identify what procedure is to be carried out prior to surgery, gain written consent and mark the appropriate site/side for surgery using the correct Trust recognised paperwork and protocol.

- *To ensure the appropriate treatment is prescribed and the patient is aware of the risks and benefits of treatment.*
- *To ensure that the patient is fully aware of the treatment plan and the viable alternatives.*

8.2 Once in theatre, the patient will be identified, surgical procedure correlated against the patient surgical safety checklist and the consent verified with the patient and the theatre team.

- *The WHO safety check list provides a basis to verify the patient and the treatment plan.*

8.3 The size of the graft required is outlined on the skin with a marker pen.

- *To ascertain the size of graft that needs to be harvested.*
- *The fat of the graft is positioned in the orbit to mimic the anatomical location of the pre-aponeurotic fat.*

8.4 The DFG is harvested from the lower abdominal wall left or right iliac area or the upper outer quadrant of the buttock.

- *This area will, for many patients, have an appropriate amount of fat to harvest safely.*

8.5 Saline is injected into the epidermis by the practitioner to create a peau d'orange appearance.

- *This delineates the planes between the epidermis and the dermis.*

8.6 The practitioner will use a 15 blade to make an incision through the dermis, and the epidermis is then removed from the marked graft area. The dermis should appear white. Then a small incision is made through one edge of dermis with the blade. The underlying subcutaneous fat will appear, and the rest of the incision is completed along the edge of the dermis, using Stevens scissors.

- *The epidermis is not required as it is removed.*
- *The Stevens scissors are more suitable for the thicker dermis.*

8.7 The underlying fat, which is connected to the harvested dermis, is dissected to a depth of 2–3cm, depending on the indications.

- *The amount of fat required will depend upon its use.*

8.8 The graft is carefully removed and safely stored in a moistened swab.

- *To protect the graft from drying out.*

8.9 The harvest site will be assessed and any bleeding vessels will be cauterised using diathermy (as per protocol 4.0).

- *To control the bleeding.*

8.10 The donor site will now be closed with subcutaneous interrupted 4/0 Vicryl sutures and interrupted 4/0 Nylon for the skin closure (following suturing protocol 3.0).
- *The skin will be closed to allow the wound to heal by primary intention.*

8.11 The skin is cleaned and a simple dressing will be applied.
- *To allow the wound to heal and prevent infection.*

KNOWLEDGE REQUIRED:
- Anatomy and physiology of the skin.

Competency must be demonstrated in the following areas:
- Dermis fat harvesting technique
- Marking the graft site
- Injecting the site with saline to create the peau d'orange effect
- Identification of risk factors
- Identification of contraindications
- Identification of complications
- Understand the actions to be taken in all of the above.

BOUNDARIES OF PRACTICE
The surgeon will always be present to provide direct supervision.

LIMITATIONS OF PRACTICE:
Any situation where the practitioner does not feel competent or comfortable to provide the appropriate level of expertise, and finds the provision of this particular practice is beyond their level of competence.

References

Leatherbarrow, B. (2019). *Oculoplastic surgery.* 3rd edn. USA: Thieme.

Competency will also need to have been achieved for the following protocols:
1.1 Preparation and draping of the surgical patient
2 Infiltration and administration of subcutaneous local anaesthetic into the eyelid and/or surrounding area to enable minor operative procedures to be performed
3 Suturing of subcutaneous layers, stapling or suturing of the skin
4 Applying diathermy for haemostasis.

9. Harvesting of an autologous scleral patch graft from an enucleated eye for use in an enucleated socket

EXPECTED OUTCOME:

The practitioner will be able to demonstrate the ability to harvest an autologous scleral patch graft from an enucleated eye. This will include being able to identify an appropriate area to harvest the graft, and safely and competently removing the patch graft for reuse in the enucleated socket.

PERFORMANCE CRITERIA:

The practitioner will be able to:
- **i.** Demonstrate a good knowledge of the anatomy and physiology of the eye
- **ii.** Demonstrate an ability to mark the appropriate size patch graft from the enucleated eye
- **iii.** Demonstrate an ability to prepare the sclera of the enucleated eye
- **iv.** Demonstrate an ability to competently prepare the sclera, once harvested
- **v.** Demonstrate an ability to safely harvest the scleral graft, using the appropriate instrumentation
- **vi.** Discuss the potential risk factors associated with harvesting the graft
- **vii.** Discuss what is involved in dealing with the remaining enucleated eye, i.e. histopathology.

INDICATIONS:

In patients who have an increased risk of post-operative implant exposure, particularly those who have the potential for conjunctival wound dehiscence (Leatherbarrow 2019). To provide an additional barrier to reduce the potential risk of expulsion/rejection of the orbital implant, particularly when there is a reduced amount of conjunctiva/Tenons layers available to completely cover the implant.

EQUIPMENT:

- Oculoplastic/orbital instrument tray
- Metal graft board
- Marker pen
- Absolute alcohol 1–2ml
- Cotton buds/ Q-tips
- Forceps
- 15 blade and Bard Parker handle
- Blunt-tipped Westcott Scissors

ACTIONS AND ASSOCIATED RATIONALE:

9.1 Identify what procedure is to be carried out prior to surgery, gain written consent and mark the appropriate site/side for surgery using the correct Trust recognised paperwork and protocol.

- *To ensure the appropriate treatment is prescribed and the patient is aware of the risks and benefits of treatment*
- *To ensure that the patient is fully aware of the treatment plan and the viable alternatives.*

9.2 Once in theatre, the patient will be identified, surgical procedure correlated against the patient surgical safety checklist and the consent verified with the patient and the theatre team.

- *The WHO safety check list provides a basis to verify the patient and the treatment plan.*

9.3 The practitioner will have donned suitable scrub attire, mask, protective glasses and sterile gloves.

- *To prevent cross-infection and to act as a barrier.*

9.4 Once the eye/globe has been enucleated and it has been ascertained by the surgeon that an autologous scleral patch graft will be required, the practitioner will prepare the eye by cleaning it with sterile water. It may also be necessary to remove any unnecessary tissue that is still attached to the globe, using forceps and Westcott scissors.

- *To remove any extraneous material that may cause infection or inflammation.*

9.5 Using a marker pen, the practitioner will then outline the extent of the graft that is to be harvested. This is approximately 10mm x 20mm, and this will be confirmed by the operating surgeon. Prior to harvesting the scleral graft, the marking will be checked with the operating surgeon.

- *It will be necessary to ascertain the correct size of graft so that it gives complete coverage of the orbital implant.*

9.6 Then, using Parfique forceps and a 15 blade, the scleral patch graft will be excised, ensuring that only sclera is removed and not the underlying choroid layer. It may also be necessary to use Westcott scissors to facilitate this.

- *To reduce the possibility of infection and contamination of the socket*

9.7 Once the scleral patch has been harvested, it will also require further cleaning, using absolute alcohol and Q-tips, particularly on its inner surface.

- *The use of absolute alcohol will ensure that the surface of the sclera is adequately cleaned and that all remnants are removed.*

9.8 Once ready for reuse, the sclera will be wrapped in a saline gauze and given to the scrub nurse until required.

- *Once harvested, it is important to safely maintain the integrity of the sclera until it needs to be used by wrapping it in a saline-infiltrated gauze.*

9.9 The remaining enucleated eye will be transferred into a histology pot.

- *The remaining enucleated globe will (as is routine) be sent for histopathology and will therefore need to be transferred into a specimen pot with preservative.*

KNOWLEDGE REQUIRED:

- Anatomy and physiology of the eye
- Handling of the surgical instruments to facilitate the safe and competent removal of the autologous graft.

BOUNDARIES OF PRACTICE

The surgeon will always be present to provide direct supervision.

LIMITATIONS OF PRACTICE:

Any situation where the practitioner does not feel competent or comfortable to provide the appropriate level of expertise, and finds the provision of this particular practice is beyond their level of competence.

References

Leatherbarrow, B. (2019). *Oculoplastic surgery.* 3rd edn. USA: Thieme.

Further reading

During the writing of this book and throughout my career, I have referred to several key texts and books again and again. As an oculoplastics practitioner, I have found these publications invaluable. I have also included a couple of my own papers that you may find useful in your practice.

Bartalena, L., Baldeschi, L., Dickinson, A. et al. (2008). Consensus statement of the European group on Graves' orbitopathy (EUGOGO) on management of Graves' orbitopathy. *European Journal of Endocrinology.* **158**(3), 273–85.

Cooper, J. (2009). Undergoing enucleation of the eye. Part 1: preoperative considerations. *British Journal of Nursing.* **18**(22), 1386–90.

Cooper, J. (2010). Undergoing enucleation of the eye. Part 2: Post-operative considerations. *British Journal of Nursing.* **19**(1), 28–35.

Craig, J.P., Nelson, J.D., Dimitri, T.A. *et al.* (2017). TFOS DEWS II Report Executive Summary. The Ocular Surface. http://dx.doi.org/10.1016/j.jtos.2017.08.003 (last accessed 6.11.2019).

Douglas, G., Nicol, F. & Robertson, C. (eds) (2013). *Macleod's clinical examination.* 13th edn. Churchill Livingstone Elsevier.

Gray, H. (2015). Gray's anatomy: *The anatomical basis of clinical practice.* 41st edn. (originally published 1858). USA: Elsevier.

Kanski, J. & Bowling, B. (2011). *Clinical ophthalmology: A systematic approach.* 7th edn. USA: Elsevier.

Leatherbarrow, B. (2019). *Oculoplastic surgery.* 3rd edn. USA: Thieme.

Nerad, J. (2001). *Oculoplastic surgery: The requisites in ophthalmology.* USA: Mosby.

Platts, M., Cooper, J. & Cook, A. (2012). Acknowledging the contribution the nurse can make to patients with thyroid eye disease. *International Journal of Ophthalmic Practice.* **3**(4), 156–60.

Platts, M., Danial, S., Cook, A. & Cooper, J. (2014). A review of the management options for periorbital basal cell carcinomas. *International Journal of Ophthalmic Practice.* **1**(5), 23–28.

Poulson, D. (2010). *Histology and cell biology: Examination and board review.* 5th edn. McGraw-Hill Medical.

Index

acoustic neuroma surgery *212*
acrochordon *83, 286*
actinic keratosis (solar keratosis) *84*
advanced nurse practitioner roles *1–3*
advanced practice *1–3*
advanced practice in ophthalmology *3–6*
advancing practice *2*
allergies *188*
anaesthetic, local, subcutaneous infiltration and administration of *265–269*
aneurysm *42*
animal bite wounds *204*
anti-thyroid agents *151*
apex, orbital *227*
aponeurotic ptosis *43*
aqueous layer *122*
assessment, pre-operative *93*
Assistant Surgical Practitioner (ASP) competencies *244–264*
auscultation *192*
azathioprine treatment *154*

basal cell carcinoma (BCC) *88, 89, 90, 172, 287*
Bell's palsy *211, 214, 215*
Bell's palsy, ophthalmic nursing considerations *216*
Bell's phenomenon (palpebral oculogyric reflex) *49, 149*
bi-canalicular stent *135*
bi-lobed flap *99*
blepharitis *109, 111, 112, 113, 122*
blepharitis treatment *115, 116*
blepharophimosis *44*
blepharoplasty *63*
blepharoplasty, nursing care considerations for *66*
blepharoplasty surgical procedure *64*
blepharoptosis *35*
blink mechanism *124*

blood tests *149, 190*
botulinum toxin brow lift *65*
brow lift, direct *63*
brow lift, endoscopic *64*
brow lift, endotine transblepharoplasty *65*
brow ptosis *62*
brow ptosis procedure *62–66*
brow ptosis surgery, nursing care following *67*
burns *208*
burns, treating *209*
burns, types of *209*

canthal ligaments *10*
cantholysis *97, 207*
canthotomy *97, 207*
chalazia, incision and curettage of *280–288*
chalazion *78, 79, 283*
chronic progressive external ophthalmoplegia (CPEO) *40*
colour vision *148*
comedo (comedone/blackhead) *82*
computerised tomography (CT) scan *150, 190*
ectropion, congenital *13*
ptosis, congenital *44*
consent *92, 236*
corneal surface *50*
corticosteroid treatment for orbital inflammation *153*
cranial nerve (CN) examination *230*
cutaneous horn *287*
Cutler-Beard reconstruction *99*
cyst of Moll (hidrocystoma, sudoriferous cyst) *80, 81, 284*
cyst of Zeis *81*

dacryoadenitis *231*
dacryocystorhinostomy (DCR) *132, 133, 134*
dacryocystorhinostomy (DCR), endo-nasal *137*
dacryocystorhinostomy (DCR), post-operative care *136, 138*
dacryoplasty *132*

delayed reconstruction *95*
Demodex *112, 116*
dermatochalasis *44, 45, 62*
dermis *78*
dermis fat graft from the abdomen or buttock, harvesting of *318–320*
dermoid cyst *231*
diabetes *42*
diathermy for wound haemostasis, applying *273–275*
distichiasis *103*
double triangle (Crawford) procedure *61*
drain, surgical *239, 240*
draping prior to surgical intervention *244–248*
droopy upper eyelid *35*
dry eye disease (DED) *109, 110*
dry eye disease risk factors *110*
dry eye disease, treatment of *114*
dystonia *324*

ectropion *9, 11, 12*
ectropion, cicatricial *13, 21*
ectropion, involutional *13*
ectropion, mechanical *13*
ectropion, non-surgical treatment of *14–18*
ectropion, paralytic *13*
ectropion, presentation of *14*
ectropion, surgical treatment of *18–26*
ectropion, types of *13*
electrolysis *106, 276*
electrolysis procedure for trichiasis *276–279*
emergency ophthalmic care *185*
entropion *9, 27*
entropion, cicatricial *30, 31*
entropion, involutional *27*
entropion, presentation of *27*
entropion, treatment of *27*
enucleation *159, 163*
enucleation, surgical approach to *166*
epidermal inclusion cyst *285*
epidermis layers *37, 77*

325

ethmoid bone 225
everting sutures (Quickert's procedure) 28
everting sutures for the correction of involutional entropion 294–297
evisceration 159, 163
evisceration, surgical approach to 165
excision, Mohs micrographic 94
excision under frozen section 95
exenteration 171, 172
exenteration, post-operative care 181
exenteration, pre-operative considerations 176
exenteration, psychosocial considerations 173
exenteration, sub-total 179
exenteration surgery 178
exenteration, total 178
exophthalmometry 191, 229
extraconal space 228
Eye Emergency Department (EED) 186
eye removal, cosmetic impact of 162
eye removal, indications for 159
eye removal, post-operative care 168
eye removal, pre-operative considerations 162
eye removal, psychological impact of 160
eyelash anatomy 101
eyelash growth 102
eyelash hygiene 108
eyelash removal 104
eyelashes 101–108
eyelashes, assessment of 103
eyelid eversion 50
eyelid lacerations 197
eyelid lesions 75–100
eyelid lesions, examining 75, 76
eyelid, lower, anatomy of 9, 11
eyelid massage 15, 16
eyelid measurements 149
eyelid retraction 149
eyelid skin anatomy 77
eyelid skin lesions, removal of 289–293

eyelid skin, upper 48
eyelid swelling 148
eyelid taping 28
eyelid, upper, anatomy of 36, 63
eyelid weight 217
eyelids and blink mechanism, functions of 39, 40
eyelids, blood supply of 39
eyelids, innervation of 39
eyes, assessment of the 189

facial palsy 205, 211–219
facial palsy, causes of 212
facial palsy, clinical examination 212, 213
facial palsy, non-surgical therapy for 218
facial palsy, psychosocial effects of 218
facial synkinesis 214
fascia lata 59, 62
fatigue test 49
fibroepithelial polyp 83, 286
fistula, arteriovenous 233
floppy eyelid, assessment and history-taking 70
floppy eyelid syndrome 14, 69–74
floppy eyelid syndrome (FES), caring for patients with 74
floppy eyelid syndrome (FES) treatment 72
fluorescein dye disappearance test (FDDT) 130
forceps, holding tissue with 256–258
frontal bone 223
frontalis suspension 58
full-thickness skin grafts 22, 23, 97, 314
full-thickness skin graft (FTSG) harvesting procedure 314–316

glands of Moll 78, 102
glands of Zeis 78, 102
Graves' disease (see also thyroid eye disease) 143, 145
Graves' orbitopathy, classification of stage and activity of 150
grey-line 101

haemangioma, capillary (strawberry naevus) 86
haemangioma, cavernous 232
haematoma, retrobulbar 205
head bandage 202
Hering's law of equal innervation 48
history taking 187, 188, 212, 228
Horner's syndrome 42
Hughes procedure 99
hyaluronic acid (HA) injections 18
hyperthyroidism 144
hypothyroidism 144
hypothyroidism, radioactive iodine treatment for 152
hypotropia 45

inferior retractor reinsertion (IRR) or advancement 29
internal brow lift 65
intraconal space 228
intra-ocular pressure (IOP) 188
lacrimal apparatus, ballooning of the 132
lacrimal apparatus, stenting of the 132
lacrimal bone 226
lacrimal gland tumour 232
lacrimal gland 120
lacrimal sac 126
lacrimal scintillography 130
lacrimal system 119, 120, 130
lacrimal system, damage to the 140
lateral tarsal strip procedure (LTS) 18, 25
lentigo (lentigines) 88
lesion, excision of (see also eyelid skin lesions) 94–95
lesion, malignant, nursing considerations 92
lesions, benign 78–88
lesions, malignant 88–92
lesions, orbital 233, 234
Lester Jones tube (LJT) 138, 139
levator aponeurosis advancement (LAA) procedure 52–57

levator aponeurosis advancement, posterior approach 58
levator function (eyelid excursion) 46
levator palpebrae superioris muscle 38
lid eversion 190
lipid layer 121
LTS/MS procedures, nursing considerations with 19
lubricants 15, 27
Lyme disease 212
lymphoma 231

madarosis 103
magnetic resonance imaging (MRI) scan 191
malignant tumours 172
Manchester Orbital Exenteration Wound Assessment Tool (MOEWAT) 177
Marcus-Gunn jaw-wink 44
marginal reflex distance (MRD) 46
mattress suture 73
maxillary bone 226
medial spindle (MS) procedure 19
meibomian cyst 78
meibomian gland dysfunction (MGD) 109, 111, 113
meibomian gland dysfunction (MGD) treatment 115, 116
meibomian gland lipogranuloma 78
meibomian glands 10, 78
melanoma 91, 173
Merkel cell tumour 91
metastases 232
milia 84, 285
molluscum contagiosum (water warts) 84
mucin layer 122
mucous membrane graft 31, 32
Müller's muscle 38
Müller's muscle resection 56, 57
Mustarde flap 100
myasthenia gravis (MG) 40, 49

myotonic dystrophy (MD) 41
naevi 286
naevus (acquired 87
naevus (congenital) 88
nasal endoscopy 306–309
nasolacrimal duct 126
neurofibroma 85
neurogenic ptosis 41
non-specific orbital inflammatory disease 231
nursing roles, specialised 1, 2

obstructive sleep apnoea (OSA) 71
ocular cicatricial pemphigoid (OCP) 30
ocular pulsation 229
oculocardiac reflex 167, 178
operative procedures, comparison of minor 283
ophthalmic ultrasound B scan 191
optic nerve sheath meningioma 232
orbicularis oculi muscle 9, 38
orbit 221–242
orbit, bones of 222, 223
orbital assessment and examination 228
orbital biopsy 233
orbital cellulitis 193–195, 231
orbital decompression surgery 154–157
orbital exenteration – see exenteration
orbital floor fracture 195–197
orbital implants 164, 165
orbital lesions, surgical approach to 233, 234
orbital prosthesis 182
orbital surgery, discharge after 241
orbital surgery, nursing considerations in relation to 234–241
osteology 221

palatine bone 227
palpebral fissure (PF) 46
pentagon (Fox) procedure 59, 60

periorbita 227
periosteum, orbital 227
phenylephrine test 49
poliosis 103
post-operative care 94
post-operative care (LTS) 25
pretrichial brow lift 64
prolene sutures 59
proptosis 143, 149, 191, 229
prosthetic eye, care of 169, 170
pseudoptosis 44
ptosis 35
ptosis examination and assessment 45
ptosis, mechanical 43
ptosis, myogenic 40–41
ptosis surgery, post-operative 55–57
ptosis surgery, pre-operative nursing considerations 51
ptosis, surgical approaches 52
ptosis treatment and management 50–62
ptosis, upper eyelid, causes and aetiology of 40
puncta 125
punctal cautery 302–304

reconstructive surgery 96
reflex epiphora 129
relative afferent pupillary defect (RAPD) 188
retractor muscle 10
rhabdomyosarcoma 232
rhomboid flap 98
Rundle's curve 145, 146

sac washout test (SWO) 126, 127
Schirmer's test 123, 124, 214
scleral patch graft, harvesting of 321–323
sebaceous cell carcinoma (SGC) 91, 173
sebaceous cysts 82
sebaceous glands 78
seborrhea 112
seborrhoeic keratosis (basal cell papilloma) 83, 84, 286
selenium treatment for thyroid

eye disease *147*
silicone sling *59*
silicone stents, removal of *310–313*
skin crease *47*
skin layer of the eyelid *37*
skin preparation prior to surgical intervention *244–248*
skin tag *83, 286*
sleep apnoea *69*
smoking and thyroid eye disease *146*
sphenoid bone *224*
sphenoid wing meningioma *233*
SPIKES template *175*
split-thickness skin graft (STSG) *180*
squamous cell carcinoma (SCC) *90, 173, 287*
squamous papilloma *83, 286*
squint *45*
stapling or suturing of the skin *270–272*
steroid treatment *15*
Stevens-Johnson syndrome (SJS) *30*
stye (external hordeolum) *80, 283*
subcutaneous layers, closing of *270–272*
suction, applying to the operating field *253–255*
superior tarsal muscle *38*
surgery, nursing considerations during *93*
suture-cutting *262–264*
sympathetic ophthalmia *162*

tarsal plate *10*
tarsorrhaphy, temporary suture *17*
tear break-up time (TBUT) *122*
tear layers *121*
tear production *121*
tear types *122, 123*
Tenzel flap *100*
theatre-operating microscope, use of *259–261*
third cranial nerve (CN) palsies *41, 42*
thyroid eye disease *143–157*
thyroid eye disease, initial assessment for *147*
thyroid eye disease, ophthalmic assessment for *148*
thyroid eye disease, symptoms of *145*
thyroid gland *144*
thyroid hormones *144*
thyroxine *144*
tissue retraction *249–252*
titanium orbital implants *183*
toxic epidermal necrolysis (TEN) *30*
trauma *42*
triage *186*
trichiasis *103, 104, 276*
tumorous lesions, characteristics suggesting *77*
tumour *42*

Valsalva manoeuvre *229*
vascular lesions *233*
vasculitis *42*
vertical palpebral aperture (PA) *46*
visual acuity (VA) *148, 187*
visual assessment *188*

wedge excision, lower eyelid *19*
white-line advancement *58*
Whitnall's ligament *38*

xanthelasma *86, 284*
xanthelasmata, application of trichloroacetic acid 90% (tca) to *298–301*
x-rays *191*

zygomatic bone *227*